AF531671

CANCER VACCINE

ENCYCLOPAEDIA OF CANCER

Vol. II

CANCER VACCINE

By

Dr. Amita Sarkar

Dept. of Zoology
Agra College
Agra (U.P.)
(India)

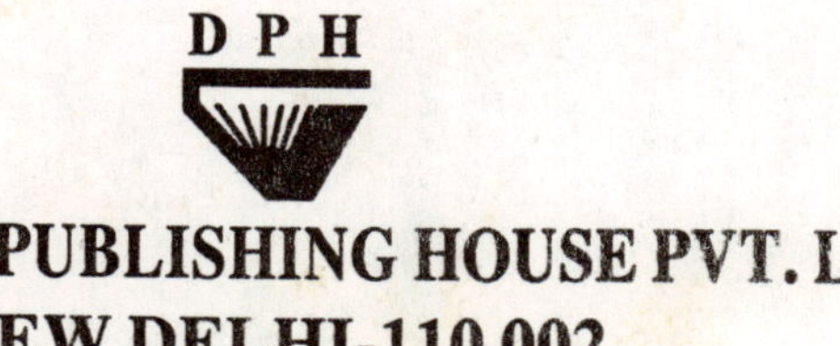

DISCOVERY PUBLISHING HOUSE PVT. LTD.
NEW DELHI-110 002

First Published-2008

ISBN 978-81-8356-356-7 (Set)

Published by:

DISCOVERY PUBLISHING HOUSE PVT. LTD.
4831/24, Ansari Road, Prahlad Street,
Darya Ganj, New Delhi-110002 (India)
Phone: 23279245 • Fax: 91-11-23253475
E-mail: dphbooks@rediffmail.com
dphtemp@indiatimes.com
Website: www.discoverypublishinghouse.com

Printed at:

Preface

Over the past 20 years, technological advances in molecular biology have proven invaluable to the understanding of the pathogenesis of cancer. The application of molecular technology to the study of cancer has not only led to advances in tumor diagnosis, but has also provided markers for the assessment of prognosis and disease progression. The aim of *Encyclopaedia of Cancer* is to provide a comprehensive collection of the most up-to-date techniques for the detection of molecular changes in cancer.

This book is intended to provide a relatively short overview of important concepts and notions on the molecular biology of human cancers, including many facts essential to find one's way in this field. It is, however, not meant to be compreshensive and probably cannot be, as our knowledge is rapidly growing.

The salient feature of this book is that it covers a wide range of molecular techniques and provides a source of information to readers at all levels. Although several books on cancer have been published in the last decade, most of either very shallow or cover few areas in depth. Rarely do they cover the broad spectrum of topics which would provide enough information for understanding the subject or provide simple protocols for execution of molecular change. In my opinion, this book can help the reader to easily understand the subject and also excecute the experiments very efficiently.

There can be no claim to originality except in the manner of treatment and much of the information has been obtained from the books and scientific journals available in the different libraries.

The author expresses his thanks to his friends and colleagues whose continue inspirations have initiated him to bring out this book.

The author is painfully aware of the shortcomings, errors and misprints that have crept in, and shall be greateful to receive suggestion for improvement of the next edition from all the readers.

The author expresses his gratitude to Mr. Wasan and staff of M/s Discovery Publishing House for their whole hearted co-operation in the publication of this book.

Author

Contents

1

INTRODUCTION

What is commonly called '*human cancer*' comprises in fact more than 200 different diseases. Together, they account for about one fifth of all deaths in the industrialized countries of the Western World. Likewise, one person out of three will be treated for a severe cancer in their life-time. In a typical Western industrialized country like Germany with its 82 million inhabitants, >400,000 persons are newly diagnosed with cancer each year, and ≈200,000 succumb to the disease. Since the incidence of most cancers increases with age, these figures are going to rise, if life expectancy continues to increase.

If one considers the incidence and mortality by organ site, while ignoring further biological and clinical differences, cancers fall into three large groups. Cancers arising from epithelia are called '*carcinomas*'. These are the most prevalent cancers overall. Four carcinomas are particular important with regard to incidence as well as mortality. Cancers of the lung and the large intestine (*colon* and *rectum*) are the most significant problem in both genders, together with breast cancer in women and prostate cancer in men. A second group of cancers are not quite as prevalent as these '*major four*' cancers. They comprise carcinomas of the bladder, stomach, liver, kidney, pancreas, esophagus, and of the cervix and ovary in women. Each accounts for a few percent of the total cancer incidence and mortality. Each of them is roughly as frequent as all leukemias or lymphomas taken together. They are rarely lethal, with the important exception of melanoma. Cancers of soft tissues, brain, testes, bone, and other organs are relatively rare; but can constitute a significant health problem in specific age groups and geographic regions. For instance, testicular cancer is generally the most frequent neoplasia affecting young adult males, with an incidence of $>1\%$ in this group in some Scandinavian countries and in Switzerland.

The health situation in less-industrialized countries differs principally from that in the highly industrialized part of the world because of the continuing, recurring or newly emerged threat of infectious diseases, which include malaria, tuberculosis, and AIDS. Nevertheless, cancer is important in these countries as well, with different patterns of incidence and often higher mortalities. Cancers of the stomach, liver, bladder, esophagus, and the cervix are each endemic in certain parts of the world. Often, they manifest at younger ages than in industrialized countries. Conversely, of the major four cancers in industrialized countries, only lung cancer has the same impact in developing countries.

This snapshot view of present-day cancer incidence of course conceals changes over time. For instance, large-scale industrialization and the spread of cigarette smoking are generally associated with an increased incidence of lung, kidney, and bladder cancer. On the positive side, improvements in general hygiene and food quality may have contributed to the spectacular decrease in stomach cancer incidence that is continuing in industrialized countries. On the negative side, prostate and testicular cancer appear to have increased over the last decades. In prostate cancer, a slight increase in the age-adjusted incidence is exacerbated by the overall aging of the population. In some regions, the incidence of melanoma has escalated in an alarming fashion. This increase is not related to the aging of the population, but perhaps to life-style factors.

One important aim of molecular biology research on human cancers is to understand the causes underlying the geographical and temporal differences in cancer incidence. This understanding is one important prerequisite for cancer prevention. Obviously, the prospects for prevention are brightest for those cancers that exhibit large geographical differences or the great changes over time in their incidences. To give just one example: The incidence of prostate cancer of East Asia residents may be 10-20-fold lower than that of their relatives who grow up in the USA. It is easy imagining the potential for prevention, if the causes for this difference were understood.

Unfortunately, overall, neither incidence nor mortality of human cancer have been much diminished by conscious human intervention over the last decades. The mainstay of treatment of the '*big four*' cancers and of the carcinomas in the second group outlined above remain surgery, radiotherapy, and chemotherapy, as they were 30 years ago. Surgery and radiotherapy are often successful in organ-confined cases, and chemotherapy is moderately efficacious for some advanced cancers. In general, only modest improvements have been made in cure and survival rates for these. Importantly, the quality of life for the patients is now widely accepted as a criterion for successful therapy. Modern cancer therapy recognizes that not every malignant tumor can be cured by the means presently available. So, treatment needs to be carefully chosen to maximize the chance for a cure while retaining a maximum of life quality. Providing a better basis for this choice will perhaps constitute the most immediate application of new insights on the molecular biology of cancers. In addition, palliative treatments have become more sophisticated and pain medications are less restrictively administered. Nevertheless, the treatment of metastatic carcinomas remains the weakest point of current cancer therapy and a crucial goal of cancer research.

Great steps towards successful treatment have been made with specific cancers, unfortunately mostly from the third group above. These improvement have had little effect on the impact of cancer on the overall population, but have helped many individuals, often young people and children. Formerly incurable leukemias and lymphomas can now be successfully treated by chemotherapy and/or stem cell transplantation, particularly in children and young adults. Likewise, the rise in testicular cancer incidence is stemmed by highly efficacious chemo- and radiotherapy, with cure rates exceeding 90%. Obviously, there is a need to understand why these cancers, but not others respond so well to the chemotherapeutic drugs currently available. It is hoped that a better understanding of the molecular and cellular basis underlying this difference will eventually open the door to successful treatment of the major carcinomas, as will the development of novel drugs and novel therapies based on the results of molecular biological cancer research.

Causes of Cancer

Since the genetic constitution of mankind hardly changes within a century and differs only moderately between human populations in different parts of the world, the changes in the incidences of individual cancers over time and their geographical variation to a large extent reflect environmental effects. Cancers are caused by exogenous chemical, physical, or biological carcinogens. They act on humans who, however, vary in their ability to cope with them due to differences in their genetic constitution and – not to forget - their psychological, social, and economic conditions. Endogenous processes in the human body also contribute to the development of cancer, on their own or by interacting with exogenous agents.

The mechanisms of carcinogenesis in humans are often multifactorial and complex. Different factors may act by different mechanisms and at different stages of tumor development. In experimental animals carcinogens can be applied in a controlled fashion and the individual steps and interactions can therefore be analyzed more precisely. It is, e.g., possible in some cases to distinguish between initiating and promoting agents as well as complete carcinogens, or between carcinogens and co-carcinogens. In these laboratory models, initiating carcinogens are usually mutagens, while promoting agents act by facilitating the expansion of cells with altered DNA.

These distinctions are more difficult to apply in real human cancers. For instance, tobacco smoke is a human carcinogen, without a shade of doubt. In fact, it contains a variety of different carcinogens, some of which may act as initiators and some as promoters, and some as both. Nicotine itself is almost certainly not a direct carcinogen, but a potent alkaloid which acts not only on the central nervous system, but also influences cell signaling and cell interactions in the airways and in the lung. So, it would have to be classified as a co-carcinogen. Similarly complex interactions take place during skin carcinogenesis caused by UV radiation. Moreover, the actions of carcinogens and co-carcinogens are modulated by genetic differences in the human population, which is outbred, unlike many laboratory animals.

As a consequence, it is often difficult in humans to elucidate exactly by which mechanism a potential carcinogen acts, even though it is clearly identified as being associated with a specific cancer by epidemiological data. Attempts at prevention must therefore often be started before the relationship between a carcinogen and cancer development is fully understood. Nevertheless, precise elucidation of the mechanisms is helpful and insights from molecular biology are beginning to contribute to improved prevention of cancer.

Many carcinogens have been established as important in human cancer, in one or the other way. Exogenous carcinogens can be classified into chemical, physical, and biological agents. For some carcinogens the evidence is very strong, while for others the notion '*carcinogen*' has to be applied in a broader sense. Another type of classification issued by the World Health Organization groups human carcinogens by the level of available evidence.

Table 1.1. Types and examples of human carcinogens

Type of carcinogen	*Examples*
Chemical carcinogens	Nickel, cadmium, arsenic, nitrosamines, trichloroethylene, arylamines, benzopyrene, aflatoxins, reactive oxygen species
Physical carcinogens	UV ırradiation (specifically UVB), ionizing radiation
Biological carcinogens	Human papilloma virus (e.g. strain), Epstein-Barr-Virus, Hepatitis virus B, Helicobacter pylori, Schistosoma mansoni
Endogenous processes	DNA replication, metabolic reactions generating reactive oxygen species, chronic inflammation

Chemical carcinogens come from different sources and comprise very different chemicals. Inorganic compounds like nickel, cadmium, or arsenic are encountered in the workplace or are present as contaminants in water. Organic compounds acting as carcinogens can be aliphatic, like nitrosamines, which occur in smoked and pickled foods, or trichloro-ethylene, which is used for cleaning. Nitrosamines are thought to contribute to stomach cancer, in particular *Aromatic compounds* like benzopyrenes and arylamines are generated from natural sources by burning, and are among the many carcinogens in tobacco smoke. They also present a danger in the workplace, e.g. during coal processing and dye production and use, respectively. Arylamines are thought to cause bladder cancer, in particular. Polyaromates like benzopyrene are also released into the environment by burning of coal and fuels. Natural compounds produced by plants and molds can be highly carcinogenic. Aflatoxin B1 is implicated as a carcinogen in liver cancer and is the most infamous of many chemically diverse compounds in this group. Medical drugs can be carcinogenic, notably those used in cytostatic tumor therapy like cyclophosphamide, nitrogen mustards, and platinum compounds. Various hormones and hormone-like compounds from natural and pharmaceutic sources also influence the development of cancers in specific tissues, e.g. in the breast and prostate. Doubtless, the most abundant exogenous carcinogen is oxygen. The form present in air, dioxygen, is relative inert and, of course, safe when fully reduced towards H_2O. However, partially reduced oxygen or dioxygen activated towards its singlet state are highly reactive and can be mutagenic. Reactive oxygen species are formed at low levels during normal metabolism and are produced at increased rates during certain physiological processes such as immune defense and inflammation. Their concentrations can also be increased during the metabolism of some exogenous compounds, e.g. quinones, and by pathophysiological states such as iron overload.

Table 1.2. Classification of human carcinogens according to the WHO/IARC

Group	*Definition*
Group 1	The agent is carcinogenic in humans. The exposure circumstance entails exposures that are carcinogenic to humans.
Group 2A	The agent is probably carcinogenic to humans. The exposure circumstance entails exposures that are probably carcinogenic to humans.
Group 2B	The agent is possibly carcinogenic to humans. The exposure circumstance entails exposures that are possibly carcinogenic to humans.
Group 3	The agent (or exposure circumstance) is not classifiable as to carcinogenicity in humans.
Group 4	The agent (or exposure circumstance) is probably not carcinogenic to humans.

Physical Carcinogens

Any energy-rich radiation can in principle act as a carcinogen, depending on dose and absorption. Visible light is not usually carcinogenic, unless it is absorbed by '*photosensitizing agents*' which generate reactive oxygen species. UVB irradiation is an important carcinogen in the skin, and its effect is augmented by UVA. In contrast, UVC is strongly absorbed in the non-cellular protective layers of the skin and does not usually act as a carcinogen. γ-Radiation from natural, industrial, and iatrogenic sources (e.g., used in X-ray diagnostics) can penetrate into and through the body. It is carcinogenic to the extent to which it is absorbed, damaging DNA and cells by direct absorption but also indirectly by generating reactive oxygen species. Damage and carcinogenicity by γ-radiation therefore depend on the concentration of oxygen and also on the repair capacity. Radioactive β-radiation and specifically α-radiation is most dangerous when nuclides are incorporated, e.g. of cesium, uranium, and plutonium. The effect of radioactive isotopes depends also on their distribution in the body. For instance, radioactive iodine is accumulated in the thyroid gland and therefore causes specifically thyroid cancers, whereas radioactive cesium isotopes tend to become enriched in the urinary bladder. The potential carcinogenicity of microwave and radio wavelength electromagnetic radiation are, of course, the subject of public debate.

Biological Carcinogens

Certain viruses and bacteria act as biological carcinogens in man. Specific strains of *human papilloma viruses* (HPV16 and HPV18) are established as causative factors in cervical and other genital cancers. They also influence the development of cancers of the skin and of the head and neck, and perhaps others as well. Papovaviruses like SV40 (simian virus 40) cause cancers in animals and partially transform human cells in vitro, but whether they actually cause human cancers is a controversial issue. The best evidence exists for mesothelioma, a rare cancer which may be caused by the combined action of SV40 and asbestos. Specific herpes viruses can also act as carcinogens or co-carcinogens, e.g. *human herpes virus* 8 (HHV8) in Kaposi sarcoma or *Epstein-Barr virus* (EBV) in lymphomas. The *hepatitis B virus* (HBV) with its DNA genome is certainly involved in the causation of liver cancer, although in a complex fashion, as is the *hepatitis C virus* (HCV) which has an RNA genome. Human retroviruses such as HIV facilitate the development of cancers mostly by interfering with the immune system, but HTLV1 (*human T-cell leukemia virus*) causes a rare leukemia by direct growth stimulation of T-cells.

While there are many speculations on a carcinogenic role of bacteria, definitive evidence exists for a relationship between *Helicobacter pylori* infection and stomach cancer. More generally, bacterial infections may contribute to inflammation which can promote cancer development. Schistosoma trematodes also cause cancer in humans, mostly in the urinary bladder.

Endogenous Carcinogens

How effective exogenous carcinogens elicit cancer in a specific person depends strongly on an individual's exposure, specific responses, and general health. So, endogenous processes are in any case involved in cancer development through modulation of the response to exogenous carcinogens. However, cancers may also be caused by strictly endogenous processes:

1. Normal metabolism generates carcinogenic compounds such as nitrosamines, aromatic amines, quinones, reactive aldehydes, and – as mentioned above – reactive oxygen species. The concentration

of these potential carcinogens may vary depending on factors like diet or physical activity, but a minimum level is associated with any level of metabolic activity and any type of diet. Potent protective and detoxification mechanisms exist for many of these compounds, but they can never be perfect.

2. In the same vein, damage to cells and specifically DNA occurs at a minimum rate spontaneously and particular during cell proliferation, e.g. by errors in replication or by spontaneous chemical reactions of DNA bases. The potentially huge number of such errors is kept at bay by very efficient DNA repair mechanisms specifically directed at typical errors of this kind. In addition, damaged cells are removed by apoptosis and other mechanisms. These protective mechanisms, however, cannot be perfect, either.
3. There is, consequentially, some evidence that damaged DNA and cells accumulate with age and that protective mechanisms may become less efficient in the course of a human life. These factors may contribute to the increase of cancer incidence with age, although it is not clear, to which extent.
4. While each of the above processes takes place in any human anytime, the risk of carcinogenesis is certainly higher during specific phases, e.g. when tissues proliferate after incurring damage. A period in human life with particularly high proliferative activity is, of course, fetal development. Genetic and even epigenetic errors occuring during this period may lead to cancer in children, but also favor cancer development much later in life.
5. Some pathophysiological conditions may increase the risk of cancer development. Chronic inflammation, in particular, is associated with increased cancer risk in many organs, e.g. colon or stomach. Several factors are involved, including an increased production of mutagenic reactive oxygen species by inflammatory cells as well as secretion of proteases, cytokines, and growth factors by various cell types in the tissue that favor the growth and spreading of tumors. So, tissue regeneration in general is associated with an increased cancer risk, but particularly, if it involves remodeling as in liver cirrhosis or in cystic kidneys. Some carcinogens have, in fact, been proposed to act simply by stimulating tissue growth and rebuilding without being actually mutagenic.

In summary, both endogenous and exogenous factors can be responsible for human cancers. In many cancers, they interact so intricately that their contributions are difficult to discern. In some cases, the involvement of specific carcinogenes can be identified by characteristic mutations. In other cases, the absence of such '*fingerprints*' and the epidemiological evidence point to a predominance of endogenous processes. On this background, estimates of 5% of all human cancers being due to occupational carcinogens or 15% being caused by viruses have to be taken with more than one grain of salt. They do provide, however, rough estimates of how much could be achieved by prevention.

Characteristic Properties of Cancer and Cancer Cells

In spite of their diversity, human cancers share several fundamental properties. Different cancers display each of these to different extents. Moreover, these properties may be acquired step by step and become evident at various stages during the progression of a cancer. Most of these properties individually are also found in other diseases and some are even exhibited during physiological adaptive responses. However, the combination of uncontrolled cell proliferation, altered differentiation and metabolism, genomic instability, and invasiveness with eventual metastasis is unique to and defines cancer.

Table 1.3. Characteristic properties of human cancers

Property
• Increased cell proliferation (often autonomous)
• Insufficient apoptosis
• Altered cell and tissue differentiation
• Altered metabolism
• Genomic instability
• Immortalization (growth beyond replicative senescence)
• Invasion into different tissue layers and other tissues (with disturbed tissue architecture)
• Metastasis into local lymph nodes and distant tissues

Increased and Autonomous Cell Proliferation

The most obvious property of tumors is growth beyond normal measures. In fact, the term '*tumor*' when used in a broader sense designates every abnormally large structure in the human body, also including swellings or fluid-filled cysts. More precisely, then, cancers belong to those tumors caused primarily by increased cell proliferation, i.e. a permanent and continuing increase in cell numbers. Increased cell proliferation as such is also observed during tissue regeneration, adaptative tissue growth, and in some non-cancerous diseases. For instance, atherosclerosis can also with some right be regarded as a tumor disease. In general, an increased number of cells in a tissue is designated '*hyperplasia*'. Extensive hyperplasia or hyperplasia with additional changes such as altered differentiation ('*dysplasia*') is considered a '*benign*' tumor. Dysplasia often precedes malignant tumors and in such cases is regarded as a '*preneoplastic*' change. Substantial alterations in the tissue structure and in particular the presence of tumor cell invasion define a malignant tumor or cancer. The borderlines between hyperplasia, benign tumors, and cancer are often evident from microscopic or even macroscopic inspection, but in some cases additional criteria or markers have to be employed to make the distinction. Hyperproliferation in cancers is brought about by an altered response to exogenous growth regulatory signals. On one hand, cancers are often hypersensitive to growth-stimulatory signals, and some cancers become largely independent of them. On the other hand, sensitivity to growth-inhibitory signals is usually diminished or abolished. Together, these altered responses result in the growth autonomy that characterizes cancers. Moreover, it typically increases during their progression.

Insufficient Apoptosis

Cell proliferation in cancers may be caused by a combination of three factors: (1) The rate of cell proliferation is enhanced by an increase in the proportion of cells with an active cell cycle, i.e., a higher '*proliferative fraction*', and/or by a more rapid transit through the cell cycle, together resulting in increased DNA synthesis and mitosis. (2) The rate of cell death is often decreased by relatively diminished apoptosis. In some cancers, this is in fact the driving force for increased proliferation. In others, the rate of apoptosis is enhanced compared to normal tissue; but not sufficiently so as to compensate for the increase in mitotic activity. (3) In normal tissues, successive stages of differentiation are typically associated with progressively decreased proliferative capacity and/or with apoptotic death of the fully differentiated cells. Thus, a block to differentiation is in some cases sufficient to confer an increased proliferation rate.

Altered Differentiation

Many cancers consist of cells which resemble precursor cells of their tissue of origin and have not embarked on the normal course of differentiation, whereas others show properties of cells at intermediate stages of differentiation. Some cancers, however, do consist of cells with markers of full differentiation, with the crucial difference that they continue to proliferate. In these cancers, it is not difficult to identify the cell of origin, which is important for diagnosis. Many cancers, however, express markers that do not occur in their tissue of origin. Frequently, cancer cells express proteins which are otherwise only found in fetal cells. Such proteins, e.g. carcinoembryonic antigen in colon carcinoma or alpha-fetoprotein in liver cancer are called '*oncofetal*' markers. Other proteins expressed in cancers are never synthesized in the original cell type, e.g. '*cancer testis antigens*' in melanoma and various peptide hormones in small cell lung cancer. This phenomenon is called '*ectopic*' expression. Some cancers change their phenotype to resemble cells from a different tissue in a process called '*metaplasia*'. One might think that this is a clear hallmark of cancer, but metaplasia occurs also in some comparatively innocuous conditions. Metaplasia can, in fact, precede cancer development, e.g. during the development of a specific type of stomach cancer. In some other carcinomas, metaplasia may be a late event. Other changes of cell differentiation obliterate the original cellular phenotype so strongly that it can be difficult to distinguish from which primary site a metastasis originates. Two such '*generic*' cell types are a small epithelial-like cell with a large nucleus to cytoplasm ratio and a spindle-shaped cell resembling a mesenchymal fibroblast. These cell types are end points of cancer progression in some carcinoma cases, typically found in aggressive cases and therefore also in metastases.

So, altered differentiation confers properties to cancer cells that are otherwise found in tissue precursor cells, fetal cells or cells of other tissues. Moreover, altered differentiation is also related to increased proliferation. As pointed out above, the control of proliferation and differentiation are intimately linked in normal tissues. The final stages of differentiation of many normal tissues are associated with an irreversible loss of replicative potential or even with cell death. This process is therefore called '*terminal differentiation*'. For instance, differentiated cells in keratinizing epithelia crosslink with each other, dissolve their nuclei, and become filled with structural proteins. This way, a steady state between cell generation and loss is maintained which breaks down, if differentiation fails in a cancer.

Altered Metabolism

Cell proliferation, whether normal or abnormal, requires according changes in cell metabolism. Most evidently, DNA synthesis requires deoxynucleotides, so enzymes required for nucleotide biosynthesis, and specifically of deoxynucleotide biosynthesis, are induced and activated in proliferating cells. Further cell components such as membranes and organelles also need to be duplicated. For this reason, lipid biosynthesis is increased in cancer cells, likely because they cannot obtain enough fatty acids, phospholipids and cholesterol from lipoproteins supplied by the gut and liver. As a consequence, expression and activity of key enzymes like fatty acid synthase and hydroxymethylglutaryl-coenzyme A reductase are increased in cancer cells. Porphyrin biosynthesis is also often increased. As Warburg already noted in the 1930's, many tumor cells switch from aerobic to anaerobic glucose metabolism.

A key requirement for cell growth is increased protein synthesis, which is apparent at several levels by enhanced size and number of nucleoli, increased expression of transcription initiation factors and enhanced phosphorylation of ribosomal proteins. A particularly strong boost in protein synthesis may be required during invasion and metastasis.

Overall, cancer growth poses an enhanced energy demand on the patient, which increases with the tumor load. Moreover, cancers release the waste products of their metabolism, such as lactate, with which the body has to cope. These are, unfortunately, only some of the systemic effects of cancers. Cancers also secrete enzymes and hormones that act on the host, some of which are toxic. In particular, cytokines like tumor necrosis factor α can elicit a general break-down of metabolic function with visible wasting, termed '*cachexia*', and suppression of the immune system, thereby facilitating '*opportunistic*' infections. Other tumor products, such as FAS ligand, can damage sensitive organs such as the liver, and ectopically produced hormones can interfere with homeostasis. For instance, calcitonin production by small cell lung cancers may cause life-threatening variations in calcium levels. Such indirect disturbances of the body homeostasis by cancers, designated as '*paraneoplastic*' symptoms, can be as problematic for the well-being and survival of a patient as the malignant growth per se.

Genomic Instability

A clear distinction between cancerous and non-cancerous cell proliferation lies in genomic instability. Cancer cells as a rule contain multiple genetic and epigenetic alterations. Polyploidy, an increase in the number of genomes per cell, can be ascertained by measuring cellular DNA content. Aneuploidy, i.e. a change in the number and structure of individual chromosomes, is revealed by cytogenetic methods. These aberrations are often already revealed upon microscopic observation of tumor tissues by altered size and shape of the nuclei in the cancer cells and aberrant mitotic figures. Other cancers remain diploid or nearly so, but contain point mutations and/or altered DNA methylation patterns.

As cancers progress, the numbers of alterations in their genome tend to increase. Therefore, cancers, even if outwardly homogeneous, usually consist of cell clones that differ at least slightly in their genetic constitution. The variant clones are continuously selected for those proliferating fastest, tolerating adverse conditions best, capable of evading immune responses, etc., with the best-adapted cell clone dominating growth. This variation becomes particularly evident during tumor treatment by chemotherapy which exerts a strong selection pressure for those cell clones carrying alterations that allow them to survive and continue to expand in spite of therapy.

There is some debate, whether some cancers have simply accumulated many mutations during their development or whether all exhibit genomic instability leading to an increased rate of chromosome alterations, point mutations, and/or epigenetic defects. This is not an academic question, because cancers with genomic instability will display greater variation and a higher risk of developing resistance. It seems indeed possible that true genomic instability develops in some cancers during progression, e.g. in CML. Genomic instability in cancer cells can be derived from several sources, e.g. from defects in DNA repair and in mechanisms checking genomic integrity.

Immortalization

Many cancer cells are '*immortalized*', which means they are capable of a theoretically infinite number of cell divisions. Most human cells can undergo only a finite number of divisions, likely up to 60-80, before they irreversibly lose their ability to proliferate. Obviously, the cells constituting the germ line are exempt from this restriction and so are tissue stem cells. For instance, hematopoetic stem cells in the bone marrow can be successively transplanted across several recipients and still remain capable of reconstituting the entire hematopoetic system, blood and immune cells. Immortality in stem cells is maintained by specific mechanisms such as expression of telomerase, which is also found in cancers. Moreover, some human cancer cells can be maintained in tissue culture or as transplants in animals, designated '*xenografts*', over many generations, as far as we can tell, infinitely many. On a note of caution, it is not certain that all human cancers are immortalized, since many cannot be grown in tissue culture or as xenografts. Even telomerase expression is not universal. To become life-threatening, however, a cancer does not need to consist of cells with infinite growth potential. Starting out from a single cell, 50 replications would yield up to 2^{49} tumor cells, which must be compared to something between 10^{13} and 10^{14} normal cells in a human. Lethal cancers are much smaller than that.

Invasion and Metastasis

A property more directly evident in human cancers is their ability for invasion and metastasis. Invasion and metastasis are the definitive criteria which distinguish benign from *malignant tumors*. Moreover, invasion and metastasis, with tumor cachexia and immune suppression, account for most of the lethality of human cancers.

During invasion, cancers spread from their site of origin into different layers and parts of the same tissue, eventually growing beyond it and into neighboring structures. Invasion involves multiple steps and often substantial rebuilding of the tissue structure by the tumor cells, by other cells in the tissue responding to signals from the tumor cells, and by immune and inflammatory cells. Typically, in carcinomas, the basement membrane separating epithelium and mesenchyme is destroyed and tumor extensions push through the connective tissue and muscle layers. From some cancers, cells separate and migrate through the neighboring tissues, as single cells, in an Indian file pattern or as small, adherent cell clusters. Invasion is often accompanied by inflammation, so lymphocytes, granulocytes and macrophages are present in the invaded tissue and in the tumor mass.

An important component of malignant growth is *neoangiogenesis*. The nutrient and oxygen supply from preexisting blood vessels is usually not sufficient to support growth of tumors beyond a size of a few mm. Therefore, cancers, but also some benign tumors, induce neoangiogenesis, which comprises the growth of new capillaries, and the rebuilding of existing blood vessels. Lymph vessels can also be remodeled or newly formed.

During metastasis, cancer cells separate from the primary tumor and migrate by the blood or lymph to different organs where they form new tumors. Depending on the route, '*hematogenic*' metastasis, which usually leads to metastases at distant organ sites, is distinguished from '*lymphogenic*' metastasis, which leads initially to the formation of metastases in lymph nodes draining the region from which the cancer emerges. Like invasion, metastasis is really a multistep process. Thus, many more cancer cells enter the blood or lymph than actually form metastases. Important barriers are posed by the necessity to leave the blood stream at capillaries which carcinoma cells cannot pass ('*extravasation*') and to survive and resume proliferation in the micro-environment of a different tissue. In fact, individual cancer cells or small groups may end up in a different tissue only to survive over long periods without net growth. These '*micrometastases*' are not detectable by current imaging techniquew, although they may be biochemically detectable by proteins secreted by the cancer cells. Over time, they may adapt to their new environment and expand to larger metastases that threaten the patient's life. This may occur several years after the primary tumor has been removed. Cancers differ in the extent and the sites to which they metastasize. Generally, preferred organs for metastasis are those with extended microcapillary systems such as liver, lung, and bone.

Characterization and Classification of Cancers in the Clinic

Many properties of cancers described in the previous section are reflected in the terms and methods used in the clinic and in diagnostic histopathology to describe and classify cancers as a prequisite for appropriate treatment and for prognosis. For these purposes, as well as for cancer research using specimens of human cancers, it is mandatory to obtain as exact as possible descriptions of the extension of the tumor, of its degree of malignancy and of its histological subtype.

Staging

The extension of a tumor is described by '*staging*'. Prior to surgery or if none is performed, a clinical stage is defined by visual inspection, palpation and various imaging techniques. These techniques use a.o. ultrasound, X-rays, scintigraphy, computer tomography, magnetic resonance, and positron emission tomography. Some imaging procedures detect changes in tissue shape and density, whereas others react to changes in metabolism and blood flow in cancers. If surgery is performed, a more precise delineation of the extension of the tumor can be made by inspection of the tumor site and by histopathological investigation of the specimen. The stage defined in this fashion is called *pathological stage*. It is denoted by a 'p' prefix to distinguish it from clinical stage, which is denoted by a 'c'.

Several staging systems are employed. The most widely used and systematic staging system is the TNM classification, while others remain in use for specific cancers. In the TNM system, the extent of the primary tumor is normally described by T1-T4, where increasing numbers describe larger and/or more invasive tumors. The system varies for different tumor sites. The presence of cancer cells in lymph nodes is denoted by N0, N1, and in some cancers also N2, with N0 meaning none detected. The presence of metastases is indicated by M0 meaning none detected, M1, or in some cancers also M2. After surgery, it is also important to know whether all of the local tumor growth has been removed. This is designated by the R value. R stands for resection margin, so R0 means that the tumor seems to be wholly contained within the removed specimen. In all categories, the affix 'x' is used for '*not determined/unknown*'.

Grading

The degree of malignancy of a tumor is further estimated by grading systems. Again, several systems are in use for different tumors and in different countries. To different extents they score the degree of cellular and nuclear atypia and/or the degree of tissue disorganization in tumor sections, biopsies, or even single tumor cells. The most prevalent system is G grading, which usually ranks from G0 to G4. The designation G0 typically denotes normal differentiation and no cellular atypia, as would be found in a benign tumor. At the other end, G4 would be assigned to cancers with a cellular morphology completely different from the normal tissue and pronounced atypia of the cells and nuclei. The grades G1-G3 are called well-differentiated, moderately and poorly differentiated. It is important to be aware that the use of '*differentiation*' in this context is different from that in cell or developmental biology. This can be confusing, the more so as in modern pathology grading based on morphology is sometimes supported by staining for specific markers of cell differentiation or of cell proliferation. For instance, immunohistochemical staining against PCNA, a subunit of the DNA replisome mainly expressed in S-phase cells, and Ki67, a protein essentially restricted to actively cycling cells, can be used to estimate the proliferative fraction in a tumor, in addition to estimating the proliferative rate by counting mitotic figures.

Histological Classification

The location of a tumor is the first clue to its classification. It is, of course, not sufficient, since (1) a tumor mass may represent a metastasis or the extension of a cancer originated in a neighboring organ. Moreover, (2) several different kinds of cancer may develop within one tissue, often with very different properties, clinical course and treatment options. Therefore, a tumor must be histologically classified from samples acquired by biopsy or from surgical specimens. Several of the designations used in this context have already been introduced in this chapter. Histological typing of tumors is performed by evaluating their morphology. Routine procedures use a variety of specific stains developed over centuries in anatomy and pathology to highlight particular cell types as well as extracellular structures like basement membranes, fibers or mucous. Increasingly, tumor classification by histopathological investigation is being improved by specific molecular markers. Immunohistochemical staining with antibodies directed against specific antigens of the presumed tissue of origin, e.g. cytokeratins, or tumor-specific antigens, e.g. carcino-embryonic antigen, is often performed. For leukemias, analysis of subtypes can be determined by antibody staining followed by flow cytometry. Analyses at the RNA or DNA level for specific patterns of gene expression or specific genetic alterations are not standard yet, but are employed by specialized institutions. Similarly, cytogenetic techniques are becoming more widely used, particularly for the classification of hematological cancers.

Insights into the molecular biology of human cancers have begun to improve staging, grading, and histological classification. These improvements have an immediate impact on cancer therapy, because in most cancers the choice of therapy is contingent on these parameters. Even now, a tumor in the kidney, e.g., will be treated quite differently, if it is a malignant renal carcinoma at an early or at an advanced stage, a benign tumor of mesenchymal origin, a melanoma metastasis, or a lymphoma. However, recent and future molecular markers are expected to go far beyond such distinctions. They may reveal differences between cancers that look morphologically the same, but represent different diseases, as do certain leukemias. They may reveal previously unrecognized subclasses within one disease, as may be the case with breast cancer and may predict different clinical courses for morphologically similar tumors. Moreover, molecular insights should allow selection of certain cancers for treatment with drugs tailored to specific targets and may allow to predict how well a patient tolerates cancer treatment by radiotherapy or cytostatic medication.

Treatment of Cancer

In principle, a range of different therapies is available for the treatment of human cancers. Surgery, irradiation or drugs can be employed, or a a combination of these. Which therapy is chosen depends strongly on the classification of the cancer by the criteria described in the previous section.

Surgery or radiation are treatment choices for localized cancers. In contrast, leukemias, lymphomas, and metastatic or locally advanced carcinomas and soft tissue cancers require drug chemotherapy, which is in some cases supplemented by radiotherapy or surgery of primary cancers or metastases. Conversely, surgery can be followed by chemotherapy or irradiation to attack residual local tumor or metastases. This is called '*adjuvant*' treatment. Accordingly, chemotherapy applied before surgery to shrink the tumor mass and facilitate its complete resection is often called '*neo-adjuvant*' treatment. The standard chemotherapy regime for a cancer is usually designated as '*first-line*', if it fails, '*second-line*' therapy can be attempted. The efficacies of chemotherapy and radiotherapy are extremely dependent on the tumor type. Some cancers, e.g. some testicular cancers and certain lymphomas, are highly sensitive, whereas others, e.g. renal cell carcinoma, appear to be overall less sensitive than many normal tissues.

In cancer chemotherapy a wide range of different drugs are employed. Some drugs are aimed at the cancer itself, but other medications are employed to stabilize specific body functions in the patient or for pain relief. The most important component in the treatment of many cancers is cytotoxic drug therapy, often simply called *chemotherapy*. In this kind of therapy, chemical compounds are employed that block DNA synthesis, transcription, and/or mitosis in the cancer cells, often driving them into apoptosis. A different type of anti-cancer drugs summarized as '*biological agents*' bind to receptor molecules in the cancer cells that are not directly involved in DNA replication or mitosis, but regulate them. Examples for this type of drugs are hormones and antihormones used in the treatment of breast cancer and prostate cancer and retinoids used for several cancers, especially a specific acute leukemia, promyelocytic leukemia. Since the advent of recombinant DNA biotechnology, cytokines and growth factors can be produced at reasonable cost and sufficient purity to be used in cancer therapy. In some cases, they act directly on the cancer cells, in other cases, they stimulate the immune response against the cancer, and in still another application, they stabilize the hematopoetic system of the patient against the effects of the cancer and the treatment. Interferons and interleukins used in the therapy of leukemias and renal carcinoma are examples for the first two applications. Erythropoetin stimulating erythrocyte production and GM-CSF enhancing hematopoesis more globally are examples for the third type.

Several different types of radiation can be used in cancer radiotherapy and even particles and radioactive isotopes. Most widely used is ionizing radiation in the form of high energy γ-radiation. It damages cancer cells by direct effects on cellular macromolecules or by generating reactive oxygen species, as during carcinogenesis. Typically, radicals are induced which initiate chain reactions that lead to DNA double-strand breaks which prevent further cell proliferation or induce apoptosis. The radiation dose that can be applied is limited by its effects on normal tissues. Modern techniques allow an improved focussing of the radiation or use radioactive isotopes implanted into the tumor. However, these improvements are mostly useful for the treatment of localized cancers. In some cases, the tumor cells can be sensitized towards the radiation. For instance, the fact that many tumors have a higher rate of porphyrin biosynthesis than normal tissues is exploited in photodynamic therapy. In this technique, intense light with a wavelength near the absorption maximum of protoporphyrins is applied by a laser beam to generate reactive oxygen. In other cases, the preferential uptake of radioactive isotopes by the cancer can be exploited, e.g. in the therapy of well-differentiated thyroid cancers by radioactive iodine.

Even where the full range of modern cancer therapies is available, many cancers cannot be cured today. In not too few malignant diseases, state of the art therapies are at best palliative, i.e. symptoms caused by the cancer are alleviated, but survival is not or only slightly prolonged. Novel cancer therapies are urgently required. Therefore, cancer therapy is the area, in which expectations are highest for the applications resulting from insights into the molecular biology of cancers. Indeed, novel drugs have been developed based on such insights. Moreover, the understanding of established therapies like cytotoxic chemotherapy and radiotherapy has also been deepened. These developments are beginning to have a significant impact on cancer therapy. Evidently, it is hoped that completely novel therapies may emerge. Immunotherapy is already being applied in some cancers, albeit with highly variable efficacy. Since the causes for its successes and failures are becoming gradually elucidated, it may be more broadly used in the future. Gene therapy of cancer also carries high hopes and several hundred clinical trials have been performed or are underway. At this stage, however, it is a purely experimental therapy.

2

Cancer Diagnosis

Evolving Scope of Molecular Diagnostics

There is widespread agreement that insights into the molecular biology of human cancers will make their most rapid impact in the area of cancer diagnosis. As described in the previously, implementation of cancer prevention is not only impeded by our limited knowledge of the complex causes of cancer, but also by a host of socioeconomic factors. The development of molecular-based cancer therapies is also hampered by scientific as well as general factors. In contrast, translation of research results into routine diagnosis is underway and is favored by scientific and general factors.

1. Other than in cancer therapy, the techniques used in research laboratories can be applied in diagnostic laboratories with relatively little additional effort. In general, techniques need to be further standardized and additional controls must be introduced. Often, procedures are developed to make them amenable to automatization.
2. The translation of molecular biology results into diagnostic procedures can built on the existing infrastructures provided by pathology and clinical chemistry laboratories in the clinic. These laboratories are already accustomed to performing biochemical and immunochemical assays and are now adding molecular biology techniques to their repertoire.
3. Similarly, the production of standardized and validated reagents for molecular diagnostic techniques has been taken up by companies that have previously marketed diagnostic kits for immunohistochemical or biochemical assays or by new biotech companies.

4. Molecular biology techniques fit well into an ongoing trend towards individualized therapy, as discussed later in this chapter.

Molecular biology techniques can be applied for a wide range purposes in cacer diagnosis.

Table 2.1. Applications of molecular diagnostic techniques for cancer detection and classification

Purpose
Detection of cancer predisposition
Detection of preneoplastic changes
Cancer detection
Tumor staging
Tumor grading
Differential diagnosis
Subclassification
Prognosis of spontaneous clinical course
Prognosis of response to therapy

Tumor Staging, Grading, and Differential Diagnosis

The first applications that come to mind concern differential diagnosis of tumors before therapy. Here, assays for proteins and nucleic acids in body fluids and tissue samples supplement diagnostic procedures relying on imaging techniques and '*classical*' histopathology. Routine histopathology increasingly makes use of molecular markers at the protein, RNA and DNA level. After all, it is not a big leap from traditional staining methods for tissue samples to immunohistochemistry to detect specific protein markers, RNA-in-situ-hybridization to detect specific mRNAs, or fluorescence-in-situhybridization to detect chromosomal aberrations. Nevertheless, a new specialty is emerging, labeled '*molecular pathology*'.

It is important to be aware that, as developments in molecular biology are changing histopathology, developments in physics and information technology are revolutionizing imaging techniques. Modern computing power, e.g., allows the reconstruction of virtual dynamic 3D images from tomography data to detect and precisely localize very small tumors by non-invasive techniques. The combination of modern imaging techniques with molecular markers, such as labeled antibodies, is a rapidly developing field of applied medical science. This combination may eventually be used to localize even micrometastases consisting of a few tumor cells, to monitor the distribution of therapeutic molecules, and to improve the targeting of radiotherapy.

While modern imaging techniques can excellently circumscribe the extent of a tumor and thereby help to determine its stage, they yield little information on its histology and its biological properties, which determine its further clinical behavior. This information is also required for the choice of therapy. Traditionally, the tumor subtype was determined by its morphology, usually determined by staining of tissue sections. More recently, immunohistochemistry, e.g. for cell type-specific cytokeratins in carcinomas or CD surface proteins in leukemias, has entered routine practice and improved differential diagnosis. In general, the precise identification of the tumor type already provides a great deal of information on the likely future course of the disease (i.e. the prognosis of the patient) and a basis for the choice of the most appropriate treatment. In routine histopathology, additional information on the aggressiveness of a tumor is obtained by grading, which relies on subjective estimates of the degree of tissue disorganization as well as cellular and nuclear atypia.

Like the determination of the tumor type, this estimation of its '*character*' has in many cases been improved by the use of antibodies. These can help, e.g., to measure the proliferative fraction of the tumor or to ascertain the intactness of the basement membrane separating a questionable carcinoma in situ from the underlying connective tissue. In spite of these improvements, classification, staging and grading of many tumor types by current methods are far from perfect in predicting prognosis and the response to specific therapies. Molecular diagnostic techniques will thus be helpful for the determination of tumor stage, e.g. by allowing detection of tumor cells in the blood or in the bone marrow.

Cancer Subclassification

A major impact of molecular diagnostic techniques is expected in the subclassification of tumors with respect to prognosis and response to therapy. In several cases, particularly in hematological cancers, molecular analyses have revealed that a disease which appeared uniform by morphological criteria can be further differentiated. In other instances, e.g. renal cancers or breast cancer, molecular classification has corroborated previous suspicions that different subclasses of the disease exist and may need different treatments. Yet another situation is found in some cancers that are morphologically and molecularly similar, but in which progression depends on specific molecular alterations. For instance, mutation of *TP53*, as detected by accumulation of the mutant protein in the tumor cell, may predict a worse prognosis in several cancers, including Wilms tumors and bladder cancer.

Prediction of Response to Specific Therapies

The advent of cancer therapies directed against specific molecular targets has advanced these developments one step further. Previously, cancer therapy was directed against one type of cancer in general, e.g. against breast cancer, exploiting what was seen as general properties of cancer cells, such as increased DNA synthesis or increased sensitivity to ionizing radiation. As therapy increasingly targets specific molecular changes which are present in a subclass of cancers of one histological type, diagnosis has to follow suit. So, increasingly, molecular diagnostics is required to determine which cancers express the targets for specific molecular therapies. In this way, the introduction of molecular diagnostics into the clinic strengthens the already established trend towards individualized cancer therapy.

Early Detection

Although imaging and histopathology have become more sophisticated, they are limited by the size of a cancer. Molecular diagnostics holds the promise of detecting cancers at even earlier stages. This can be applied in several circumstances, particularly in cancer prevention and screening. Another application is in the monitoring of therapy efficacy and of recurrences.

Detection of Predispositions

Specifically, molecular diagnostics can be used to identify populations at risk for the development of a cancer. This is often not possible by traditional methods. Importantly, the definition of risk conferred by inherited mutations is unique to molecular diagnostics.

Molecular Diagnosis of Hematological Cancers

Arguably, molecular diagnostics is presently best established in hematology, of all subspecialties within oncology. Molecular techniques are used to ascertain the initial diagnosis and to determine the exact subtype among morphologically similar leukemias and lymphomas as a basis for prognosis and therapy selection. They are applied to assay autologous bone marrow and stem cell transplants for residual tumor cells and to match allogenic donor transplants to the recipient patient. During and after therapy, they are employed to monitor its success and to detect residual tumor cells and recurrences at an early stage.

Since many hematological cancers are characterized by specific cytogenetic aberrations, typically translocations, cytogenetic techniques are well suited for differential diagnosis. In addition, detection of surface markers by antibody staining is used, since cells at various stages and sublineages of the hematopoetic lineage express specific cell membrane proteins.

Burkitt lymphoma (BL) invariably carries one of three translocations which bring the *MYC* gene under the control of immunoglobulin gene enhancers. These translocations can be detected by karyotyping of tumor cell metaphases, which is best performed on cultured tumor cells. For the direct investigation of tissue sections, interphase two-colour FISH is more convenient. Tissue sections are hybridized with two DNA probes, one each from the *MYC* locus at 8q and an immunoglobulin locus (initially for *IGH* at 14q, which is most often involved), labeled by different colours. In normal cells, the loci are on distinct chromosomes and located at some distance from each other in an interphase nucleus. Even in BL cells, one pair of signals corresponding to the normal chromosomes 8 and 14 remains apart and serves as an internal control. In contrast, the signals from the translocation chromosome appear close to each other. While this apposition may occur by chance in an occasional cell, its regular appearance in a lymphoma tissue proves the presence of this particular translocation chromosome and confirms the diagnosis of Burkitt lymphoma.

This kind of technique can be used in general to detect translocations, including those in *chronic myeloid leukemia* (CML). However, while the translocations in BL cause the overexpression of MYC mRNA and protein, whose structures are not necessarily altered, the characteristic translocation in CML generates a novel fusion gene, *BCR-ABL*, with a transcript and a protein that are unique to tumor cells. This provides further opportunities for detection. The rearrangement creating the *BCR-ABL* gene can be detected by Southern blot or PCR analysis. In principle, translocations in BL could also be detected by these methods, but the detection is more straightforward and reliable in CML, since the breakpoints occur within restricted regions in both genes. They therefore create a limited number of different mRNA forms, none of which is present in a cell without a translocation. All can be detected by RT-PCR using a few pairs of PCR primers, one primer each from the *BCR* and *ABL* gene. This detection can be performed qualitatively to verify the diagnosis or quantitatively to estimate the number of tumor cells. Moreover, RT-PCR can be made extremely sensitive by nesting and real-time techniques allowing the detection of one tumor cell in a billion. Therefore, this method is much more sensitive than cytogenetic or morphological detection of tumor cells.

Thus, owing to the development in molecular diagnostics, CML therapy can be monitored at several levels by a set of techniques with different sensitivities. '*Clinical remission*' remains an important criterion. The improvement of symptoms in a treated patient and the disappearance of morphologically detectable tumor cells ('*hematological remission*'), however, are not sufficient to predict whether a recurrence will occur. Indeed, in some cases with clinical improvements and lack of obvious tumor cells, cytogenetic techniques can still detect translocation chromosomes indicative of '*minimal residual disease*'. Without additional therapy, such patients as a rule relapse. The prognosis is much better, if '*cytogenetic remission*' is achieved and no cells with translocation chromosomes can be detected. However, some of these patients still experience recurrences. Indeed, RT-PCR analyses can detect residual tumor cells in the bone marrow and even in blood. In fact, these methods can be made so sensitive as to detect tumor cells in every treated patient and even in some healthy individuals. Therefore, quantitative methods are employed and cut-off values are defined to determine which patients are very unlikely to experience recurrences.

Molecular monitoring in CML is not only important to determine the efficacy of treatment. It is also helpful in the choice of therapy, particularly to decide which patients need stem cell transplantation, and when. This treatment can have serious side-effects, such as graft-versus-host disease. Therefore, the definitive exclusion of residual disease by molecular diagnostic techniques can identify those patients for whom transplantation can be deferred. Of course, the selection of donors and cells for transplantation is also aided by molecular techniques.

In a similar fashion, molecular diagnostics can help in the choice of *acute promyelocytic leukemia* (APL) therapy. Cytogenetic or molecular diagnostics can identify patients that carry the t(15;17)(q22;q21) translocation generating the *PML-RARA* fusion gene. These can then be treated with all-trans retinoic acid, which has little effect in other acute myeloid leukemias and even in some cases of APL that are not caused by this particular translocation.

Unfortunately, the predominance of *MYC* translocations in BL, of *BCR-ABL* fusion genes in CML, and of *PML-RARA* fusions in APL are the exception rather than the rule in hematological cancers. More often, acute leukemias and lymphomas with similar phenotypes can be caused by several different genetic alterations, i.e. different translocations or other characteristic chromosomal alterations. Moreover, not all leukemias and lymphomas are characterized by specific single chromosomal changes or gene mutations. In carcinomas, this is the rule. Phenotypically similar diseases caused by different translocations can exhibit large differences in their spontaneous clinical course and in their response to specific treatments. So, determining the correlation between specific translocations and clinical behavior is a continuing effort in hematological oncology that leads to a steady progress in adapting the treatment to the individual patient's cancer.

The problem is of course exacerbated in those hematological cancers that do not show specific chromosomal aberrations. Such cases represent a significant fraction of acute lymphocytic leukemia. Here, advances are expected from '*gene expression profiling*'. Initial studies using these techniques showed that is feasible to distinguish ALL from AML (*acute myeolid leukemias*) by analysis of mRNA expression patterns. This is rarely a problem in the clinic, because protein markers for the myeloid and lymphatic lineage can be used, if the morphology of the tumor cells is not already distinctive. Indeed, the mRNAs that showed the most pronounced differences in the expression profiles were those encoding such protein markers. More importantly, the technique can distinguish different subtypes among AMLs lacking conspicuous chromosomal changes.

Another pressing clinical problem is the distinction between different subtypes of follicular lymphomas and large cell lymphoma. They exhibit similar morphological and biochemical markers, but some subtypes are rather indolent, while specific ones are aggressive, and therefore require a different therapy. This distinction can also be made by expression profiling. In other cases, expression profiling has suggested new protein markers for detection of minimal residual disease of specific subtypes.

Molecular Detection of Carcinomas

Molecular diagnostics of carcinomas is less straightforward than that of leukemias and lymphomas. The first additional complication lies in obtaining material for analysis. For leukemia diagnostics, blood samples are in many cases sufficient to detect the presence of a leukemia and even establish an initial differential diagnosis. In some cases or later in the diagnostic procedure, bone marrow aspirates or other biopsies are additionally required. Even solid types of lymphomas often present as relatively accessible swellings.

In contrast, samples from carcinoma can often be obtained only through more invasive procedures, which may carry a risk of inadvertently spreading tumor cells, e.g. in the peritoneum. So, often, only limited amounts of useful material from a carcinoma are available until surgery has been performed. This may be one reason why molecular biology of human carcinomas is not as advanced as that of hematological cancers. Another reason is that molecular alterations in carcinomas are often more complex and more heterogeneous than in hematological cancers.

Table 2.2. Important criteria in the use of molecular diagnostic assays in the clinic

Criterion
Minimal sample required
Applicable with samples obtained by non-invasive or minimally invasive methods
Speed of result
Stability of molecule assayed
Cost effectiveness
Reliability
Specificity
Sensitivity
Reproducibility
Compatibility with existing expertise, procedures, and equipment

A diagnostic assay applicable in a clinical setting has to fulfil several requirements. (1) It should require as little material as possible, e.g. from biopsies. This is a strong point of many molecular assays, in particular of PCR techniques. (2) Ideally, an assay should be able to use samples obtained by non-invasive methods. Saliva, sputum, urine, and stool samples can be obtained by completely non-invasive routes. Blood samples also present few problems. In some organs, e.g. the urinary bladder, washes can be performed which yield '*lavage*' fluids containing cells and molecules from tumors. (3) PCR techniques have also, in general, made molecular assays more rapid, which is a further requirement in many clinical situations. (4) A more problematic requirement is the stability of the molecule to be assayed. Some proteins and RNA in general are not very stable in tissue samples, unless these are quickly frozen or fixed. Therefore, assays based on DNA or on more stable proteins are generally preferable. RNA instability is even more of a problem, if quantitation is required. This is one factor withstanding the use of expression profiling techniques in clinical routine. (6) Another factor in this case, as in general, is cost-effectiveness. Cost, however, is relative. Using an expensive assay to determine the correct therapy in a small number of patients is a different issue from using an assay for screening a large population. (7) Assay sensitivity and specificity are of course crucial, although again, the required levels depend on the intended use. (8) Last not least, an assay has to be reliable, which means that it measures the parameter it is supposed to measure, not only in a laboratory situation, but also with clinical samples.

Specificity and cost are the major hurdles when a molecular assay is designated for screening larger groups or populations. Such assays also have to be essentially non-invasive, i.e. no more invasive than taking a small blood sample. In the application of molecular diagnostic techniques for carcinomas in the clinic, sensitivity and cost effectiveness most often represent the crucial issues. It is at these points, where the complexity and heterogeneity of molecular alterations in carcinomas become relevant.

The problem of sensitivity arises mainly, because there are only few instances, in which a single molecular alteration is found in every cancer of one type. This is particularly true for carcinomas. For instance, while almost every colon carcinoma shows constitutive activation of the WNT pathway, these are brought about by different genetic changes. In most cases, both copies of the *APC* gene are inactivated, while in a smaller fraction activating mutations in *CTNNB1* (β-Catenin) are responsible. In still another, albeit small fraction of colon carcinomas, neither of these genes is affected. This would probably not compromise sensitivity overly. More problematic is that the alterations in *CTNNB1* and *APC* are not homogeneous, either. Mutations that activate β-Catenin are restricted to a small region of the protein, but are not uniform. *APC* inactivation is worse, since it occurs by different mechanisms which include small and large deletions as well as point mutations at many different sites in the gene. Since most lead to a truncated protein, alternatively a protein assay could be envisioned that employs an antibody against the carboxy-terminus of the APC protein. This assay could be applied to colon cells obtained by biopsies or from faeces. This method would miss the (rare) cases with missense mutations, in addition to all those not caused by APC mutations. More problematic is that this is a '*negative marker*' assay. Assays that detect the disappearance of a marker tend to yield lower sensitivities and specificities. Hopes are placed in a microarray technique that detects all possible mutations in *APC* and *CTNNB1* (and perhaps *AXIN1*).

In contrast to loss of a protein, point mutations in DNA represent '*positive*' markers that can be detected in spite of a background of DNA from non-tumor cells in samples obtained by non-invasive methods (e.g. stool samples). Therefore, some approaches for the molecular detection of colon cancer have pursued detection of *KRAS* mutations. While these occur only in 40-60% of all colon cancers, they are strictly limited to the three codons 12, 13, and 61. These mutations can be highly sensitively detected by appropriate PCR techniques. Of course, as *KRAS* mutations mostly develop during the progression of colon cancers, this assay would detect carcinomas rather than adenomas. In theory, then, a sensitivity of 40-60% could be achieved, with a specificity approaching 100%. In practice, neither figure has been reached. The reasons for this disappointing outcome are under investigation. One might speculate that sensitivity is limited by the amount of tumor DNA entering the gut lumen and surviving the passage. There are furthermore indications that specificity is lowered by an unexpectedly high fraction of false positives, i.e. mutations detected in persons without carcinomas. Perhaps, mutations in *KRAS* sometimes occur in normal cells or arise in DNA as it travels through the gut.

A straightforward place to look for molecules originating from a cancer is blood. A number of serum protein markers are employed for the detection and monitoring of specific cancers.

Some carcinomas, including those of the colon, can be detected by increased levels of *carcino-embryonic antigen* (CEA) in the blood. This protein marker can be determined very reliably and at moderate cost by a routine immunoassay. Unfortunately, the assay is not very sensitive, since only a fraction of cancers express this oncofetal antigen, and not very specific, a.o., because several cancer types express CEA. However, once a cancer has been found to express CEA, the marker can be used to monitor the success of the therapy.

A similar immunoassay for *prostate-specific antigen* (PSA) is used to monitor prostate cancer therapy. Detection of PSA has several advantages that have led to its almost ubiquitous use. (1) Prostate epithelial cells are the only significant source of PSA in males.

Therefore, any increase in serum must be due to a process in this tissue. (2) Only few prostate carcinomas cease to synthesize the protein, often only at a very late stage when this is no longer clinically important. (3) The PSA level is roughly related to the tumor volume. Following removal of the prostate harboring the cancer, PSA declines. Ideally, the protein should become undetectable (<0.1 ng/ml) and stay so, if the cancer has been cured. A nadir in the ng/ml range typically indicates that the local tumor has not been completely removed. In that case, one would consider adjuvant radiotherapy or anti-androgenic therapy. Recurrences caused by micrometastases are usually announced several years in advance by a slow increase of serum PSA from zero levels. In late stage systemic disease, values >1000 ng/ml may be reached.

PSA levels can also be employed in clinical and experimental studies. The presence and size of primary and metastatic tumor masses is an important parameter to determine the efficacy of a new drug or the significance of a molecular marker. However, metastases in prostate cancer can often only be detected with difficulty, least their size be measured. So, in prostate cancer the success of a new therapy is often monitored via the PSA level, which is used as a '*surrogate parameter*' of cancer extension. In general, a 50% decrease is taken as evidence of remission. While PSA assays are thus helpful, they do have downsides, on the scientific as well as on the psychological side. On the scientific side, PSA synthesis is induced by androgens. Therefore, treatments that influence androgen signaling may decrease PSA levels much more than they affect tumor growth. On the psychological side, as PSA plays such a dominant role in the treatment of prostate cancer, not only patients, but also doctors and scientists are tempted to ascribe more value to a PSA level than it is worth.

While PSA is an excellent marker for monitoring of prostate cancer, its specificity for the initial detection of the carcinoma is limited. Here, additional molecular diagnostic assays might be helpful, which detect cancer cells in prostate biopsies or blood, or cancer-specific markers in blood, urine, or ejaculate.

As in colon cancer, genetic alterations in prostate cancer are heterogeneous, if anything, much more so. In some patients, tumor cells can be detected in the blood, e.g. by an RT-PCR assay for prostate-specific mRNAs such as PSA mRNA. Detection of PSA mRNA is a more specific indication of cancer than detection of PSA protein, because the protein is secreted, whereas its mRNA can only be dectected if prostate epithelial cells are present in the circulation. These are in most cases cancer cells. For a while, this method was even thought to be useful for the distinction of metastatic from organ-confined cancers, i.e. for '*molecular staging*'. However, this may not prove to be true.

Other assays are based on DNA alterations in tumor cells. In many tumor patients, increased levels of DNA are found in blood plasma, which is cell-free. Its source is not entirely clear, but much of it appears to be derived from tumor cells, perhaps released from cells dying in the circulation. Typical mutations present in cancer tissues can also be detected in this circulating DNA, e.g. *KRAS* mutations from a colon or pancreatic carcinoma.

In prostate cancer, specifically, no characteristic mutations occur regularly enough to be exploited for this kind of assay. However, alterations of DNA methylation are highly prevalent, in particular hypermethylation of the *GSTP1* gene, which may occur in >80% of all prostate carcinomas. Since DNA hypermethylation affects CpG-islands which are unmethylated in normal tissues, its detection is very specific and sensitive because of a negligible background from normal tissues. Moreover, while hypermethylation of some genes is also found in aging tissues or early preneoplastic lesions, the hypermethylation of *GSTP1* appears to be cancer-specific, or at least restricted to late preneoplastic lesions in addition. So, detection of *GSTP1* hypermethylation in blood or prostate fluid may provide a valuable technique to supplement PSA assays.

DNA hypermethylation is also found in many other cancers and similar assays are being developed for their detection. Unlike in the case of prostate cancer and *GSTP1*, in most cancers, hypermethylation assays must be performed for several genes, since each is hypermethylated in only a fraction of cancers. Moreover, hypermethylation of *GSTP1* is relatively specific to prostate cancer. It is otherwise only found in a smaller fraction of renal carcinomas and hepatomas. These cancers are relatively straightforwardly excluded in prostate cancer patients. In contrast, another gene, *RASSF1A*, is hypermethylated in prostate cancer, but also in many others and even some precursors. This property could make *RASSF1A* hypermethylation useful as a general sensitive tumor marker, but limit its specificity.

Tumor DNA in plasma can also be assayed for mutations or for allelic imbalances. As in general, the sensitivity of these assays is limited by the heterogeneity of genetic alterations within the tumor type. Some current research therefore aims at developing assays which detect every mutation in one gene, e.g. in *TP53*. These assays would, however, still miss alternative pathways of TP53 inactivation, such as MDM2 over-expression. The sensitivity of assays for allelic imbalances is in addition limited by the extent to which tumor DNA is diluted in the plasma by DNA originating from normal cells.

A hotly debated question in the use of plasma DNA for tumor detection is how its overall presence and amount relate to tumor stage. A similar question pertains to the issue of tumor cells found to circulate in the blood. If DNA from a tumor is present in blood, it appears to have gained access to the circulation, which is almost certain, if tumor cells are encountered in blood outside the tumor tissue. So, while early stages of tumor development can perhaps not be discovered by assays using blood samples, the detection of tumor-specific DNA alterations or even of tumor cells may yield information on how far the cancer has advanced. This approach may therefore yield a chance to achieve a '*molecular staging*'. Alternatively, the type of mutations and allelic imbalances might be used for '*molecular staging*', if they can be assigned to specific stages of tumor development.

Molecular Classification of Carcinomas

Detection of a cancer is only the first step towards therapy. Whether and which therapy is administered, depends on a further, more precise classification of the cancer. Traditionally, cancers were assigned to different histological subtypes by their morphology and further classified by stage and grade by imaging techniques and histopathological examination. Experience and carefully collected observational data were used to assess the prognosis of the cancer and select the most appropriate therapy.

The criteria underlying tumor staging, in particular, are not arbitrary, but have usually been chosen to correspond to those steps in tumor progression, at which the prognosis and accordingly, the most appropriate treatment changes. Such steps may be evident, such as beginning invasion of outer layers in a tissue or growth beyond an organ, or they may have to be determined by careful follow-up of large numbers of patients. For instance, renal carcinomas rarely metastasize unless they exceed a certain volume, but are as a rule incurable, once metastases have developed. Accordingly, the criteria for staging of renal carcinomas have been changed back and forth based on observational data relating the course of disease to the diameter of the tumor. In this case, prognosis additionally depends on the specific histological subtype, with some histological subtypes metastasizing more readily than others. Therefore, knowledge on the histological type of the tumor is important for the determination of prognosis. More recently, identification of characteristic chromosomal alterations for each subtype of renal carcinomas has been introduced to aid in the classification of ambiguous cases.

There are many carcinomas, in which the '*classical*' trias of histology, staging, and grading does not consistently yield sufficient information for optimal selection of therapy. It is not at all exceptional for carcinomas with identical stage, grade, and histology to take divergent clinical courses. The most severe problem in general is that micrometastases escape detection by current imaging methods. Therefore, staging is not really precise and the extension of the primary tumor as well as its histology and grade only yield an estimate on the presence of micrometastases. These are responsible for recurrences and patient death, even if the primary tumor can be completely removed or destroyed. Thus, the decisions on how to deal with the primary tumor and whether to apply an adjuvant therapy (and which, if there is a choice), are based on probabilities rather than definitive information. A large set of empirical data has been collected for each cancer type which can be used in these decisions. In some cancers, algorithms and nomograms taking all known relevant parameters into account have been introduced as a help for patients and doctors. Nevertheless, the overall situation is far from satisfactory.

In a sense, progress in therapy has aggravated this dilemma. Since a larger choice of treatments has become available, criteria are needed to determine which patients will respond to which therapy. In addition, therapies differ with respect to their side-effects and their costs, which can often not be neglected.

For these reasons, improvements in the classification of carcinomas are a major goal of current molecular research. Breast cancer may represent a major carcinoma, where this type of research is advanced and is translated into the clinic at a rapid pace. Molecular assays are increasingly used in this cancer as supplements to staging, grading and histology.

As in other carcinomas, prognosis in breast cancer depends on tumor size, tumor grade, and the histological subtype. Neither unusually, breast cancers in young patients tend to be more aggressive. More specific to breast cancer, prognosis and therapy differ before and after menopause. The single most significant prognostic factor in this cancer is the extent of lymph node involvement. Less than 30% of cancers without detectable tumor cells in the lymph nodes recur, whereas >75% of cancers with several positive lymph nodes have progressed to systemic disease and will recur, if only the primary tumor is destroyed. So, almost all patients with lymph node involvement receive adjuvant therapy. Moreover, since recurrent breast cancer is rarely curable, chemotherapy or anti-estrogenic therapy is also administered to most of the patients with no positive lymph nodes as well, unless additional favorable factors are found, such as small tumor size or low grade, or a rarer less aggressive histological subtype is present. This means that overall ≈60% of breast cancer patients unnecessarily receive an unpleasant and toxic therapy, but it is difficult to determine, whether this is so for each individual patient.

Some molecular markers are already in routine use to help with this decision. Low concentrations of the plasminogen activator uPA and its inhibitor PAI-1 indicate a favorable prognosis, at least in cancers that are well or moderately differentiated. Patients with cancers designated ER+/PR+ that express both the estrogen and progesterone receptors also fare better, as a rule. More recently, determination of the ERBB2 status by immunohistochemistry and FISH analysis has been introduced. In general, breast cancers with ERBB2 overexpression caused by gene amplification are more likely to have metastasized. However, determinations of the ER/PR and ERBB2 status are employed primarily for the choice of therapy rather than for the determination of prognosis. Cancers that are ER+/PR+ tend to respond well to anti-estrogenic therapy, whereas cancers that do not express the steroid hormone receptors or that overexpress ERBB2 do not. Instead, some cancers with ERBB2 over-expression can be treated more successfully by a combination of chemotherapy, including anthracyclins, and an antibody directed against ERBB2, trastuzumab.

Overall, >100 individual molecular markers for the prognosis of breast cancer have been suggested over the last years. Promising candidates that may make it into clinical routine are the proliferation markers Ki67 and PCNA, which are also useful in several other cancers. They can be detected in a semi-quantitative manner by immunohistochemistry. Similarly, the cell cycle regulator Cyclin E is overexpressed in more aggressive breast cancers, and $p27^{KIP1}$ is accordingly down-regulated.

It is generally presumed that no single clinical or molecular parameter may be sufficient for an optimal prognosis of breast cancer.

Rather, several are already in use and further ones are being added. Considering appropriately all the known factors and their complex relationships becomes increasingly difficult. Therefore, algorithms and nomograms have been introduced that help to take into account the relative importance of each information obtained, including histology, staging, grading, patient age, and various molecular markers, and their relationship to each other. These can help in the choice of therapy, which ultimately rests with the doctor and the patient. As more and more interacting factors become known and can be assayed, computer programs are being developed that calculate the risks associated with each treatment strategy. Learning algorithms and neuronal networks are particularly suited to this task, as they can improve with their 'own' experience and integrate information from new clinical studies.

In a sense, therefore, expression profiling using microarrays is a logical continuation of a development that is already underway in breast cancer diagnosis. Analysis of the expression levels of a large number of genes indeed allows to classify breast cancers into ER+ and ER- types. It distinguishes previously unrecognized luminal cell-like and basal cell-like subtypes, with ERBB2+ cancers representing a distinct subclass within the basal-cell-like subtype. Cancers arising in patients with inherited mutations in the BRCA genes also exhibit characteristic profiles. Most importantly, metastatic cancers appear to show distinct expression patterns from those still growing locally.

The next step therefore will be to verify these profiles in larger groups of patients in prospective studies. A large population study of this kind is underway in the Netherlands. If these studies are successful, the technical and cost problems that currently prohibit routine use of expression profiling in the clinic are likely to not present serious obstacles in the long run. In parallel with these studies, much smaller sets of genes that are decisive for the distinctions provided by microarray data will be assayed for their potential as prognostic markers. For prostate cancer, e.g., a set of just four genes has been proposed for this purpose. Expression of all four can be followed by immunohistochemistry, facilitating the introduction of these markers into routine laboratories.

Prospects of Molecular Diagnostics in the Age of Individualized Therapy

The examples of breast cancer and leukemia described in the previous sections illustrate a general development in cancer diagnosis and therapy. Cancer therapy has moved towards individualization. This development began actually quite independently of the availability of adequate molecular markers and any in-depth understanding of the molecular basis of cancer pathophysiology. Already, surgery, chemotherapy and radiotherapy are administered contingent on histopathological parameters and on the patient's general state of health and psychosocial circumstances. A vast amount of empirical data can serve as a basis for the decision in each individual case ('*evidence-based medicine*'). This individualization helps to achieve optimal therapeutic results, to minimize suffering not only from the cancer, but also from the treatment, and to avoid unnecessary expenses. In this situation, molecular markers come in handy to continue an ongoing development in all subdisciplines of oncology.

However, the potential of molecular markers in the diagnosis of cancer goes beyond providing better distinctions between subclasses of one cancer and serving as prognostic markers. It is captured in the novel notions of '*pharmacogenetics*' and '*pharmacogenomics*'.

In a sense, pharmacogenetics is also a continuation of an existing trend, since it has been known for quite a while that individual patients can react very different to some drugs.

NAT2

'*Slow*' and '*fast*' acetylators, e.g. not only metabolize carcinogenic arylamines at a different rate, but also a variety of drugs in medical use. Therefore, this phenotype influences susceptibility to cancer as well as the response to therapy. The '*slow*' and '*fast*' acetylator phenotypes are due to polymorphisms in genes encoding N-acetyl-transferases, mostly in *NAT2*.

UGTA1

Individuals with Gilbert syndrome, like slow acetylators, are otherwise asymptomatic, but excrete certain drugs more slowly than others. These can therefore accumulate to dangerous levels. The molecular basis of Gilbert syndrome is a polymorphism in the promoter of the *UGTA1* gene encoding UDP-glucuronyl-transferase A1. The promoter contains a variable number of TA repeats. The allele *UGT1A1*1* with six repeats yields maximum expression, whereas a frequent polymorphic allele containing seven repeats, *UGT1A1*28*, is associated with diminished expression. The UGTA1 enzyme transfers glucuronic acid to hydroxyl groups of endogenous or exogenous compounds, which increased their solubility in aquous solution and facilitates their excretion. In cancer therapy, this polymorphism is most relevant for the metabolism of irinotecan, a topoisomerase inhibitor used a.o. in the treatment of colorectal and lung cancers. Severe toxicity of the compound is observed predominantly in persons homozygous for the *UGT1A1*28* allele.

TS

The promoter of the *TS* gene encoding thymidylate synthetase is likewise polymorphic. It contains either two or three repeats of a 28 bp tandem repeat. The respective alleles are designated *TSER*2* and *TSER*3*. The *TSER*3* alleles lead to increased expression of the enzyme that is crucial for the synthesis of dTTP required for DNA replication. Increased expression of TS diminishes the effect of inhibitors, such as 5-fluoro-uracil, which are employed in the treatment of many different cancers.

TMPT

Thiopurine methyltransferase (TPMT) metabolizes and detoxifies purines containing a thiol group, especially the drug azathioprine, which is used in the chemotherapy of leukemias. About 1% of all individuals lack enzyme activity due to a genetic polymorphism. In these persons, administration of thiopurine drugs at the standard dose can be lethal. Heterozygotes for the *TPMT* polymorphism tolerate intermediate doses.

ATM

Sensitivity to radiotherapy, likewise, is influenced by genetic polymorphisms, as exemplified by individuals heterozygous for mutations in the *ATM* gene. This gene encodes a protein kinase controlling the cellular response to DNA damage by ionizing radiation, but also to other forms of DNA damage. Pharmacogenetics, thus, is the systematic study of all genetic variation that determine the individual response to drugs. Of course, pharmacogenetics is not restricted to drugs used in cancer therapy, and as indicated by the case of *ATM*, genetic polymorphisms are also relevant to therapies other than drugs.

In current clinical practice, pharmacogenetics is rarely used explicitly. Rather, it is implicit in the way drugs are administered. Patients are asked about known hypersensitivities and are observed for adverse reactions known to occur with specific compounds. New drugs are monitored for side effects while being developed and are continued to be monitored for side effects after their introduction to the general market. This latter monitoring is important, since some polymorphisms are present in only a few individuals or are only prevalent in specific subpopulations. Drug trials can never be comprehensive in this respect. While these general procedures are well established, specific genetic analysis for polymorphisms influencing drug sensitivity are currently only used in selected circumstances. For instance, some institutions have an *TPMT* assay set up routinely.

The reasons for this are practicability and cost to a much greater extent than a lack in understanding of individual variabilities in the reaction to drugs. For many drugs in current use, the mechanisms underlying different toxicities are in fact well elucidated. However, the genetic polymorphisms underlying individual variabilities are often complex and assaying them is currently more expensive than relying on careful observation in a trial-and-error fashion.

The '*slow*' and '*rapid*' acetylator phenotypes, e.g., are brought about by quantitative interactions between >10 different *NAT2* alleles. To predict the phenotype from the genotype, a range of polymorphisms must be tested. So, observing the patients or monitoring the excretion of a test drug dose, is more practical. Similarly, individuals with low UDPGTA1 expression can usually be identified by a slight elevation of serum bilirubin in the absence of other signs of liver disease, as determined by routine clinical chemistry. A molecular genetic assay is preferred for assaying *TPMT*, because the genotype/phenotype relationship is straightforward and the polymorphisms are relevant for a clearly defined class of drugs administered for selected diseases.

This situation may change radically in the future. One factor driving the change is the continuing automatization of techniques for molecular genetic analysis which reduces expenses. Many in the field envision a chip-based assay, which at one stroke detects all polymorphisms relevant for drug metabolism in an individual. This analysis could be performed once and for all for each person and drugs could be prescribed accordingly. However, not everybody is enthusiastic about this scenario, for diverse reasons. One concern is safeguarding of individual genetic data. It is one thing to determine the genetic properties of an individual responsible for the sensitivity to one particular drug administered against a deadly disease, but it is another to record many polymorphisms influencing the response to a variety of medical and other drugs. There are also purely scientific concerns. As the example of the acetylator phenotype shows, the relationship between genotype and phenotype is often not straightforward. The individual reaction to most drugs is determined by several factors, of which only some are determined by the DNA sequence assayed in molecular tests. Even if genetic factors predominate, several genes may be involved and their interactions can be complex.

The issue is different, if not adverse reactions, but positive response to a drug or treatment are at stake. A substantial number of otherwise efficacious drugs have failed in early clinical trials (i.e. in phase I or phase II) or have not even proceeded to being tested in humans (i.e. to phase I) because they display intolerable sideeffects. Others seem efficacious in a subset of patients too small to warrant their further development for the general market. If one could predict which patients tolerate or respond, respectively, to such drugs, they could still be used in selected patients. This would extend the range of individualisation of therapy.

The notions of '*pharmacogenetics*' and '*pharmacogenomics*' are still pretty fresh and are often used rather loosely, so some confusion has arisen. In fact, prediction of positive responses to therapy is one area in which pharmacogenetics and pharmacogenomics meet and overlap. The precise distinction should be that pharmacogenetics deals with the patient's reactions to specific therapies, whereas pharmacogenomics considers the therapeutic targets specific for a disease. A broad definition of pharmacogenomics would therefore encompass almost the entire molecular biology of human cancers. In everyday use, the term '*pharmacogenomics*' more specifically denotes the investigation of drug targets in specific cancers.

A good illustration of the purpose of pharmacogenomics is the case of ERBB2. In a specific subclass of breast cancers, ERBB2 is overexpressed, typically as a result of gene amplification. Determination of ERBB2 expression and of amplification of its gene gives a very good indication of whether cancers will respond to an antibody directed against the protein. This may sound like an issue for pharmacogenetics, but it is a genetic property of the particular tumor and not the individual patient that provides the basis of the treatment.

As more and more therapeutic agents become available that are targeted to specific molecules in specific tumors, pharmacogenomic testing will become more important.

Moreover, other than in pharmacogenetics, prediction of the response of a cancer to a drug typically relies on an molecular assay. Obviously, the response of a breast cancer patient to an anti-ERBB2 antibody cannot be predicted from her previous experience with everyday drugs. Similarly, the simple strategy of applying the drug and monitoring the response is inefficient and costly, since the treatment is expensive and is efficacious in only a fraction of the patients. So, the molecular assay has to precede the application of the drug. The necessity of pharmacogenomic tests is underlined by failed efforts to extend the use of ERBB2-targeted therapy to other cancers. Amplification and over-expression of ERBB2 are rare in prostate and bladder cancers and clinical trials with the antibody directed against the protein were by and large unsuccessful.

In contrast, imatinib, an inhibitor of the BCR-ABL protein kinase, was found to induce remissions not only in chronic myeloid leukemia, which is driven by this fusion protein, but also in other cancers. In gastrointestinal stromal tumors, its effect could be related to the inhibition of the KIT receptor tyrosine kinase, already known as an alternative target of the drug from in vitro assays. However, among these, only those cancers in which KIT was activated by a mutation responded. This experience makes a strong argument in favor of pharmacogenomical approaches to therapy. However, further cancer types, without KIT activation, have responded to imatinib. In these, the effect of the drug is ascribed to inhibition of the receptor tyrosine kinase PDGFR (*platelet-derived growth factor receptor*).

Pharmacogenetics and pharmacogenomics are two specific areas which may be representative for the overall direction that molecular diagnostics in oncology is taking. It is expected that molecular diagnostic techniques will supplement the established methods of tumor diagnosis, rather than replace them. The main impact of innovation will be to better tailor therapy to each individual patient and to each individual cancer.

3

CANCER PREVENTION

Less than 60% of all cancers can be cured by current therapies, even though these are often burdensome with serious side effects. Therefore, the best strategy would seem to prevent cancers in the first place. Moreover, strategies focusing on cancer prevention could circumvent the increasing economic problems in the health systems of Western industrialized countries, where treatment costs are felt to have become exuberant and ressources are strained. In some developing countries, with health care budgets of down to $1 per person and year, cancer preventive strategies are plainly the only realistic option.

While these arguments are in principle conceded by everybody, in practice cancer prevention measures are slowly implemented. The scientific literature, too, rarely yields the impression that cancer prevention is high on the list of research priorities. The reasons for this discrepancy are manifold. Political and socioeconomic factors may be dominant. More pertinent to the theme of this book, the science behind prevention is also anything but trivial. Cancer prevention requires a multidisciplinary approach with contributions from many fields, from molecular biology, infectiology, and pharmacology through psychology to health system economy. The scientific basis for successful prevention is not convincing for many cancers. Nevertheless, many programs have already been successfully implemented and further developments are underway. The prime task of molecular biology research in this context is to identify the causes of cancers as precisely as possible and to define the most appropriate stage and optimal means for intervention. Both are different for different cancers. Moreover, in many cases the implementation of cancer prevention hinges on progress in diagnostics and therapy. Several different types of cancer prevention are distinguished, mostly according to the stage of cancer development at which they are applied.

Table 3.1. Types of cancer prevention

Type of cancer prevention
Primary prevention (avoidance of exposure to carcinogens)
Chemoprevention
Dietary changes
Detection of preneoplastic changes and early cancer stages
Prevention of cancer after preneoplastic changes
Prevention of recurrences and second cancers
Prevention in individuals with inherited high-risk predisposition to cancer

Primary Prevention

Ideally, a cancer can be prevented by eliminating or avoiding the responsible carcinogens. These can be chemical compounds such as aromatic amines in bladder cancer, physical agents such as UV radiation in skin cancer, or biological agents such as the virus HBV in liver cancer and the bacterium *H. pylori* in stomach cancer. Obviously, cancers arising overwhelmingly from endogenous processes, which may include many cases of colorectal cancer and prostate carcinoma, will require a different approach for prevention.

Even in those cancers, in which a responsible carcinogen has unequivocally been identified, the implementation of prevention is not generally straightforward. Arguably, the most tragic case is that of tobacco smoking and lung cancer. A causal relationship has been established at every conceivable level from epidemiological data down to the molecular detail of detecting major carcinogens from cigarette smoke covalently bound to precisely those bases in the *TP53* gene of bronchial epithelial cells, at which mutations are most often observed in lung cancers. Moreover, while addiction to tobacco smoking is difficult to heal in many afflicted persons, tobacco use is not necessary for human life and could principally be avoided. The inability to prevent a large fraction of lung cancers (and others caused by tobacco smoke carcinogens) is hardly due to a lack of scientific insight.

Not all these arguments apply to UV radiation, which is the established major cause of different types of skin cancer. The relationship between the carcinogen and the disease can be considered proven. An important piece of molecular evidence is that mutations in *TP53* and other tumor suppressor genes like *PTCH1* in skin cancers bear the signature of induction by UV radiation. However, while unreasonable exposure to UV radiation during leisure activities might be avoided, complete avoidance of the carcinogen is not realistic for people with outdoor occupations. Even more importantly, up to a certain dose sunlight with its UV component is beneficial and even necessary for human health.

The critical level, at which danger surpasses benefit, differs between individuals and populations. It depends strongly on genetic polymorphisms that determine the intensity of skin pigmentation. In addition, a smaller number of individuals are oversensitive to UV radiation or sunlight, e.g. as a consequence of defects in DNA repair in xeroderma pigmentosum patients. Thus, skin cancer prevention requires an individualized approach. It is pursued by a combination of campaigns aiming at the general public and individual counseling by general practitioners and dermatologists.

A different dilemma is posed by chemical carcinogens in the workplace, illustrated by the case of aromatic amines causing bladder cancer in humans. Like in the above cases, the relationship is well established and consequences have been drawn. Today, a situation like that encountered by Ludwig Rehn when he went to investigate why so many of his patients developed bladder cancers, is - hopefully - not found anywhere anymore. Yet, it was not a century ago, when one third of the employees in another German chemical plant manufacturing benzidine developed bladder cancers. However, after a retreat battle vividly described by Robert Proctor in "*Cancer Wars*", these experiences have led to the establishment of strict regulations in the production and use of chemicals that are established or likely carcinogens in man. Unfortunately, many carcinogenic chemicals are necessary and cannot reasonably be eliminated completely. Therefore, it is in the end a political decision which amounts should be produced and which levels should be accepted. Chemical plants and laboratories can be fitted to minimize the risk for those working there, whereas the environment and the population at large cannot. Therefore, the acceptable levels of chemical carcinogens are not only determined from the angle of occupational risk, but also by their presumed impact on the environment and the general population.

In many cases, however, the responsible carcinogens are not known sufficiently precisely for intervention. For instance, epidemiological studies consistently demonstrate an increased risk of bladder cancer in the plastics and rubber industry, but it is not entirely clear which compounds are responsible and which measures could be taken to avoid exposure to them.

Another complication stems from the fact that most cancers have different and potentially interacting causes. Consider the (realistic) case of a bladder cancer patient, who has been employed in a tire factory, has been a long-time smoker, is an amateur painter, and regularly takes (too much) phenacetine against his recurrent headaches. This person has likely been exposed to four different sources of chemical carcinogens that each could cause bladder cancer, and it is not unlikely that they synergize. With the exception of smoking, none of these exposures is completely preventable in a real world.

As in the case of UV exposure, there are substantial differences in the way individuals react to chemical carcinogens. In the case of exposure to aromatic amines, several polymorphisms in enzymes responsible for their activation, metabolism, and excretion have been found to modulate a person's risk of cancer and other adverse reactions. Their combined effects are not small. Thus, among the employees that developed bladder cancer after occupational exposure to benzidine-related compounds, the vast majority where '*slow acetylators*', while few '*rapid acetylators*' were affected. These phenotypes are due to polymorphisms in the *NAT2* gene.

In the general population, all different combinations of such polymorphisms are represented. It is tempting to select more resistant persons from this heterogeneous group for the inevitable production of arylamines needed for dyes and drugs by testing for their *NAT2* and further genotypes. There are, of course, serious ethical problems associated with this approach, since it might lead to a sort of '*genetic selection*'. Proponents point out that this approach is already used in protecting more sensitive persons, e.g. pregnant women are prohibited from working with radioactive materials. Certainly, one would not like to expose an over-sensitive person to a dangerous chemical compound either? On the other hand, a person's genotype can be considered a part of his or her privacy. If it is revealed to employers, who else could be barred from that information? In addition, choosing a vocation is certainly an important constitutent of individual freedom. A general concern is that genetic testing for susceptibility to carcinogens in the workplace might lead to a lowering of the established standards for prevention of occupational carcinogenesis and might eventually endanger the population. Clearly, this issue requires a public consensus as a basis for political decisions. It also requires solid data and excellent counseling for informed choices to be made.

The problem of balancing economic necessities with disease prevention reemerges in the wider context of exposure of the entire population towards chemical carcinogens. Unlike in the workplace, special protective measures are not feasible here. Moreover, the population is even more heterogeneous than the employees in a chemical plant, encompassing not only healthy adults, but also children or people with disabilities or largely increased susceptibilities. Moreover, while the release of synthetic chemical compounds into the environment can often be controlled, many natural sources of carcinogens cannot. It is hardly surprising, therefore, that issues such as the allowable levels of carcinogenic benzene in fuel or of carcinogenic arsenic in drinking water have not only stirred up scientific but also political debates.

These two cases illustrate different kinds of problems that complicate the scientific evaluation of such issues. Benzene causes leukemia after being oxidized to phenolic and quinoid metabolites in the bone marrow. Its carcinogenicity appears to be limited by the activity of a specific quinone reductase, NAD(P)H:quinone oxido-reductase 1 (NQO1). The *NQO1* gene is polymorphic in man, and $<2\%$ of Central Europeans, but $>20\%$ in some Asian populations are homozygous for an allele encoding an unstable and essentially inactive enzyme. These homozygotes are likely more susceptible to the carcinogenic effect of benzene. So, which level of sensitivity should be chosen?

Arsenic, too, is established as a human carcinogen by epidemiological data and case studies. It causes primarily cancers of the skin and the bladder. Its mode of action, however, is not at all clear, so all estimates of its impact have a large error margin. It does not induce point mutations, but appears to cause epigenetic changes and perhaps acts by indirect mechanisms as a clastogen, e.g. it favors chromosomal instability. Moreover, the uncertainty is exacerbated by evidence pointing to substantial differences in arsenic metabolism between individuals, whose molecular basis is neither elucidated.

While many controversies surround the issue of prevention of chemical carcinogenesis, prevention of carcinogenesis by infectious agents is almost unanimously accepted. Theoretically, elimination of the infectious agents by chemotherapy or vaccination could have major effects. Its potential is illustrated by the geographical differences in the incidence of liver cancer (more precisely: hepatocellular carcinoma) caused by HBV or HCV and the decline of stomach cancer in industrialized countries, which is ascribed largely to the decreasing prevalence of *H. pylori*.

Indeed, vaccination programs against HBV appear to be highly effective. For instance, in countries where the virus is endemic, such as Taiwan, even children develop hepatocellular carcinoma. Since the introduction of vaccination for young children, the incidence of such cases has plummeted. Hopefully, this trend will continue in the future. Since HBV appears to act synergistically with aflatoxins from contaminated food in countries with a humid climate, protection against viral infection might be complemented by programs improving the quality of food storage. Like the actual implementation of vaccination programs, however, this may be less of a scientific than of an economic problem.

The RNA virus HCV is likewise implicated as a cause of liver cancer and could be the next target for a vaccination campaign. In Western countries, where this virus is responsible for a slow, but persistent increase in the incidence of hepatocellular carcinoma, efforts are made to advertise a recently developed vaccine against HCV in risk groups.

Several other viruses, mostly DNA viruses, are implicated in human cancer. The relevance of the papovaviruses SV40, BK, and JC for human cancer is controversial, although (or perhaps, because) chronic infection with BKV, in particular, is highly prevalent. The herpes virus EBV is very likely involved in some human cancers, but its mode of action is unclear and the majority of the population lives without adverse effects. Apparently, its cocarcinogenic effect is mostly exerted in immuno-comprised persons. This is almost certainly so for another member of the herpes virus family, HHV8/HKSV, which is the causative agent in Kaposi sarcoma. For both viruses, preventing or improving the immunodeficiency seems the most practical strategy.

Therefore, the current prime candidates for cancer prevention by antiviral vaccination are the oncogenic strains of *human papilloma virus* HPV. Vaccination against HPV is expected to lead to a huge decrease in cervical cancer incidence, but it might also diminish the incidence of other cancers, notably of squamous cell carcinomas of the head and neck.

The most clear-cut case of a bacterium causing cancer in humans is that of *H. pylori* in stomach cancer. Quite certainly, the continuous decrease in stomach cancer incidence in most Western industrialized countries is in part due to eradication of the bacterium by antibiotic treatment and increased hygiene. Other factors have very probably contributed. They include lower exposure to nitrosamines from smoked and pickled foods and the increased availability and consumption of protective fruit and vegetables. Since it is considered difficult to eradicate *H. pylori* completely, progress in prevention of this cancer, which worldwide remains one of the most lethal diseases, may also come from improvements in general hygiene and nutrition. There are some concerns that in the absence of accompanying measures, the eradication of *H. pylori* by antibiotic treatment or vaccination might result to some extent in a shift of cancers from the lower parts of the stomach to the cardia and the esophagus.

How strongly pathogenic *H. pylori* acts in an individual person depends on genetic variation among the bacterial strains and on genetic polymorphisms in the host. Together, these determine whether the bacterium behaves as a symbiote protecting against reflux disease (and perhaps other infections and obesity) or as a carcinogenic agent. In an ideal world with unlimited ressources, one would like to understand these interactions as fully as possible, determine the genotypes of bacterium and host alike and then choose how to proceed for each individual. This is, however, not even practical in a rich industrialized country, least in a $1 per year and person health system. A more realistic strategy is targeting of high-risk strains of *H. pylori* in populations known to carry a high risk overall. Another approach relies on the assumption that carcinogenesis in the stomach can be reversed even at the stage of gastritis and intestinal metaplasia by antibiotic treatment against *H. pylori*. This is in fact the approach that is now pursued, more or less deliberately, in countries with a well-functioning health system. Strictly argued, this type of strategy does not fall into the category of '*primary prevention*'. Instead it is a case of '*secondary prevention*', because the primary carcinogen is eliminated only after carcinogenesis has begun, but at an early stage.

Cancer Prevention and Diet

In most human cancers, carcinogens are not so clearly defined that they can be eliminated or avoided. Even the carcinogens discussed in the previous section are not the only causes of the respective cancers. Thus, more careful exposure to sunlight will prevent many, but not all skin cancers. Vaccination against HBV (and eventually HCV) is expected to prevent liver cancers resulting from chronic viral infection, but not those resulting from alcohol-induced cirrhosis. Only a fraction of bladder cancers is prevented by strict regulations of arylamine use in the workplace. Nevertheless, primary prevention in these cancers is feasible and is successfully pursued.

Among the four major lethal cancers in Western industrialized countries, in only one, lung cancer, a large fraction of the cases is associated with exposure to a clearly defined exogenous agent, i.e. tobacco smoke. As mentioned above, primary prevention in lung cancer has proven frustratingly difficult in spite of the evident relationship between carcinogen and cancer. In the other three major cancers, colorectal carcinoma, breast cancer and prostate carcinoma, there is certainly no single major exogenous carcinogen. Therefore, early dectection of localized tumors and preneoplastic lesions is the main option for reducing their mortality.

However, in epidemiological studies, all three cancers show associations with a more or less clearly defined '*Western life-style*'. While several aspects of this lifestyle have come under scrutiny, the most convincing arguments point to diet as a major factor. This is not to say that the Western diet is thought to contain a high level of contaminating carcinogens. Rather, diet appears to modulate the risk for these three cancers by affecting endogenous carcinogenic processes. The potential for prevention by changes in the diet is illustrated by the order of magnitude difference in the incidence of prostate cancer between East Asia and North-West Europe, and even more impressively, by the same difference emerging in successive generations of Asian immigrants into the USA. The incidences of the three cancers in Southern Europe and in the Near East are typically intermediate, so a '*Mediterranean life-style effect*' has been postulated. Of note, diet may be only one of several factors responsible for these differences. The difficulty with prevention at the level of life-style is illustrated by the case of tobacco smoking. If prevention of a cancer caused by a clearly defined recreational drug is frustrating, prevention of cancers by insufficiently defined factors in the everyday diet could prove impossible.

This difficulty may be one reason, why much research on prevention of these major cancers has focussed on single components in the diet. Ideally, one might be able to identify one responsible dietary component that could be added as a supplement to staple foods (e.g. folate to flour) or offered as a drug (e.g. soy extracts). This '*micronutrient*' component could either be low in the Western diet or be specifically present in East-Asian foods. In fact, candidates for both types of factors have been proposed.

Compared to '*Westerners*', East Asians eat on average fewer calories. This difference in absolute calories is relatively small, whereas the difference in calories provided by animal fat is huge. Typical '*Western*' diets are reach in red meat, which has a high fat content, and in dairy products. In contrast, typical '*Eastern*' diets provide a higher fraction of calories from grains and legumes. There are also differences in the amount and type of vegetables and fruit consumed as well as in the proportion of fish in the diet. These differences are, however, almost as large within the '*East*' and '*West*' each as between these regions, and do probably not account for the difference in cancer incidence in general. There are more factors of this sort. For instance, selenium deficiency predisposes to several cancer types in some regions of China as well as some in Europe. Selenium deficiency compromises protection against reactive oxygen species, since enzymes such as glutathione peroxidase require this trace element for their catalytic activity.

Among the components discussed to be lacking in the typical Western diet are some that are thought to protect against reactive oxygen species. Carotenoids and related compounds are contained in many vegetables and fruits, and their levels in blood correlate with the consumption of yellow/red vegetables. According to such measurements carotenoid supply may indeed have been low in more traditional Western diets. In particular, the main carotenoid of tomatoes, lycopene, has been proposed as a major protective factor in the Mediterranean diet. Several large prospective longitudinal cohort studies, which are among the most reliable tools of epidemiology, have indeed confirmed the presumed relationship between consumption of vegetables and risk for the major cancers. Variously, significant decreases in cancer risk were found between consumption of vegetables overall, of yellow/red or green vegetables. In contrast, intervention studies using pure β-carotene were unsuccessful and in some cases even increased the rates of cancer. Taken together, these results could mean that a combination of compounds rather than a single compound in vegetables and fruit protects against cancer.

Several further compounds contained in fruits and vegetables may synergize with carotenoids to protect against cancer. Vitamin C (*ascorbate*) and vitamin E (*tocopherol*) are also antioxidants. Unsaturated fatty acids contained in vegetable oils and seeds are essential for cell membrane function and the synthesis of paracrine factors regulating tissue homeostasis and function as well as immune responses.

Table 3.2. Dietary components proposed to influence cancer risk

Increasing risk	*Decreasing risk*
High fat (saturated animal fat)	Carotenoids (e.g., β-carotene, lycopene)
High total calory intake	Vitamin C (ascorbic acid)
Alcohol consumption	Vitamin E (tocopherol)
Pickled and salted foods	Vitamin B_{12}
Smoked and burnt meats	Folic acid
Phytoestrogens	Unsaturated fatty acids
Mold toxins (e.g., aflatoxins)	Phytoestrogens
	Flavonoids, isoflavonoids (e.g. genistein, resveratol, epigallo-catechin-3-gallate)
	Sulphoraphane

Flavonoids and isoflavonoids are also antioxidants, but may exert additional effects. Some are weak estrogens and may modulate hormone metabolism. This may influence the development of breast cancer and prostate cancer, although the evidence is vague. Some of these compounds are kinase inhibitors and, at least at pharmacological doses, are capable of inhibiting the proliferation of tumor cells or induce apoptosis. Genisteine from soy beans, resveratol from grapes and wine, and epigallocatechin-3-gallate (EGCG) from green tea belong to this group. Flavonoids and isoflavonoids are present at higher levels in East Asian and Mediterranean diets than in typical Western diets. Accordingly, quantitative, albeit not striking differences in their blood levels are observed between different geographic regions.

It is nevertheless unlikely that concentrations of such compounds sufficient to inhibit a receptor tyrosine kinase are reached by consuming typical Eastern or Mediterranean diets. It is also questionable whether consuming these compounds as purified dietary supplements will prevent cancer. More likely, in a well balanced diet they may synergize to impede the early development or progression of cancers. Notably, these compounds are excellent '*leads*' for the development of specific cancer drugs.

Dark green vegetables contain specific compounds, in addition to carotenoids, which could affect cancer development. For instance, sulforaphane contained in several kinds of cabbages, especially in broccoli and brussel sprouts, is a potent inducer of glutathione transferases and other phase II enzymes of xenobiotic metabolism. Induction of such enzymes would be thought to accelerate the inactivation of electrophilic carcinogens from exogenous and endogenous sources and prevent mutagenesis.

Dark green vegetables are also an important source of bioavailable folic acid, which is limited in some traditional Western diets and in modern low-quality ('*junk*') foods. Deficiencies in folic acid are known to synergize with deficiencies in vitamin B_{12}, with deficiencies in methyl group donors such as choline and methionine, or with extensive consumption of alcohol to cause cardiovascular disease and developmental defects such as spina bifida. These deficiencies may also advance the development of several human cancers.

Folate deficiency acts by two related pathways. Folate is an essential coenzyme for one-carbon metabolism, prominently for the biosynthesis of thymidine and of purine nucleotides. In an initial reaction, the hydroxymethyl-group of serine is transferred to *tetrahydrofolic acid* (THF) yielding N^5,N^{10}-methylene-THF. This is used in the *thymidylate synthase* (TS) reaction to derive dTMP from dUTP. The TS reaction is rate-limiting for dTTP biosynthesis and under some conditions for the synthesis of DNA. This is exploited in chemotherapy by 5-fluorouracil and related compounds. In the absence of cytostatic drugs, the thymidylate synthase reaction can be suboptimal, when folate or methyl group donors are insufficiently available. As a result, more dUTP becomes incorporated into newly synthesized DNA. Uracil in DNA is removed by uracil glycohydrolase and replaced by thymine via short-patch repair. So, as a consequence of folate deficiency, the number of DNA strand-breaks and the potential of errors during DNA replication increase. An alternative reaction catalyzed by *methylene tetrahydrofolate reductase* (MTHFR), directs N^5,N^{10}-methylene-THF towards the '*methyl cycle*'. Its product is N^5-methyl-THF. This can be used by methionine synthase to regenerate the otherwise essential amino acid methionine from homocysteine in a reaction that also requires coenzyme B_{12}. Following conversion to *S-adenosylmethionine* (SAM) by SAM synthetase, the methyl group can be used in a variety of methyltransferase reactions, including the methylation of lipids, RNA, proteins and DNA. In each case, S-adenosylhomocysteine (SAH) is formed, which is hydrolyzed to adenosine and homocysteine by SAH hydrolase, thereby completing the '*methyl cycle*'. SAH is a product inhibitor of methyltransferase reactions, including the DNA methyltransferases. Therefore, the efficiency of DNA methylation depends on the SAM:SAH ratio. Deficiencies in folate, vitamine B_{12}, methionine or other methyl group donors can therefore compromise the correct establishment of DNA methylation patterns, and perhaps also the methylation of RNA and of proteins.

The extent to which such deficiencies become relevant also depends on genetic factors. Several enzymes involved in one-carbon metabolism and in the '*methyl cycle*' are polymorphic in man, most prominently MTHFR. Among several polymorphisms in the *MTHFR* gene, the most prevalent is an exchange of alanine for valine at codon 677. Since the valine variant is less stable, MTHFR activity varies between individuals. Depending on the genotype, limited amounts of methylene tetrahydrofolate are therefore shuttled preferentially towards nucleotide biosynthesis or towards the methyl cycle, thereby compromising either DNA synthesis or DNA methylation. Indeed, the *MTHFR* genotype and folate deficiency have been shown to synergize in causing defects in DNA replication and DNA methylation. Moreover, several epidemiological studies have shown cancer risk to increase, e.g. in the colon, most strongly in individuals with specific *MTHFR* genotypes who consume, a diet deficient in folate and vitamin B12 and consume large amounts of alcohol.

Popular accounts of these studies and others demonstrating similar interactions for cardiovascular disease have labeled this effect '*methyl magic*'. There is, in fact, little magic involved. A diet with a good supply of folate and vitamin B_{12} is all that is needed. Current nutritional recommendations such as '*Take 5*' (meaning: per day servings of fruit and vegetables) are based on the insights into methyl group metabolism, antioxidant action, and effects of other plant ingredients described above. In some countries, folate is even added to staple foods. Recommendations such as these could lead to a gradual decrease of the incidence of major cancers, even more when they are supported by overall changes in life-style. For instance, immigrants from Southern Europe and the Near East have introduced a greater variety of Mediterrean fruits and vegetable dishes into the Central European diet. Tomatoes, e.g., are now common in the 'Western'diet. Because of the complex interactions involved, the precise causes of changes in cancer incidence that result from such cultural developments will be very difficult to trace.

While individual ingredients of the diet certainly influence cancer risk, and may synergize with each other, the most consistent difference between '*Eastern*' and '*Western*' diets is the amount of saturated fat consumed, particularly of animal fat. For breast and prostate cancer each, and to a lower degree for colon cancer, the cancer incidence in a country is proportional to the amount of saturated fat consumed. The molecular basis of this relationship is not understood. Conspicuously, the risk for these three cancers, among all malignancies, also increases in adipose (obese) persons. Obesity is caused by an interplay of genetic predisposition, cultural factors, overnutrition and lack of exercise that in itself is extremely complex. Even *H. pylori* may feature in this relationship by influencing the levels of hormones secreted by the stomach that regulate satiety. So, the relationship between adipositas and cancer is not expected to be straightforward.

An important component in this complex relationship may be insulin-like growth factors. While IGF2 acts mostly locally as a paracrine factor, IGF1 circulates as a hormone in the blood, supporting the growth of several tissues. It also regulates glucose metabolism, but much less so than insulin, which in turn is a weaker growth factor. Increased expression of IGFs is thought to contribute to a wide range of human cancers, including breast and prostate cancers. Normally, IGF1 levels in blood peak during the adolescent growth phase and decline later on. They remain significant, however, and are regulated by nutrition and by exercise, similar to those of insulin. So, in adipose persons, insulin levels are often enhanced, leading to a pre-diabetic state and often to diabetes, but IGF1 levels too are supraphysiological. Indeed, the level of IGF1 in mid-life has been found to predict the risk of prostate cancer which appears several decades later. The action of IGFs is controlled by binding proteins (IGFBPs). These are likewise subject to regulation by nutrition and by insulin. The levels of IGFBPs in serum also appear to correlate with the risk for breast and prostate cancers. While these relationships are intriguing, they are certainly only part of a complex relationship that needs to be elucidated to define the best approach to addressing obesity as a cause of cancer.

Prevention of Cancers in Groups at High Risk

Recommending dietary changes such as 'Take 5!' is a cancer prevention strategy that addresses the overall population. This strategy is unproblematic. No adverse effects are to be feared and the same changes in diet supposed to decrease the risk of major cancers very likely diminish the risk of cardiovascular disease and diabetes, to a perhaps even greater extent. It is similarly unproblematic to pursue cancer prevention by vaccinating an entire population against HBV or HCV, which likewise has the additional benefit of preventing acute and chronic liver disease. There are risks involved in vaccination, since a few individual show adverse reactions, but they are much lower than the risks associated with actual infections. Moreover, as HBV does not seem to possess an animal reservoir, there is hope that this virus may not only be contained, but eventually be exterminated by vaccination. No foreseeable downside would be associated with its demise.

A bit more problematic is the handling of *H. pylori*, since many strains of the bacterium may actually constitute symbiotes rather than pathogens, even though others present a considerable risk to susceptible humans. Therefore, a vaccination strategy would have to take these considerations into account. As described above, one way out of this dilemma is to restrict anti-bacterial treatment to the susceptible part of the population and/or to those carrying high-risk strains. Ideally, one would identify these persons by molecular diagnosis, but more realistically, patients with gastritis will be identified and treated before ulcers and cancer have a chance to develop.

This is an example of identifying a population at increased risk for a specific cancer. In the case of stomach cancer associated with *H. pylori* infection, there is the added advantage that treatment is available and can usually be admitted without severe side effects and at moderate cost. Moreover, it is not too difficult to identify a precancerous state, viz. gastritis or ulcers, because it is symptomatic. Each of these factors is generally important for the successful prevention of cancers in risk populations, i.e. straightforward delineation of the population at risk, availability of an achievable specific treatment with few or no side effects, and easy identification of preneoplastic or early tumor stages by symptoms or simple and affordable assays. Unfortunately, instances such as stomach cancer associated with *H. pylori* infection represent the exception rather than the rule.

Table 3.3. Prerequisites for successful cancer prevention in risk groups

Criterion
Clear identification of population at risk
Sensitive, specific, reliable, and inexpensive assay
Detection of significant preneoplastic or early cancer stage
Efficient and affordable treatment with acceptable side effects

Important tasks during cancer prevention in populations at risk are monitoring and – as in the case of stomach cancer – education and information of health professionals and the affected population. This can be very successful, if the population exposed to a specific cancer risk is clearly defined, e.g. in the workplace. In occupations with hazards from radiation or chemicals, regulations aiming at minimizing exposure are put in place and controlled, regular instruction meetings are instituted, and regular examinations are performed to detect early signs of cancers such as aberrant cells in the blood or urine. Monitoring in such instances can be improved by molecular-based techniques for the early detection of cancers or preferably of preneoplastic changes.

Like exposure to defined carcinogens, inheritance of mutations in high-risk genes predisposing to cancer is a risk factor in a specific part of the population. Insights from molecular genetics now allow a better definition of this population by identification of those individuals within affected families who carry high-risk mutations. Since monitoring is likewise warranted in these persons, techniques for early detection of cancers are being developed. One might feel intuitively that preventing inherited cancer today should be a straightforward task. It is unfortunately not, for a variety of reasons.

One complication is encountered in cancer syndromes inherited in a recessive mode. These are typically rare diseases caused by mutations in genes involved in DNA repair and become manifest during childhood or during adolescence. This means that familial clustering occurs only to a limited extent. In most cases, only siblings of the first child affected (the '*index patient*') are also at risk, unless the family belongs to a religious or ethnic group with frequent intermarriage. These diseases often comprise a wider range of symptoms, some of which may precede the manifestation of cancers. This can provide an advantage in so far as monitoring for cancers can be begun after the disease has been identified by other symptoms and has been confirmed by molecular genetic diagnostics.

The major problem then is how to avoid and treat the cancers that develop. In spite of being aware of the risk, and even of understanding the involved mechanisms as precisely as in the hypersensitivity of xeroderma pigmentosum patients towards UV, this can be exceedingly difficult. Another problem may arise during therapy, because patients with these afflictions may be hypersensitive to commonly used treatments such as radiation therapy (in ataxia teleangiectasia) or to crosslinker cytostatic drugs such as cis-platinum (in *Fanconi anemia*). So, each case requires a careful, individualized approach. As a practical consequence patients with this sort of diseases are often referred to specialized centers. There, experience can be gathered and therapy can be improved with each case. Some diseases in this group are candidates for gene or stem cell therapy, e.g. *Fanconi anemia*, where predominantly the hematopoetic system is at risk for cancer.

The second, larger group of inherited cancers comprises autosomal-dominantly inherited diseases with an increased incidence of benign and malignant tumors, typically in young adults or in middle age. Cancer predisposition in these cases is not necessarily associated with conspicuous symptoms characteristic of a syndrome. Instead, the diseases often run within families, affecting not only siblings of an '*index*' patient, but also second and third degree relatives. Almost all are caused by an inherited mutation in a tumor suppressor gene. *Familial adenomatous polyposis coli* (FAP) predisposing to multiple colorectal adenomas and eventually carcinoma and hereditary breast cancer are prominent examples.

The first hurdle encountered when trying to prevent cancer in affected persons can be awareness. FAP is very distinctive and the emergence of multiple polypous adenomas typically precedes the development of a cancer. Therefore, patients are usually identified, even if the familial background is unknown. A familial background in a disease like FAP may seem hard to overlook, but as families become smaller and mobility increases, family history is not always trivial to ascertain.

This problem is more severe in patients with hereditary breast cancer, since malignancies are generally the first manifestation of the disease, except in patients with more generalized cancer syndromes, e.g. *Cowden disease*. Awareness of hereditary breast cancer may have increased since the discovery of the *BRCA* genes was widely reported in medical journals and in the lay press. Perhaps, the following controversies about how to apply the new knowledge may have increased awareness further. These controversies relate to the most crucial problems in cancer prevention within selected groups mentioned above, viz. delineation of the population at risk, availability of achievable specific treatments with few or no side effects, and the identification of preneoplastic or early tumor stages.

FAP is not only phenotypically distinctive, but is also essentially a homogeneous disease at the genetic level. Almost all cases are caused by mutations in the *APC* gene and many of these occur in hot spots within the gene. So, molecular genetic confirmation of the disease is feasible at moderate cost. Within a family, the mutation identified in one person can be specifically sought in relatives, or closely linked genetic markers, e.g. microsatellites, can be used. Moreover, a reasonably good correlation exists between the location of the mutation and the severity of the disease. So, molecular diagnostics can be helpful to choose an appropriate preventive approach.

Nevertheless, problems remain. The first one is ethical. Diagnosing the disease in one person reveals an information on all relatives, particularly if diagnostics is performed by linkage analysis. In the case of FAP with its very high penetrance, this is mostly a problem concerning children, since asymptomatic adults are rare. Nevertheless, people have a right to to know or not to know. So, adequate counseling is absolutely necessary. Because of the nature of the disease in FAP, this issue is not as problematic as in some other diseases, including breast cancer.

In everyday practice, the most serious problem is how to proceed after an *APC* mutation has been verified. One option is preventive surgery by partial colectomy, i.e. removal of the segment of the gut most susceptible to adenomas and carcinoma, usually in young adults before multiple polyps have developed. This diminishes the cancer risk, but does not exclude cancers in other parts of the colon and rectum. Thus, monitoring for carcinomas is regularly performed.

More recently, chemoprevention has been introduced. Non-steroidal antiinflammatory drugs, i.e., inhibitors of COX2 such as celecoxib, diminish colon cancer risk not only in patients with inflammatory bowel diseases, but also appear to be efficacious in FAP patients.

Thus, overall early diagnosis of FAP allows to diminish the risk of lethal cancers and extends the life of affected individuals. This is achieved with considerable effort and costs, in life quality of the patient and in economic terms.

Similar, but also additional issues are to be considered in the prevention of hereditary breast cancer. One additional problem is the identification of the population at risk. Unlike FAP, hereditary breast cancer has no distinctive morphological features and worse, no distinctive precursor stage preceding actual cancer. So, before the advent of molecular techniques, it was not possible to discern whether a familial clustering of breast cancers was accidential or caused by a predisposition inherited in the family.

This distinction can now often be made, but the disease is genetically heterogeneous. While the majority of hereditary cancers appears to be caused by inherited mutations in *BRCA1* or *BRCA2*, some cases are due to mutations in other known genes. However, a sizeable fraction of familial cases cannot be ascribed to a specific gene. Most likely, no single '*BRCA3*', but several genes are involved.

So, verifying a hereditary predisposition toward breast cancer in a family with several '*index*' cases can still constitute a considerable problem. Moreover, the *BRCA* genes are pretty large and germ-line mutations are spread throughout the genes. The task of identifying mutations is in some cases facilitated by the occurrence of other cancers in a family. For instance, frequent ovarian carcinomas suggest *BRCA2* as the prime candidate. Also, in some populations founder effects have caused a predominance of specific mutations whose presence or absence can be tested before a larger screening procedure is undertaken. In clinical routine, if a mutation is found in a *BRCA* gene in a member of a family, a hereditary predisposition can be assumed, if none can be found, it cannot be excluded. This is rather unsatisfactory for everybody involved.

If a *BRCA* mutation is detected, the next problem arises from another difference towards FAP. While the penetrance of FAP is generally very high and the exceptional cases with attenuated disease can be defined with some certainty (i.e. by mutations at the 5'-end of the gene), considerable differences have been observed in the penetrance of hereditary breast cancer caused by various mutations in BRCA genes. Unfortunately, very few of these differences are consistent enought to allow a prediction of the risk for an individual patient. This means that – by and large – patients with a life-time risk of 20% for development of breast or ovarian cancer have to be treated like those with a life-time risk of 80%. Again, this is not satisfactory for anybody involved, the more so, since the options for cancer prevention are also rather limited.

As in FAP, surgery is the primary option and has been shown to diminish the risk substantially. Oophorectomy not only strongly diminishes the risk of ovarian cancer, but also that of breast cancer, likely because estrogen levels are decreased. Mastectomy in various forms can be performed. An important issue is when to perform these operations. Obviously, one would like to delay them as long as possible without incurring the risk of a cancer having metastasized. Likewise, the extent of mastectomy must be balanced between risk of cancer and risks of the procedure, which are physical as well as psychological. Standard recommendations are available, but the actual decision should be made by the patient after counseling.

Monitoring can detect some breast cancers at comparatively early stages, but is not straightforward, especially in younger women. For instance, mammography has been critized as being unreliable in women below the age of 50. There is no good molecular marker for breast cancer yet, which could be used with serum or with nipple aspirates. However, research on this issue is very active.

Brighter prospects emerge from newer developments. Chemoprevention appears to be efficacious in breast cancer as well and specifically in hereditary breast cancer caused by *BRCA* mutations. NSAIDs are also tried for the prevention of breast cancer. In addition, although BRCA-associated cancers normally do not respond well to anti-estrogenic therapies, SERMs such as tamoxifen or the newer raloxifene may also be active in their prevention. However, they may delay the manifestation of the disease rather than prevent it. These drugs can have side effects, because they interfere with the normal functions of estrogens in protection of the cardiovascular system and regulation of the balance of resorption and osteogenesis in the bone. Moreover, older SERMs increase the risk of endometrial cancer.

In summary, therefore, prevention of cancers caused by inherited mutations is rarely simple and typically only to some extent efficacious, in spite of considerable efforts and costs. Not least, the quality of life is often compromised. Clearly, the task for molecular research remains to better understand the underlying pathophysiological mechanisms in order to identify more specific targets for prevention, and to improve diagnostic techniques, in particular for the early detection of cancers arising in persons at risk.

Prevention of Prostate Cancer by Screening the Aging Male Population

There can be little doubt that the considerable efforts to prevent or at least delay cancers is appropriate in small populations at high risk, such as families with inherited cancer syndromes. Likewise, drastic measures such as surgical removal of organs or long-term treatment with anti-hormonal drugs are accepted in persons known to run a high risk of developing a lethal cancer. Such measures would certainly not be acceptable for the whole population, even though one third of the population in a typical Western industrialized country will develop some kind of cancer in their life-time and one fifth will die of it. However, many different cancers in different organs contribute to this morbidity and mortality and no universal prevention scheme is at hand.

Nevertheless, for some cancers, screening of the entire population or a susceptible subpopulation could make sense, if certain requirements are met. They are similar to those defined in high-risk populations, viz. the part of the population at risk needs to be clearly defined, an affordable and reliable assay for detection of preneoplastic or early tumor stages must be at hand, and an efficacious treatment with acceptable side-effects and - in a large population - affordable costs must be available. There is a continuing debate for which cancers these requirements might be met. Obviously, the four major cancers, lung cancer, colon cancer, breast cancer, and prostate cancer are prime candidates for population screening. While according developments are underway for each of them, they are most advanced in the case of prostate cancer.

Screening for prostate carcinoma is basically a realistic option. (1) It is very prevalent with a life-time risk of up to 10% in the male population and a considerable mortality (≈3% of the male population). (2) Prostate cancer is extremely rare before the age of 50, increasing exponentially thereafter. In males over 75, the disease often takes a slower course and/or surgical treatment is not advisable. This restricts the population to be tested to males aged between 50 and ≈75. (3) A routine biochemical assay for prostate specific antigen (PSA) in serum can detect most tumors while they are still restricted to the organ. This assay has acceptable sensitivity, although its specificity is only moderate. In most cases, a definite diagnosis of prostate cancer can be achieved by further molecular assays, by imaging and by histological investigation of biopsies. (4) Organ-confined prostate cancer can be successfully treated by surgery or radiotherapy. In advanced cases, progression can be delayed by anti-hormonal treatment.

For these reasons, PSA screening of the male population starting from the age of 50 has been introduced in several countries. In smaller regions within Austria or Canada systematic attempts have been made to screen the entire male population and treat all those with detectable cancers. Indeed, the mortality rates of prostate cancer and meanwhile even its incidence have declined. Not all Western countries have followed suit, however, again for several reasons.

1. Prostate cancer is biologically heterogeneous. While a sizeable fraction of prostate cancers take an aggressive course, many remain relatively indolent, and will not cause clinical symptoms, least death in the age group at risk. In contrast, treatment by surgery or radiation can cause considerable morbidity such as incontinence

and impotence and carries even a (low) risk of mortality. Moreover, while the introduction of PSA assays has dramatically reduced the fraction of cases that have metastasized at the time of detection, some still are and cannot be cured.

At present, while a combination of biochemical and morphological parameters can predict the prognosis of a specific patient quite well, the distinction between indolent, aggressive, and already metastatic cases can rarely be made with certainty. This means that on one hand a fraction of patients are unnecessarily treated, while on the other hand in some cases treatment is useless. As one might expect, the debate on the relative sizes of the three fractions rages. A study in Scandinavia, where '*watchful waiting*' rather than therapeutic intervention is the favored strategy, has suggested that radical prostatectomy prolongs life in only one out of seventeen patients treated. This is likely an underestimate. Nevertheless, it raises doubts about the usefulness of a population-wide screening and intervention approach. Moreover, opponents of screening point out that the incidence and mortality of prostate cancer are also declining in countries where no screening/intervention has been introduced. One way out of the dilemma would be the development of molecular markers that allow to stratify prostate cancers into groups with very high, moderate and low risk.

2. PSA screening is more expensive than it looks at first sight. The PSA assay itself is relatively inexpensive, but is not highly specific. While it yields relatively few false negatives, i.e. misses few cases of prostate cancer being present, it has a relatively high rate of false positives. Specifically, men with benign prostatic diseases such as prostatitis or extensive benign hyperplasia often test positive. In these cases, further diagnostics has to be performed and - although some of these men may indeed have to undergo treatment for their benign diseases - there are considerable costs associated with the diagnostic procedure. Because taking of biopsies is an invasive procedure, a slight risk of serious infections is incurred. All this would not matter much in a small population at risk, but if an entire population of older males is screened, costs are magnified and very slight risks become significant. Consider an assay with 95% specificity (which is an excellent value) used in a population of one million males over 50. It means 50,000 men having to undergo the following more extensive diagnostical procedures unnecessarily. Combined with the uncertainty on the

clinical significance of a cancer detected in an individual, this leaves room for doubt.

3. Moreover, if 10% of all males eventually develop clinically significant prostate cancer and are all detected at an early stage, can they all be treated by current methods? In the fictious example population, 100,000 men would be diagnosed with prostate cancer. Currently, many cases are only detected, after the cancer has progressed. Before the advent of PSA assays, most cancers were highstage, often metastasized and incurable. With optional PSA assays, cases are more often diagnosed at an organ-confined stage at which they can be cured. Not so rarely, they are diagnosed in men older than 75 years or suffering from other - typically cardiovascular - diseases prohibiting surgery. In many of these men, rather slow-growing prostate carcinomas are not limiting life expectation, although the patients may eventually require palliative treatments. If screening was efficiently performed in younger men, e.g. at the age of 60, one could not predict by current methods whether many cancers detected would cause severe clinical symptoms years later or limit life expectancy. Since few males at 60 are nowadays not fit enough for surgery or radiotherapy, most of them would therefore need to be treated right away. This may be feasible in selected regions like Tyrol or Quebec, but in larger populations the ressources would simply not be available. Again, a better definition of the population at risk, more precisely, a classification of the cancers detected by PSA screening and subsequent diagnostic procedures, is required to solve this dilemma.

Evidently, an alternative approach would be chemoprevention rather than definitive therapy in men with suspicious serum levels of PSA. Anti-hormonal treatment is an option, but is problematic because of its side effects. Moreover, there are concerns that applying anti-androgenic treatment early on might spur the early development of androgen-resistant cancer cells, leaving no options if the disease recurs after surgery. Moreover, androgen independence in prostate cancer is typically associated with a more invasive and metastatic phenotype and therefore anti-androgen chemoprevention might prevent the development of less malignant cancers, while promoting the more aggressive ones. A compromise in this situation is being tried by using inhibitors of 5α-reductase. This enzyme catalyzes the formation of the more active dihydro-testosterone from testosterone in the prostate. Therefore, its inhibition has fewer side effects than anti-androgenic treatments by androgen receptor antagonists or LHRH agonists.

Moreover, the less active androgen testosterone remains present to exert beneficial effects in other tissues. As often in prostate cancer research, acquiring definitive data on the value of this approach will take many years. Intriguingly, preliminary results suggest indeed a decrease in prostate cancer incidence at the expense of a shift towards less differentiated cases.

Other Types of Prevention

Detection of prostate cancer by PSA assays can, of course, not be considered strictly as cancer prevention. PSA levels in serum increase, after the prostate epithelium has become disorganized and epithelial cells release some of their secretory products into the mesenchyme. This presupposes invasion and therefore a carcinoma by definition. Ideally, however, the cancer is detected at an early stage, while it can still be cured and systemic disease is prevented.

This is the aim of many attempts at detecting cancers early on by molecular markers. Ideally, one would detect a preneoplastic state allowing prevention of the actual malignancy. If that is not possible, detection is aspired at a stage where a cure remains possible with minimal harm to the patient.

One step further, viz. following successful therapy of a cancer, e.g. removal by surgery, another type of prevention aims at diminishing the risk of further cancers of the same type. This is prevention of secondary cancers. In contrast, adjuvant therapy by drugs or irradiation aims at eliminating residual cells of the primary cancer that might lead to recurrences.

The distinction between prevention of secondary cancers and preventing recurrences of the first cancer is clear in the prostate, which is completely removed during surgery for prostate cancer. So any cancer appearing later must have been present at the time of surgery, having spread beyond the organ.

In organs that cannot be completely removed this distinction is more difficult to make. The issue is further complicated by '*field cancerization*' occurring in many tissues. For instance, carcinomas of the oral mucosa tend to recur. Nevertheless, surgery in this sensitive enviroment must be kept as limited as possible. Therefore, in the standard procedure the cancer is removed with a margin of several cm of morphologically normal tissue around it. Some cancers recur in distant places and indeed can be shown to harbor distinct genetic alterations. Other cancers recur close to the surgical margin in tissue that was morphologically normal at the time of initial surgery. As a rule, they contain the same genetic alterations as the initial cancer. In such cases, prevention of second cancers and adjuvant therapy tend to overlap. Importantly, in each case, patients need to be closely monitored to detect recurrent as well as second independent tumors.

The main difference between adjuvant therapy and prevention of secondary cancers lies in the type of treatment used. Adjuvant therapy aims at killing tumor cells that have not been eliminated by the primary treatment, i.e. surgery or irradiation. Prevention aims at keeping normal or partially transformed cells from becoming malignant. So, it is certainly prevention to convince a bladder cancer patient treated by local surgery to stop smoking, whereas installing the moderately toxic cytostatic drug mitomycin C into the bladder is really adjuvant therapy.

In other cases, this distinction is even more blurred. For instance, anti-estrogenic therapy after partial mastectomy for breast cancer aims at both residual tumor cells and prevention of independent cancers.

Nevertheless, the distinction between prevention and adjuvant therapy is not only theoretically important. If there is a serious concern that tumor cells are still present after an attempt at definitive therapy, the side-effects of cytostatic drugs will have to be accepted. If the aim is prevention of a second cancer, they will not. For instance, if there is a concern that a bladder cancer has not been completely removed or may have metastasized, systemic therapy based on the more toxic cis-platinum will be used rather than local application of mitomycin C. Likewise, if breast cancers have spread beyond a certain stage, e.g. cancer cells are detected in multiple lymph nodes, cytostatic therapy rather than anti-estrogenic treatment will be considered.

There are several further organs, in which independent second cancers occur frequently, e.g. the skin, particularly in patients with increased susceptibilities, the epithelia of the mouth and throat, particularly in smokers, and the colon, most strongly in patients with inherited susceptibilities. Beyond regular monitoring and general preventive recommendations, such as to avoid smoking and eat a healthy diet, chemoprevention is being developed as an option for these patients. Vitamin mixtures or specific antioxidants such as β-carotene have been tried for several different tumors. For prevention of secondary colon cancers, non-steroidal antiinflammatory drugs are now the treatment of choice and they are also tried for cancers of other organs. Another group of compounds investigated for the purpose of chemoprevention are retinoids and related compounds.

4

Cancer Therapy

Today, surgery, radiotherapy, and chemotherapy, i.e. 'scalpel, ray, and pill', remain the standard tumor therapies. Novel therapies like gene therapy or immunotherapy are only administered in the setting of experimental studies. In addition, outside '*school*' medicine, a variety of '*alternative*' treatments are sought by patients and their families who do not have full confidence in standard therapies. This scepticism is, unfortunately, not entirely unfounded. With current therapies, between 30% and 40% of all cancer patients die of their disease. This average percentage conceals huge differences. Basal cell carcinoma and squamous carcinoma of the skin, e.g., are almost always detected before they metastasize and can be cured by local surgery, radiotherapy or drug application. A few formerly generally lethal tumors like testicular cancers, Wilms tumors and certain hematological cancers respond excellently to current therapies. The routine establishment of stem cell transplantation has further improved the prospects of patients with hematological cancers, most impressively of children.

On the other hand, cure rates are still abysmal for some cancers that spread early and do not respond well to chemotherapy. Mortalities exceed 95% for pancreatic carcinoma, and 85% for lung cancers beyond very early stages and some acute leukemias in adults. The rates for other common cancers fall between these extremes. As a rule, carcinomas can be cured by surgery or by radiotherapy as long as they are confined to the organ where they originate. In contrast, cure rates for metastasized carcinomas have generally remained dismal, although present-day drug and radiation therapies often alleviate symptoms and prolong survival.

Regarding this state of things, two conclusions are evident.

1. Cancer prevention is superior to cancer treatment. Therefore, prevention ought to be consigned a high priority. At the least, if cancers cannot be prevented completely, they ought be detected at an early stage, while cures are still feasible.
2. Better therapies are required, most urgently for advanced stage and/or metastatic carcinomas.

There is a general feeling that the current therapeutic concepts are approaching their limits. With the therapeutic strategies pursued till the 1990's, quantitative improvements in the therapy of major cancers may still be achieved, but no '*breakthroughs*' are expected. In a sense, therefore, the present trend towards individualization of therapy recognizes the limits of current therapies, while attempting to exploit their full potential.

Breakthroughs in cancer therapy are instead anticipated from novel '*molecular*' approaches based on the emerging insights into the molecular biology of human cancers. It is doubtful whether such breakthroughs have already been achieved. So far, only few '*new-age*' drugs developed '*rationally*' on the basis of molecular biology insights have entered clinical routine. There are, however, good reasons to believe that this situation may change. After all, the molecular biology of cancer largely a product of the late 1980's and 1990's and the establishment of a new cancer therapy requires at least a decade of development and testing. Moreover, in several cases in which initial attempts at molecular-based cancer therapy have not been successful, advances in the knowledge of cancer biology allow to understand why these failures have occurred and to improve on them. In fact, this knowledge has also elucidated the causes why current cancer chemotherapy is only efficacious up to a certain point.

Molecular Mechanisms of Cancer Chemotherapy

The cancer drugs that are most widely used today were basically developed in the 1950's to 1970's. A few novel classes of compounds have since been added, such as the taxols, and many older compounds have been chemically modified or replaced by related substances to increase their efficacy and diminish their toxicity. Most of the currently used anti-cancer drugs have been found empirically by screening synthetic and natural compounds for their effect on tumor cells, while others were designed against specific targets. Target-directed drug development, therefore, is not a wholly new invention. However, prior to the recent developments in the understanding of cancer biology, different targets/in cancers cells were regarded as important than today. Specifically, increased cell proliferation was regarded as the central property of cancers. Therefore, many '*older*' cancer drugs are directed against DNA, DNA replication, or mitosis.

Table 4.1. Some contemporary anti-cancer drugs in frequent use

Class of drugs	*Examples*
Drugs binding to DNA	cis-platinum, mitomycin C, adriamycin (doxorubicin), bleomycin, actinomycin, alkylating agents
Nucleoside analogues or nucleotide biosynthesis inhibitors	5-fluoro-uracil, cytosine arabinoside, 5-aza-deoxy-cytidine, 5-fluoro-cytosine and prodrugs, thiopurines, methotrexate, hydroxy-urea, difluoro-methyl-ornithine
Topoisomerase inhibitors	irinotecan, topotecan, etoposide, also several intercalating drugs like doxorubicin
Microtubule-binding	vinblastine, vincristine, taxols
Biological agents	antihormones (tamoxifen, raloxifen, antiandrogens), GnRH antagonists and agonists, estrogens, progesteron, retinoic acids and analogues, interferons, interleukins

Drugs Binding to DNA

A large class of anticancer drugs react directly with DNA. For instance, cis-platinum reacts with DNA bases, causing intra-strand and inter-strand crosslinks which block DNA replication and cause cell death, unless repaired. Cis-platinum is the crucial component in many drug regimes used to treat common carcinomas. It is the single most important compound in the combination of drugs that has revolutionized the treatment of testicular cancers, where cure rates of >95% can be achieved.

Nucleoside Analogs

Following conversion to nucleotides in the cell, nucleoside analogues interfere directly with DNA replication, impede it indirectly by limiting the synthesis of deoxy-nucleotide triphosphate precursors, or cause strand breaks after incorporation into DNA. 5-fluorouracil (5-FU) is a widely employed member of this class, which acts mainly by inhibition of thymidylate synthase. Methotrexate is not a nucleoside analogue, strictly spoken, but also interferes with deoxy-nucleotide biosynthesis by inhibiting dihydrofolate reductase. Thus, both compounds diminish the level of dTTP, the nucleotide precursor specifically needed for DNA replication. A special case is 5'-aza-deoxy-cytidine. It is incorporated into DNA, where it reacts with DNA methyltransferases attaching them covalently to DNA. This reaction has a double effect. It depletes the methyltransferases causing a genome-wide decrease in DNA methylation and often reactivation of genes inactivated by DNA hypermethylation. The protein-DNA complex may also interfere with DNA replication, unless removed by bulky adduct repair.

Topoisomerase Inhibitors

Etoposide exemplifies a third class of compounds which bind and inhibit enzymes involved in DNA replication. Etoposide specifically binds to topoisomerase II and blocks the enzyme at a critical stage. Topoisomerases are necessary for DNA replication (as well as for transcription), since they relax the torsional stress that is caused by the unwinding of the DNA helix. Topoisomerase I enzymes reversibly insert a single-strand break, allow the DNA strands to swivel around each other, and religate the strand-break. Inhibitors of topoisomerase I used in cancer chemotherapy comprise innotecan, irinotecan and topotecan. Topoisomerase II enzymes catalyze a more dramatic reaction, in which a double strand break is reversibly introduced and another DNA helix (or a distant part of the same helix) is passed through, before the ends are resealed by the enzyme. This is a more fundamental reaction, which in addition to relaxing torsional stress allows the untangling of DNA knots and loops. Etoposide inhibits type II topoisomerases at a crucial stage of this reaction, i.e. after the helix has been cleaved, but not yet been resealed. In this fashion, DNA replication is inhibited and DNA is fragmented, more efficiently than by topoisomerase I inhibitors.

Microtubule-binding Compounds

Taxoles are perhaps the best-known among different compounds reacting with microtubules, while vinblastine or vincristine are used for specific diseases. Some drugs of this class block the assembly of or disrupt existing microtubuli, while others block the turnover of these dynamical structures. Either way, cellular functions depending on microtubules are compromised or inhibited. The most important process affected by interference with microtubule function is mitosis, but intracellular vesicle transport and cell migration are also inhibited.

Biological Agents

The designation '*biological agents*' is sometimes used as a summary designation for a diverse group of compounds that do not directly interfere with basic cellular functions, such as DNA replication and mitosis. Rather, they act on signaling pathways controlling cell proliferation and differentiation. By activating or inhibiting receptor molecules, they redirect cancer cells in a more subtle fashion towards normal behavior. Hormones and antihormones used in the treatment of breast cancer and of prostate cancer as well as inducers of differentiation such as retinoic acid used in the therapy of acute promyelocytic leukemia can be assigned to this category. They act selectively on certain cancers since they activate or inhibit receptor proteins that are specifically required for their growth and survival. This does not automatically imply that such compounds do not have adverse side effects. However, these are typically not caused by toxicity. Rather, effects of these drugs on the proliferation, differentiation, or function of normal cells are mediated by the same receptor(s) as in cancer cells. For instance, anti-estrogens favor osteoporosis and cardiovascular disease, because they block the beneficial effects of estrogens on bone and heart tissue.

Biological agents act through specific receptors present only in certain cells, which explains their specificity. But how can drugs directed against DNA replication and mitosis, i.e. basic processes essential in many different cells of the body, or drugs reacting with DNA itself act selectively on cancer cells at all?

Table 4.2. Mechanisms responsible for the selectivity of anti-cancer drugs

Mechanism responsible for differential response of tumor/normal cells
Increased proliferative fraction and shortened cell cycle
Inefficiency or inactivation of cellular checkpoints
Defects in DNA repair
Altered apoptosis
Dependence on '*cancer pathways*'

Differences in Proliferation

Many cancers contain a higher proliferative fraction than normal tissues, and many cancer cells replicate faster than most normal cells. These differences constituted the main rationale in the early years of cancer chemotherapy development. Unfortunately, many normal tissues, too, contain fast-replicating compartments. Accordingly, treatments that aim purely at rapidly replicating cells cause damage to such tissues as well. For this reason, side effects of chemotherapy are common in organs with a rapid turnover, primarily the hematopoetic system, gut and skin. Adverse side effects of chemotherapy include leukopenia (low numbers of leukocytes), diarrhoea (as a consequence of damage to the gut mucosa), and alopecia (hair loss). These side effects can be severe and limit the dose of cytostatic drugs that can be applied. The severity of adverse effects in clinical trials and routine use of drugs is categorized from I-V for each type of effect. Grade III or IV side effects will be cause for concern and may represent the reason for termination of the treatment or for dose reduction, and grade V means a fatal outcome of the treatment.

Adverse side effects are a general problem with cancer therapy, but worse, many cancers do not confirm to the fast-replication stereotype. In many carcinomas, in particular, relatively few cells are actively proliferating at one point in time and those that are do not traverse the cell cycle very rapidly. Therefore, while cycling cells in the cancer may indeed be killed by the drug, they will later be replaced by other cells from the tumor that were not in a critical phase of the cell cycle or not cycling at all, when the drug was present. Chemotherapy of prostate carcinoma and renal cancers, e.g., is vexed by this effect. It represents, however, a wider problem and constitutes a second, specific limit to the efficacy of therapy directed at DNA and DNA replication, in addition to the first general limit provided by the toxicity of the therapy. An interesting new approach to circumwent the low proliferation problem is '*metronomic therapy*'. In this type of chemotherapy, cytostatic drugs are applied regularly at relatively low doses over longer periods than in standard regimes. Compared to standard therapy, the aim of this treatment is no longer to cure the cancer, but to slow its growth and prolong survival with minimal harm to the patient.

Defects in Cellular Checkpoints and DNA Repair

The second set of reasons why cancers are more sensitive to cytotoxic chemotherapy than normal cells was unknown when the first generation of active drugs was developed. Many cancer cells are defective in DNA damage checkpoints, e.g. as a consequence of mutations in the TP53 pathway. So, following the covalent reaction of a drug like cis-platinum with DNA, cancer cells may continue to replicate and attempt to divide in spite of the damage, with catastrophic consequences.

In addition, some cancers are defective in the repair of specific types of DNA damage, due to the inactivation of particular repair systems. For instance, some cancers lack the MGMT enzyme which removes alkyl groups from guanine, and for this reason are hypersensitive to drugs alkylating DNA at guanines. Similarly, colon carcinomas with a microsatellite instability phenotype respond on average better to chemotherapy than those with a chromosomal instability phenotype. This difference may be due to the inactivation of the mismatch repair system in cancers with microsatellite instability. In selected cancers, e.g. of the ovary, DNA crosslink repair may be compromised by epigenetic inactivation of FANC genes. Encouraged by such examples, one current line of applied cancer research aims at identifying further DNA repair defects in specific cancers and exploit them for selective therapy.

Another novel approach consists in using drugs that aggravate the checkpoint deficiencies in cancer cells, e.g. by blocking kinases involved in the control of the G2→M checkpoint. In normal cells several mechanisms ensure checkpoint control. In cancer cells, some or all of these may be deficient, rendering them more sensitive to their inhibition. Combination treatment together with compounds that interfere with DNA replication would then lead to checkpoint arrest in normal cells, but to a mitotic catastrophe in cancer cells. One compound acting in this fashion is caffeine, although at millimolar concentrations not tolerated in a human person.

Altered Apoptosis

Somewhat counterintuitively, another explanation for the selectivity of cytostatic drugs towards cancers is related to altered apoptosis. This sounds paradoxical, as apoptosis is often impeded in cancer cells. Indeed, defects in apoptotic signaling and execution can contribute to resistance against chemotherapy. However, many cancer cells can be considered as being '*poised*' for apoptosis. Inappropriate growth control, genomic instability, and nucleotide imbalances generate pro-apoptotic signals, which do not elicit apoptosis because anti-apoptotic signals prevail in cancer cells. In this critical constellation, drug treatment may add further signals that '*tip the balance*' towards apoptosis.

For instance, cancer drugs like cis-platinum, 5-FU, and etoposide lead to the induction and activation of death receptors like FAS. Others, including methotrexate, activate the intrinsic, mitochondrial pathway of apoptosis. The reaction of a cancer to drug treatment therefore depends on which defects precisely are responsible for decreased apoptosis. If the block to apoptosis is very efficient, it will protect the cell against drug-induced apoptosis as well. For instance, strong overexpression of IAP type proteins like survivin which inhibit caspases or strong overexpression of BCL2 which prohibits activation of the intrinsic pathway can also cause resistance to chemotherapy.

Loss of TP53 function also influences the response to chemotherapy in many cancers, but its effect is complex. TP53 is important for checkpoint signaling following DNA damage. So, cancer cells with TP53 loss of function tolerate more DNA damage than normal cells and continue to proliferate in spite of it. This is a questionable advantage, since they run a higher risk of mitotic catastrophes or incurring damage to essential genetic material. On the other hand, loss of TP53 certainly impedes the induction of apoptosis. Overall, therefore, cancers with loss of TP53 function tend to respond less well to chemotherapy, but there are exceptions to this rule.

From these arguments, it can be deduced why certain cancers respond well to chemotherapy, while others do not. For instance, testicular cancers respond excellently to chemotherapy and are particularly sensitive to cis-platinum. They usually contain a high proliferative fraction with rapidly replicating cells. Checkpoints in testicular cancer cells appear to be not fully functional and nucleotide excision repair, in particular, is poorly efficient. Finally, TP53 is usually not mutated and can be induced by cytostatic drugs to support the induction of apoptosis. So, in this cancer type, all pertinent factors favor therapeutic success.

Unfortunately, carcinomas in general rather resemble renal cell carcinoma. In this cancer, a low proliferative fraction, a slow, but relentless growth, and the presence of strong anti-apoptotic signals, with loss of TP53 in some cases, tilt the balance against the success of chemotherapy (as well as radiotherapy), even though checkpoints may not be fully intact and TP53 may remain functional in a subset of the cases.

These general factors that counteract successful therapy are exacerbated by specific mechanisms of chemoresistance. In renal carcinoma, the expression of the multidrug resistance protein Pgp/MDR1 and other protective proteins further limits the impact of chemotherapy, contributing to '*primary resistance*'. Expression of MDR1 is also found in other cancers, even if expression in the corresponding normal tissue is not as strong as in the kidney. In some cases, the protein becomes expressed only during therapy in resistant cancer clones, eliciting '*secondary resistance*'. High levels of the multidrug resistance protein confer resistance to hydrophobic drugs by transporting them out of the cell. Multidrug resistance ensues, since many anti-cancer drugs are hydrophobic compounds.

Multidrug resistance by over-expression of MDR1 is a general mechanism of drug resistance. Similarly, increased levels of protective proteins such as glutathione transferases diminish the sensitivity of a cancer to a range of drugs. Activation of antiapoptotic pathways, specifically of the PI3K and NFκB pathways, also contributes to decreased sensitivity against a broad range of chemical and physical therapies. Additional mechanisms confer resistance to individual drugs.

Resistance to cis-platinum, e.g., can be caused by overexpression of metallothioneines which protect cells from the toxic effects of metal ions in general. Resistance to topoisomerase inhibitors may be due to overexpression of the target enzyme as a consequence of gene amplification.

Resistance to 5-FU and related compounds targeting thymidylate synthetase is particularly complex. The response to the drug depends on properties of the tumor as well as on the genetic constitution of the patient. Resistence can be caused by altered metabolism of the drug, by mutations and amplifications in the *TS* gene, and can be favored by genetic polymorphisms in this and other genes.

Most advanced cancers are characterized by genomic instability, which can be associated with increased rates of chromosomal gains and losses, gene amplification, deregulation of gene expression, and/or point mutations. These mechanisms are not only relevant for the development of the cancer as such, but also open a variety of escape routes during drug therapy. For instance, drug targets can be rendered insensitive to inhibitors by point mutations or become less sensitive by amplification of the gene encoding the target.

In an advanced cancer, which is genetically heterogeneous, a fraction of its cells may carry an alteration leading to decreased sensitivity towards a cytotoxic drug. Administration of the drug will then select these cells from all others leading to the emergence of a new cell clone with altered properties. As a rule, this cell clone will not only be resistant to the specific drug and often to others, but also be more genetically unstable than the overall tumor before treatment.

In some cancers, the cells more responsive to drug therapy correspond to the more differentiated fraction. Induction of apoptosis and/or growth arrest in this population therefore may expose a more malignant fraction of cancer cells and sometimes release restraints on these. Such '*lurker*' cells are suspected to be responsible for the recurrent growth of breast and prostate cancer following anti-hormonal therapy. However, this phenomenon is not restricted to anti-hormonal treatment.

Worse, cancer chemotherapy may in some cases directly promote genomic instability, if it causes damage to the genome without actually killing cells or arresting their growth irreversibly. In such cases, the treatment effectively acts as a mutagen that induces a resistant cell clone, often with further genetic alterations. Outgrowth of a more malignant cancer is therefore a common observation after failed cytostatic drug chemotherapy.

Principles of Targeted Drug Therapy

One strategy to circumvent the problems associated with conventional chemotherapy is to develop drugs against more specific targets in the cancer. This is not a fundamentally novel idea. Many drugs in current use interact with highly specific targets such as microtubular proteins or topoisomerase enzymes. Their targets are not specific to cancers, though. Those drugs called '*biological agents*' in the previous section come closer to the ideal, since they act on specific receptor proteins which may occur preferentially in certain tissues, but, more importantly, are essential for the growth of specific cancers. These, then, are the forerunners of a novel drug generation.

All-trans retinoic acid, e.g., binds to receptors that are more or less ubiquitous in the body. Indeed, synthetic analogues of this tissue hormone are also used for the treatment of benign skin diseases like acne, because retinoic acid promotes cell differerentiation in the skin, as in many other epithelia. Retinoids therefore have been tried as anticancer drugs in almost every type of cancer, usually with detectable, but limited effects on tumor growth. In contrast, retinoic acid is highly active in most cases of acute promyeolocytic leukemia, out of all acute leukemias. What makes the difference towards all other cancers is that in this particular type of leukemia the causative genetic change involves the retinoic acid receptor α, whereas in other cancers changes in the response to retinoids may well occur, but are non-essential for their growth and survival.

This case, then, comes close to the ideal of target-oriented cancer therapy. Elucidation of crucial events that drive cancer growth should provide targets for therapy. Targets for rational therapy ought to be at least specific to the tumor, but better essential for its growth and survival. Elucidating these crucial events and identifying suitable target molecules are however no simple tasks.

In many hematological cancers, the presence of a characteristic chromosomal translocation points to an essential genetic event. Yet, even in leukemias and lymphomas developing a therapy from that knowledge can be difficult. *Acute promyeolocytic leukemia* (APL) is exceptional in so far as the fusion protein formed by the causative chromosomal translocation contains a receptor protein whose ligands are well characterized. Developing a therapy for *chronic myelocytic leukemia* (CML) by targeting the causative BCR-ABL fusion protein was still quite straightforward, since it contains an essential protein kinase activity.

Unfortunately, not all fusion proteins display functions that lend themselves to inhibition or activation by small molecule drugs. In the jargon of pharmaceutical research, they are not easily '*drugable*'. Furthermore, APL and CML are untypical in constituting essentially homogeneous diseases, whereas other hematological cancers may be caused by a variety of different translocations and gene fusions.

As carcinomas are characterized by multistep development with accumulation of a larger number of various genetic and epigenetic alterations, it is generally even less clear which targets are optimal. Optimists assume that many of these alterations are essential for the growth and survival of the cancer and conclude that the multitude of changes in carcinomas offer a wide choice of targets for therapy. Pessimists point out that the more alterations have already occurred, the higher the chance that some of them may be passenger alterations. Worse, a cancer with many genomic alterations is likely to develop further ones allowing escape from therapy. Likewise, optimists suggest that cancer pathways activated in specific cancers present excellent targets, as they are crucial for driving tumor growth. Pessimists point out that these same pathways are also important for normal cells which might mean a narrow '*therapeutic window*'.

In practice, potential targets for cancer-specific therapy are defined based on a variety of considerations.

Table 4.3. Molecular targets for cancer therapies

Type of target	*Examples*
Ectopic proteins	viral proteins, cancer-testis antigens
Overexpressed proteins	oncogene products, particularly receptor tyrosine kinases
Altered proteins	mutated products of oncogenes
Cancer pathway components	MAP kinases, CDKs

Ectopic Targets

An ideal drug target in a cancer would never occur in a normal tissue. Since cancer cells are derived from normal cells, one would think that such targets might be rare, but some do exist. (1) In cancers induced by viruses or cancers harboring viruses, viral proteins can be targeted. The E6 and E7 proteins of HPV are involved in carcinogenesis in several tissues. Other viruses like EBV and HBV, while not necessarily driving tumor growth, are at least present in many Burkitt lymphomas and hepatocellular carcinomas, respectively. (2) Fusion proteins in leukemias and lymphomas are composed of proteins which are also present in normal tissues, but always separately. Their fusion confers novel properties which can be exploited to target them selectively. (3) Many cancers express proteins which are otherwise only found in fetal tissues ('*oncofetal proteins*') or in a very small range of other tissues, e.g. in the testes ('*cancer testis antigens*'). These are often not essential for the growth of the cancer, but they can be used for the targeting of toxins or for immunotherapy.

Overexpressed Proteins

A second class of targets is provided by proteins overexpressed in cancer cells. Some oncofetal proteins and cancer testis antigens actually belong to this class, because they are expressed at very low levels in normal tissue. The most important group, however, of such proteins are the products of oncogenes that have become activated by overexpression, e.g. as a consequence of gene amplification.

Several strategies have been developed, e.g., to exploit the overexpression of the EGFR or ERBB2 receptor tyrosine kinases in many advanced carcinomas for therapy. An evident disadvantage of using such proteins as drug targets, though, is the very fact that they are overexpressed. This point is illustrated by the amplification of the androgen receptor gene in prostate carcinomas which have become unresponsive to anti-androgenic treatment. Accordingly, targeting an amplified protein kinase by an inhibitory drug may invite further amplification as a mechanism of resistance. Nevertheless, as the case of trastuzumab shows, overexpressed cell-surface receptor tyrosine kinases can be used for targeting by antibodies. Antibodies can also be directed at proteins that are not as essential for the growth and survival of the tumor cell as ERBB2 is for many breast cancers. Modern high-throughput proteomics and expression profiling approaches are excellently suited for the identification of proteins overexpressed in cancer cells. There is therefore no shortage of candidates for this approach.

Proteins with Altered Structures

The third class of targets are proteins whose structure is altered in cancer cells. Fusion proteins could also be assigned to this class. They are excellent targets, because their structure is different in tumors compared to normal cells and they are essential for cancer growth. The same is true for oncogenic proteins activated by point mutations, such as KRAS in colon cancer or β-Catenin in the same cancer and more often in hepatocellular carcinoma.

Even tumor suppressor proteins inactivated by point mutations deserve consideration. They could provide targets for immunotherapy, but drug therapy is not inconceivable. A favorite candidate in this respect is TP53, since it is more often inactivated by missense mutations than by deletions or promoter hypermethylation. Most missense mutations in TP53 appear to interfere with the conformational activation of the protein, which strongly accumulates in cancer cells because the mutated protein is more slowly degraded. A drug pushing the protein into an active state would therefore activate a comparatively huge amount of TP53 protein and likely elicit apoptosis.

In addition to these clear-cut cases of mutated oncoproteins, there is some evidence that cancer cells in general may harbor a larger proportion of misfolded and altered proteins than normal cells. It is not quite clear what causes this defect, but it may make cancer cells more susceptible to inhibition of chaperones and of proteasomal degradation. Inhibition of either sort of target may overload the cell with misfolded proteins, like during a heat-shock. Indeed, inhibitors of heat-shock proteins acting as chaperones have emerged as surprisingly good inhibitors of cancer growth, with few side effects. Likewise, inhibitors of proteasome function, e.g. of threonine proteases, have turned out to be surprisingly specific for cancer cells.

Cancer Pathway Signaling

The fourth category of targets comprises molecules that regulate '*cancer pathways*'. The proliferation and survival of cancer cells depend on a relatively restricted number of signal transduction pathways. In different cancers, one or the other of these are overactive or inactive. Inhibition of overactive pathways or restoration of inactivated pathways is a major goal of many current drug development.

However, the designation '*cancer pathways*' is in so far imprecise, as the same pathways also control the proliferation, differentiation, survival and function of normal tissues. So, differences between normal and cancer cells are expected to be quantitative rather than qualitative.

Hope that these differences may still be sufficient to allow improved cancer therapy is based on observations and ideas summarized by the '*addiction hypothesis*'.

Compared to normal cells, signaling pathways in cancers are thought to be 'rewired'. For instance, overactivity of pro-proliferative signals relayed through the canonical (ERK) MAPK pathway would in normal cells be counteracted by increased apoptosis. In cancer cells, this increase in apoptosis is impeded by over-activity of other pathways such as the PI3K or the NFκB pathway or by overexpression of anti-apoptotic proteins. Therefore, the survival of cancer cells is much more dependent on these anti-apoptotic activities than that of normal cells, which display more moderate and transient activities of MAPK pathways. In other words, the cancer cells have become '*addicted*' to the activity of the anti-apoptotic cancer pathway.

Of note, the addiction hypothesis predicts that inhibiting the MAPK pathway which actually drives proliferation could be less efficient than inhibiting the PI3K pathway that influences proliferation only indirectly but allows cell survival. This hypothesis may also provide an alternative explanation why cancer cells react more sensitively to inhibitors of heat-shock proteins. They may have become dependent on mutant proteins that could not be assembled in the absence of these molecular chaperones.

Targets defined by such considerations can be exploited by different kinds of therapy. Development of pharmacological therapy with small molecules is the most obvious approach. It is best suited, but not restricted to proteins with enzymatic activities. This strategy has the important practical advantage that it can build on established procedures. Nowadays, pharmaceutical companies possess compound libraries comprising ten thousands of synthetic and natural chemicals that can be screened by high-throughput methods for activating or inhibitory activity against a specific target enzyme. Even protein-protein or protein-DNA interactions can be influenced. A molecule with activity is considered a '*lead*' compound. Lead compounds can be chemically modified by a host of well established techniques and procedures to achieve increased specifity and better general pharmacological properties. Determination of the structure of the target protein by modern biophysical methods and drug design using sophisticated computer methods have further facilitated this strategy.

However, small molecule drugs are not the only option anymore. In fact, some of the most successful '*novel*' cancer drugs are antibodies against growth factor receptors. Their development, likewise, has benefited from the availability of a wide range of sophisticated molecular biology methods. For instance, therapeutic antibodies can now be detected and optimized not only in animals, but also in bacteria and phages. If an antibody is initially developed in an animal, it can be '*humanized*', i.e. the constant chains can be replaced by a human immunoglobulin sequences using standard methods of genetic engineering. This adaptation impedes the development of an immune response towards the therapeutic antibody in the patient. Without humanization, antibodies become inactive upon repeated administration or may even cause serious adverse reactions such as an allergic shock.

Application of antibodies can be regarded as a type of immune therapy, although antibodies can also be used in a similar fashion as small molecule drugs. In contrast, a suitable target molecule can be also used as the basis for a true cancer vaccine. Some modern approaches at cancer immunotherapy do indeed use defined targets.

Defined targets in cancer can also be exploited for gene therapy. In theory, gene therapy is a more straightforward approach than drug or immune therapy. However, the development of new drugs and vaccines can be pursued on a strong fundament of established procedures and long-term experience, whereas in gene therapy almost everything has to be developed from scratch. Of all the strategies contemplated and tried in gene therapy, the use of antisense oligonucleotides or siRNA against overexpressed or altered proteins in cancer most closely resembles the approach in the development of drugs. It therefore runs a good chance of becoming established in the clinic first among gene therapy approaches. There are, however, strategies that are unique to gene therapy and may in the long run prove superior. For instance, gene therapy can be used to re-introduce a tumor suppressor that has been inactivated in cancer cells or to exploit the presence of an oncogenic change to allow the replication of a cytolytic virus.

Last not least, combinations of novel therapies, drug, immune, and gene therapy, are pursued, and either type of '*novel*' therapy can be used in conjunction with established chemotherapies or radiotherapies directed at less cancer-specific targets.

Examples of New Target-directed Drug Therapies

Drug development based on target-oriented approaches is now routine. Still, the development of a new drug can take a decade from the discovery of a '*lead compound*' to routine clinical use. So, in oncology relatively few '*novel*' drug are already being used in everyday practice, although many clinical studies are underway. The experience obtained from the use of these novel drugs in clinical routine most clearly illustrates both the potential and limitations of targetoriented therapies in oncology.

Table 4.4. Selected targeted drugs employed in the clinic or clinical trials

Drug(s)	*Target(s)*	*Stage of development*
Imatinib	BCR-ABL, KIT, PDGFR(?)	routine use
Farnesyl transferase inhibitors	RAS (RHO?, RAC?)	clinical trials
Trastuzumab	ERBB2	routine use
Gefitinib	ERBB1	routine use starting

Imatinib (alias STI571, alias Gleevec or Glivec) was developed as an inhibitor of the BCR-ABL protein kinase, which is a fusion protein resulting from the characteristic chromosomal translocation in *chronic myelogenous leukemia* (CML) and is causative for this cancer. The inhibitor blocks the tyrosine kinase activity in the ABL domain of the protein that is essential for its oncogenic function. The drug is thus directed against a target largely specific to this cancer, since the normal ABL protein is not essential for growth and survival in normal somatic cells, although it is important for the control of cellular responses to DNA damage. Imatinib is now used for the therapy of CML in its chronic phase alternatively to interferon α with cytogenetical remissions in ≈70% of the patients (compared to ≈10% with former drugs). It even induces clinical remissions in many patients in which the disease has progressed into the terminal blast crisis. For these patients, no treatment was previously available.

Imatinib is relatively nontoxic, as one would hope for a targeted drug. When applied in the chronic phase of the disease, it may achieve complete cures, as indicated by molecular remission. Whether this is really so, will have to be ascertained by long-term follow-up of the treated patients. Ideally, the drug may help to spare many patients from stem cell transplantation. In blast crisis patients, however, remissions are as a rule temporary. Many cancers develop resistance against the drug. One mechanism of resistance involves amplification of the *BCR-ABL* gene. In other cases, mutations render the BCR-ABL protein less sensitive to the inhibitor. Typically, these mutations lead to changes in amino acids at the ATP binding site of the kinase where imatinib binds. So, while the drug is much more efficacious than previous treatments, it is not immune to the development of resistance. Tellingly, resistance develops more regularly in the accelerated phase or blast crisis of CML characterized by a high level of genomic instability.

Somewhat unexpectedly, imatinib was also found to be highly active against a different cancer. *Gastrointestinal stromal tumor* (GIST) is a relatively rare type of sarcoma, for which few therapeutic options beyond surgery had previously been available. A subset of these cancers responds very well to imatinib. Of note, this shows that these cancers are genetically more heterogeneous than they appear morphologically. In some cases, cures are achieved, e.g., because cancer regresses to such an extent that the primary cancer and isolated metastases can be surgically removed. In others, the progression of the disease is significantly delayed. All cancers showing remissions under imatinib treatment display activating mutations of the KIT receptor tyrosine kinase. Indeed, the drug *in vitro* also inhibits the KIT and PDGFR kinases with high affinity, in addition to the BCR-ABL kinase. In fact, the efficacy of imatinib in GIST even depends on the precise mutation in the *KIT* gene. The frequent mutations in exon 11 presage a good response, whereas a specific mutation in exon 17, D816H, is associated with a lack of response, i.e. the cancers display primary resistance. Mutations like the latter one are also found in cancers regrowing under imatinib therapy following an initial remission, i.e. displaying secondary resistance. So, clearly, this is a good case in point for pharmacogenomics.

During treatment of GIST patients with imatinib, a number of interesting observations were made which suggest that responses to novel cancer drugs may show quite different characteristics from those to standard cytotoxic chemotherapy.

1. Responses were often slow, at least when the size of the tumor was taken as a parameter. Rather than being killed, tumor cells appeared to be arrested and even to terminally differentiate. Such changes cannot be detected by many methods routinely employed in the monitoring of chemotherapy. Instead, their detection requires imaging methods based on the metabolic activity of the cancer, e.g. positron emission tomography.
2. Tumor endothelia were often severely damaged, probably as a consequence of a decreased supply of growth factors from the cancer as well as by direct inhibition of the PDGFR, which is important for endothelial cell growth. This damage may lead to

bleeding, which may contribute to the observed initial increase in tumor size after the start of treatment.

3. As the typical adverse effects of chemotherapy were not pronounced with imatinib, it appears that the clinical complications during the use of such novel drugs may be quite different from those during current cytotoxic chemotherapy.

In fact, this finding is precedented by the experience with the treatment of acute promyelocytic leukemia using all-trans retinoic acid. Here, complications can arise when a large number of cancer cells apoptose at one stroke and/or differentiate into almost normal cells (mostly granulocytes) which exhibit a range of biological activities including the secretion of cytokines.

Like protein kinases, mutated RAS proteins constitute a promising target for cancer therapy. They are overexpressed in some cancers, but more importantly, they carry mutations at very specific sites that lead to their constitutive activation in about 30% of human cancers overall. In different cancer types either HRAS or KRAS are mutated in an almost exclusive fashion, providing another potential level to achieve specificity. Even normal RAS proteins may exert an oncogenic action in some cancers by transmitting signals essential for cell growth and survival from oncogenic receptors.

The problem with targeting mutated RAS proteins by small-molecule drugs lies in the precise mechanism causing their oncogenic activation. RAS proteins are over-active in human cancers because their intrinsic GTPase activity is decreased. Mutations at very specific sites block the interaction with GTPase activating proteins (GAP), thereby prolonging the state in which RAS proteins can stimulate downstream effectors such as the kinases RAF or PI3K. So, it would probably be relatively simple to find drugs that inhibit RAS GTPase activity. However, it is more difficult to find compounds that promote GTP hydrolysis.

To circumwent this dilemma, another strategy was conceived to target oncogenic RAS proteins. RAS proteins are tethered to the inner face of the membrane by post-translational modifications that make them more hydrophobic. RAS proteins and their small GTP-binding protein relatives like RHO and RAC end in the amino acid sequence CAAX, where C is cysteine, A is an aliphatic amino acid (like alanine), and X is serine, methionine, glutamine, or cysteine. This carboxy-terminal tetrapeptide is recognized by protein farnesyltransferases that transfer a farnesyl residue to the cysteine thiol side chain. The terminal three amino acids are subsequently cleaved off by a specific protease and the new terminal carboxyl group is methylated by a protein methyltransferase. Additionally, a palmitoyl chain can be added to a penulmitate cysteine.

Related proteins and a small fraction of RAS proteins are alternatively modified through geranylation by the enzyme *geranyl-geranyl-transferase* (GGT1). The substrates for these reactions, farnesyl-pyrophosphate, and geranyl-pyrophosphate, are ubiquitous intermediates of the cholesterol biosynthetic pathway. As a consequence of these modifications, the C-terminus of the protein becomes sufficiently hydrophobic to stick to the membrane, whereas the unmodified protein is cytosolic and, importantly, inactive.

This modification, then, can be targeted by drugs. Actually, blocking cholesterol biosynthesis by statins at the level of hydroxymethyl-glutaryl-coenzyme A reductase, which is a common treatment for hyper-cholesterolemia, may have some effect on this modification as well. A more specific target for interfering with RAS function is, of course, the enzyme farnesyl transferase. A weak point of this strategy could be that it is not specific for oncogenic RAS, because normal RAS also depends on the same modification for its function. This argument can be turned around by arguing that '*upstream*' oncogenic alterations such as overactivity of receptor tyrosine kinase may depend on non-mutated RAS proteins and might be blocked by the same drugs. So, the initial idea of targeting an altered protein has in reality transformed into another approach based on the '*addiction hypothesis*', because the succes of the strategy hinges on the question whether cancer cells are significantly more dependent on RAS functions than normal cells.

Two basic types of *farnesyl transferase inhibitors* (FTIs) are available that were obtained by the two principal strategies now used in drug development, i.e. rational design based on the known structure of a target protein and its substrates and random screening of libraries of synthetic and rational compounds for inhibition (in this case) of the target activity. Rational design of FTIs was based on the structure of the tetrapeptide known to be essential for substrate recognition. This tetrapeptide was modified until optimal inhibitory specificity was obtained. Additional modifications were in this case necessary to improve solubility and uptake. In the second strategy, screening of natural compounds libraries yielded non-peptide compounds, which served as '*leads*', i.e. their basic structure was varied until pharma-cological requirements were reasonably met.

Several such compounds have been tested in clinical trials. They were found to be moderately active against some acute leukemias and some carcinomas. Efficacy has been seen against pancreatic carcinoma, in which KRAS mutations may be most prevalent among all human cancers, but in general no correlation was evident between response to FTIs and the presence of a mutated RAS protein. Moreover, some FTIs display severe side effects, e.g. in the gastrointestinal tract, which are not too different from those of traditional cytotoxic chemotherapy.

Since the idea of using farnesyl transferases as therapeutic targets was conceived, many other proteins besides RAS and related small GTPases have been shown to become farnesylated. The list of such proteins even includes major structural proteins of the cell such as lamins. It is therefore not at all clear that the anti-cancer action of FTIs results from their interference with RAS function. In some cancers, they induce apoptosis, which could be due to decreased activity of the PI3K pathway as a consequence of RAS inhibition. So, perhaps, cancers in which RAS is important for PI3K activation may be treated with these compounds. In most cancers, however, cells arrest at the G2→M border or in prometaphase, because they cannot form mitotic spindles. It is not understood, how this effect might be caused by RAS inhibition, and so it is considered to more likely result from the inhibition of a distinct protein. It is also not clear, whether the limiting toxicity of the FTIs is caused by inhibition of the normal functions of RAS proteins or by interference with that of other farnesylated proteins.

The greatest efforts in the development of novel anti-cancer drugs so far have been directed at *receptor tyrosine kinases* (RTKs). Overexpression or mutation of membrane proteins from this class contribute to the growth of many human cancers. Specifically, members of the ERBB family are over-expressed in a wide range of metastatic carcinomas, whose treatment constitutes one of the major unsolved problems in cancer therapy. The RTK superfamily also comprises proteins such as IGFRI, MET, and FGFR3 implicated in the causation of, e.g., cancers of the liver, the kidney, and the urinary bladder. In addition, the PDGFR and receptors for VEGF such as FLT1 are essential for endothelial cell growth and angiogenesis in a wide range of cancers from different tissues.

All RTKs are located at the cell membrane, making them accessible not only to drugs that can penetrate into the cell, but also to those acting on the outside of the cell and even to antibodies.

Indeed, antibodies directed at the extracellular domains of several receptor tyrosine kinases appear to provide valuable drugs. The function of RTKs, with very few exceptions such as ERBB3, depends on their intracellular tyrosine protein kinase activity. This activity is well drugable, and tyrosine kinase inhibitors in general are designated as tyrphostins.

In contrast, the ligand binding activity of the receptors located in their extracellular domain has proven a more difficult target. Antibodies are themselves proteins which recognize epitopes on other proteins consisting of several amino acids and their modifications. Binding of an antibody or a growth factor ligand to a receptor tyrosine kinase is a protein-protein interaction. This kind of interaction typically involves a large number of comparatively weak interactions (often hydrophobic or van der Waal interactions) across a relatively large surface. The binding of an enzyme substrate or inhibitor depends instead on a small number of stronger and individually more specific binding interactions (often ionic bonds or hydrogen bonding in addition to hydrophobic interactions, or even covalent bonds). In general, protein-protein interactions are therefore relatively difficult to inhibit by small molecules. For this reason, antibodies are superior to small-molecule drugs for inhibition of ligand binding to growth factor receptors. These structural requirements also provide a plausible explanation why almost all inhibitors of receptor tyrosine kinases found so far by screening approaches inhibit binding of ATP, but not of protein substrates.

While several antibodies to RTKs have proceeded to advanced stages of clinical development, the only one already widely employed in clinical routine is trastuzumab (alias '*herceptin*'), a recombinant, humanized antibody directed against ERBB2. Although it has been tested in several other malignancies, it is routinely used mainly in the treatment of breast cancer. Like imatinib in its application for the treatment of CML and GIST, trastuzumab is paradigmatic, because the rationale for its application differs from that of traditional cytostatic drugs. Herceptin is only prescribed against a specific subset of breast cancers, which is defined by a molecular marker, viz. overexpression of ERBB2 with amplification of the gene. So, while the administration of cytotoxic chemotherapy was contingent on histopathological parameters, tumor grading and staging, the application of trastuzumab therapy is dependent on the classification of the cancer as ERBB2+ (and ER-). This principle is likely to be extended to many of the target-directed novel therapies currently under development.

Administration of trastuzumab is clearly beneficial for the group of breast cancer patients with ERBB2+/ER-metastatic cancers, whose prognosis is in general dire. However, while trastuzumab extends survival in these patients and improves their quality of life, it is not a miracle drug that might lead to a cure. Administered usually in combination with a cytotoxic drug such as adriamycin, it induces apoptosis and growth arrest in many cancer cells, but does not stop their growth entirely. Moreover, some patients with ERBB2+ cancers do not show remissions or even stable disease. An important area of research is therefore to determine the precise mode of action of this therapeutic antibody in human patients as well as the mechanisms underlying therapeutic failures.

Since in the age of robotized high-throughput assays it is fairly straightforward to screen 10,000s of compounds for their ability to inhibit a tyrosine kinase, a multitude of inhibitors for receptor tyrosine kinases are now available for research purposes. However, very few are presently used in the clinic. This is, of course, because use of a drug in human requires careful testing.

Many tyrosine kinase inhibitors are now investigated in phase I or phase II studies. In phase I studies, the dose tolerated without adverse effects is established in a small number of individuals. In addition, it is determined whether the drug actually reaches levels that are sufficient to inhibit the intended target. For instance, its level can be quantitated in serum or in leukocytes and, if possible, target enzyme activities or the state of their substrates are measured. If phase I studies are performed in patients, which is the rule with cytotoxic drugs, some indication of efficacy can be gained.

However, determination of efficacy is really the formal aim of phase II studies. These involve a larger number of patients. Therefore, they provide information on whether the drug induces complete or partial remissions or at least delays the further progress of the cancer ('*stable disease*'). They also reveal a fuller range of the side effects to be expected. Due to differences in drug metabolism and general constitution, susceptibilities for adverse effects vary widely and in some cases side effects become only apparent after a large number of patients have been treated. For instance, a substantial number of novel drugs, including tyrosine kinase inhibitors, could not be further developed because they interfere with a specific cardiac ion channel, causing a state called '*long Q-T*'. This particular complication is, as a consequence, now routinely evaluated in the preclinical phase (or latest in phase I) to avoid later disappointments. Of course, novel kinds of difficulties may arise with every novel drug.

If phase II studies have been successful, with reasonable efficacy and safety, phase III studies are initiated with large numbers of patients, in a double-blinded setup. Depending on the tumor type, these studies in particular can take a long time. For instance, the period needed to determine whether a new drug aimed at preventing the development of androgen-refractory prostate cancer indeed does so, is estimated as 5 - 10 years.

A drug can be introduced into general use following phase III. However, its efficacy and safety continues to be monitored for quite a while. This is considered phase IV. Its purpose is to detect adverse reactions in smaller subsets of the population, e.g. due to genetic polymorphisms in drug metabolism and to define even better which patients exactly benefit from use of the drug.

Before cancer drugs can be entered into these phases of '*clinical development*', they have to be optimized in a '*preclinical*' phase. Part of the task is biochemical characterization. The specificity of an inhibitor has to be determined by measuring its K_i for a variety of kinases, including non-tyrosine kinases. As a rule of thumb, K_is of suitable inhibitors are in the nanomolar range for the target kinase, while other kinases are inhibited by micromolar or higher concentrations. Very few tyrosine kinase inhibitors are specific for one or a few kinases, those in clinical use like imatinib (STI571, Gleevec), gefitinib (Iressa, ZD1839), or OSI-774 are among them. The biochemical explanation for this problem is that they all bind to the ATP binding site, which is relatively conserved between many enzymes and even more so within the superfamily of receptor tyrosine kinases.

Another step in preclinical development is optimization of the pharmacological properties of the inhibitor drug. Medicinal chemists wield a large repertoire of modifications of a small molecule affecting its solubility, its ability to pass through cell membranes, its stability against metabolic degradation, its binding to carrier proteins, and its half-life in the patient and in the tumor overall. The drug entered into a phase I trial may look quite different from the lead compound emerged from a high-throughput kinase inhibitor screen and even from the compound that is used in laboratory research to inhibit a particular kinase.

Preclinical development of cancer drugs further comprises their testing in cell culture and animal models. Cell culture models include established cancer cell lines and increasingly often primary cultures of cancer and normal cells. Typical animal models are xenografts of human cancers or cancer cell lines in mice, but also transgenic or gene knockout animals. For some cancers, animal models can be used in which a cancer similar to that in humans arises spontaneously or can be induced by a carcinogen. For instance, bladder cancers that are similar to those in humans can be induced by chemical carcinogens in rats or dogs. Liver cancers, likewise, can be induced by chemical carcinogens in rats or mice. However, while these are similar in some respects to human cancer, they do not mimic well the etiology of human liver cancers through the stage of cirrhosis.

Cell culture and animal models are absolutely necessary for the development of new therapies. However, in many cases, novel therapies looked extremely promising in preclinical development, but did not live up to that promise in the clinic. This is also true to a certain degree for tyrosine kinase inhibitors. This criticism extends even to immunotherapy and gene therapy approaches. It is a very important aim of current research to understand the causes of such discrepancies and to establish better models and criteria for prediction of therapeutic efficacy in humans.

This is a complex matter, but some factors are evident. (1) The growth fraction of many '*real*' metastatic carcinomas in humans is small, whereas that of model cell lines and xenografts is larger. This can hardly be avoided, since one would not want a preclinical experiment to extend over several years. Nevertheless, this difference is at least partly responsible for the differential effect of novel target-directed drugs in models vs. in patients, as it was for the same difference seen with '*classical*' cytotoxic drugs. (2) Human cancers are very heterogeneous and the cell lines and xenografts used as models are at best representative of a subset of each cancer type. In some cancers, e.g. prostate carcinoma, they may even be exceptional, as most cancers do not grow in culture or as xenografts. (3) Animal models may not reflect certain aspects of human cancers. This may be particularly true for rodent tumors, which are most widely used at present. Only some of the differences are understood at the molecular level, such as the differences in the regulation of cellular senescence, telomeres and the *CDKN2A* locus.

Gefitinib or ZD1839, which is marketed as Iressa, is a relatively specific inhibitor of the EGFR. It was developed for application in metastatic carcinomas, exhibiting excellent efficacy in preclinical models. Indeed, the compound has shown significant activity in several cancers that so far had defied all attempts at treatment, viz. several types of recurrent and metastatic carcinomas. Adverse side effects were often moderate and rarely exceeded grade II. Not unexpectedly, they occurred in the skin and gut, where the EGFR is thought to mediate signals for tissue renewal. Indeed, in skin samples from treated patients, autophosphorylation of the EGFR was largely blocked and likely downstream effectors of EGFR activation followed suit. AKT phosphorylation was likewise decreased and $p27^{KIP1}$ became induced.

Still, the therapeutic benefits of the drug were moderate. Responses were seen in only a fraction of the patients, and the treatment usually resulted in stable disease rather than remissions. In general, overall survival was only slightly improved, if at all. So, contrary to hopes the drug has proved to be at best palliative rather than curative. Most unexpectedly, neither the presence nor the absence of responses to gefitinib were found to correlate with the expression or activity level of the EGFR in a particular cancer. Present evidence suggests that the cancers responding to the drug are those in which the EGFR is activated by mutations rather than by overexpression. If confirmed, this observation would allow a pre-selection of the patients to be treated with gefitinib.

There are several potential explanations for the unexpectedly moderate success of this novel drug, which are being explored. The most likely one is that human cancers are even more heterogeneous than previously assumed. The most worrying explanation is that the well-established over-expression of the EGFR in many metastatic cancers does not really have the presumed significance, and is not as essential for growth and survival of the cancer cells as one might have hoped.

In conclusion then, the novel cancer drugs developed against carefully selected targets are still largely at the beginning of their application in the clinic. Limited successes have been achieved, but with the exception of imatinib in chronic phase CML and some GISTs, they have not been greeted unanimously as breakthroughs. Experience with the drugs already used in the clinic and those currently or previously tested in phase I and phase II studies will certainly be helpful to generate better drugs by this relatively new approach. After all, the first generation of '*novel*' drugs was based on the understanding of cancer molecular biology of the early 1990's which today in retrospect many would consider as quite naive. Also on the positive side, drugs directed against specific targets in cancer cells have in general shown lower toxicity than the previous generation of cytotoxic drugs. What pharmacologists label ADMET parameters (for absorption, distribution, metabolism, excretion, and toxicity) remain challenges for the new drug generation as well. Most importantly, this first generation of novel target-oriented drugs has made it very clear that a thorough understanding of the molecular biology of cancers is a prerequisite to generate further therapeutic drugs that are at least as successful as imatinib.

New Concepts in Cancer Therapy: Immunotherapy

Immunotherapy is arguably the most elegant concept in cancer therapy. After all, its central idea is to harness the body's own ressources against a cancer. Furthermore, diverse evidence indicates that immunotherapy might represent an extension of anticancer immunity that prevents many cancers from developing in the first place. (1) Various lymphomas, leukemias, sarcomas, skin carcinomas and cervical carcinomas occur with increased frequencies in patients with immunodeficiency diseases, e.g. in AIDS patients. (2) Stimulation of immune reactions by interleukins and interferons is routine in the treatment of several cancers, including chronic phase CML and metastatic renal carcinoma. (3) Stem cell therapy by transplantation of hematopoetic precursor cells is thought to be active against leukemias (and even some solid tumors) through a graft-versus-tumor reaction. (4) There are a few documented cases of cancers which have spontaneously disappeared, and these are usually ascribed to a successful immune response.

Indeed, cancers as a rule do elicit an immune reaction. Antibodies to cancer-specific antigens and T-cells directed against cancer cells are found in many cancer patients. The detection of such antibodies can even be exploited for cancer diagnostics. Tumor tissue contain almost invariably infiltrating immune cells, macrophages, neutrophils and even cytotoxic T-cells that can be shown to exhibit specificity against tumor cell antigens.

However, the spontaneous immune response can evidently not contain all cancers. In late stage cancers, the patient's immune system may simply become overwhelmed by the tumor mass spreading through the body. In fact, it may cave in completely and become as well incapable of coping with unrelated bacterial and viral infections.

Even at earlier stages of cancer progression, however, the patient's immune response to the cancer often appears inefficient or muted.

Cancer cells evade the immune response by a variety of mechanims, e.g. secretion of TGFβ1, down-regulation of FAS, or the diminished presentation of antigen peptides and co-activator proteins at the cancer cell surface. Worse, in many cancers, the effect of the immune response is ambiguous. While cancer cells are being attacked, the destruction of the tissue structure associated with the immune response and the ensuing inflammation facilitate invasion and metastasis. Some cancers may even respond to cytokines and chemokines secreted by immune cells by enhanced proliferation or migration. The CXCR4/CXCL12 system, e.g., may be involved in directing metastases to the bone.

So, if immunotherapy is to be successful, it has to overcome the mechanisms that prohibit an efficient anti-tumor response by the patient's immune system. This is likely what happens in those CML and renal carcinoma patients in which immunotherapy using IFNα or IL2, respectively, causes remissions. These cytokines '*awake*' cytotoxic T-cells directed against tumor cells. Typically, the immune cells are already present at the site of the cancer, but are relatively inert. Cytokine treatment then may activate them, stimulating their proliferation and their ability to kill tumor cells.

Of note, not all patients respond to these treatments. This is very typical of immune therapy. In many immunotherapy trials, including those of novel therapies, some patients respond excellently, to the point of '*miracle cures*', whereas others show no response at all, or only adverse reactions to the treatment. So, while the results of such trials are often encouraging, they get stuck at this point, because it is incompletely understood what is responsible for the variable responses. '*Proximate*' parameters such as killing efficiency of CD8+ T-cells or the levels of cytokines in the tumor and serum can, of course, be ascertained, but why such cells become activated in one patient, but not in another, remains largely unclear.

If the lack of response can, perhaps, not be amended, it would at least be helpful to be able to predict which patients respond to a treatment. For instance, 15-30% of metastatic renal carcinomas show partial remissions after administration of a combined cytokine/cytostatic drug cocktail, while many more develop adverse effects resembling the symptoms of a severe flu. It would therefore be helpful to have some indication of which patients might benefit from the treatment, but this is not yet possible.

An alternative approach towards activating cytotoxic T-cells is to isolate them, activate them in vitro, and reintroduce them into the patient or directly into a tumor. This can be done in various ways. T-cells can be treated with cytokines. They can be incubated with professional antigen-presenting cells challenged with tumor extracts or specific antigens, which activate the T-cells by direct contact and by cytokines. In a combination of immunotherapy and gene therapy, they can be transfected or transduced with a gene encoding a cytokine, such as IL-2, which stimulates the activation and proliferation of cytotoxic T-cells. In fact, one of the first experiments in human gene therapy was exactly this one.

Meanwhile, professional antigen-presenting cells, dendritic cells, have become much better characterized and their crucial function in the activation of T-cells has become recognized. Specifically, their insufficient function in tumors was identified as another weak point in the spontaneous immune response to cancers. Moreover, dendritic cells can now be differentiated from monocyte precursors and manipulated in vitro. So, several newer attempts at immunotherapy have used dendritic cells isolated from the tumor or differentiated from blood precursors in vitro.

These dendritic cells can be exposed to tumor antigens in several different fashions. They can be exposed to specific antigens of the tumor or transfected with expression constructs for tumor antigens. They can be incubated with tumor lysates or with lysates from primary cultures of tumor cells. In still another approach, they can be fused with tumor cells. In each case, they are reintroduced into the patient, either alone or in combination with T-cells.

The procedure of treating dendritic cells in vitro with specific tumor antigens or tumor protein lysates resembles the process occurring in vivo during a vaccination. So, this is also considered a sort of vaccination. It is only one step from there towards using tumor lysates or antigens as vaccines in vivo. These vaccines must be supported by adjuvants to elicit a significant immune reaction. In fact, one such adjuvant, BCG, consisting of *Mycobacterium tuberculosis*, is used to prevent recurrences of localized bladder cancers.

Vaccination against tumor antigens could also be considered for the prevention of cancers. The prime candidates in this regard are viral proteins in cancers caused by or associated with viruses. Vaccination against HBV appears indeed to be effective for the prevention of hepatocellular carcinoma. Likewise, vaccination against HPV is expected to diminish the incidence of cervical and other cancers. It is uncertain whether such vaccines would still be beneficial once cancer are established. In the case of HBV, in particular, immunotherapy might do more harm than good.

In spite of occasional successes, overall, '*novel*' approaches at immunotherapy have not made a major impact in the clinic, yet, compared to the more established (but also not veteran) immunotherapies using cytokines or stem cell transplantation. This may have several causes that cover the range from understandable to worrysome. Novel therapies are typically tried in patients with advanced stage cancers for whom no other treatments are available. These may be the very patients, in which the immune system is on the verge of collapsing, and the chances of succeeding are therefore minimal. At the end of the range of arguments, it remains possible that some cancers manage to turn even immune therapy to their advantage, in a similar fashion as they likely distort spontaneous immune responses. An improved understanding of these interactions is certainly required, particularly in those cases in which immune therapy fails.

New Concepts in Cancer Therapy: Gene Therapy

If one considers cancer primarily as a genetic disease, it is consequent to treat it by therapy of the genes that cause cancer. Moreover, the fact that genetic alterations are essentially specific to the cancer cells ought to obliterate the problem of therapeutic selectivity that complicates other therapies, at least in theory. Since genetic alterations in cancer comprise the increased or misdirected activity of oncogenes as well as the lack or insufficiency of tumor suppressors, gene therapy can aim at inhibiting oncogenes or at restoring oncogene function. With ≈250 genes implicated as oncogenes or tumor suppressor genes in human cancers, there is no shortage of targets.

Gene therapy does not have to be addressed directly at oncogenes or tumor suppressor genes, but can exploit their altered activities indirectly. The lack of the function of a tumor suppressor may be exploited to allow the replication of a cytotoxic virus in tumor cells or the increased activity of an oncogene may permit the selective expression of a toxin gene.

Genes that are not oncogenes or tumor suppressors themselves, but which oppose or mediate their effects, can also be employed. Genes that modulate the interaction between tumor cells and immune cells can be introduced into either cell type. Genes that protect sensitive populations like hematopoetic cells from toxic therapy can be introduced, thereby allowing the administration of increased doses of drugs or radiation.

So, ideas are plenty and even experiments, to the stage of human trials. In fact, the majority of gene therapy trials conducted in humans so far have been attempts at cancer therapy. In most studies the goals were to establish the safety of the procedure and to determine whether the therapeutic gene reached the target tissues, while proving the efficacy of the treatment was not an official aim. These experiments were thus comparable to phase I studies in drug development, and usually were labeled as such. In more than a hundred trials involving thousands of patients, few, if any have been cured. It has, however, become clearer which requirements gene therapy has to meet if it is to provide the intended breakthrough in cancer therapy and what the obstacles to its clinical application are.

The limited successes in clinical trials stand in striking contrast to the results obtained in gene therapy experiments with preclinical models, such as cell cultures and animals. There, the full panoply of gene therapy approaches has been tried, with often impressive results.

Resubstitution therapy is particularly effective in such models. Introducing tumor suppressor genes that are inactivated in a specific tumor cell line or in a tumor xenograft causes growth arrest or apoptosis in all tumor cells that receive the gene. To reach as many tumor cells as possible, viral vectors are typically employed in this type of experiment. An alternative is gene transfer by liposomes or dendrimers.

The most efficacious gene for the purpose of resubstitution may be TP53. (1) It often elicits apoptosis in tumor cells with chromosomal instability. (2) It is functionally inactivated in many different types of human cancer. (3) It augments the effects of cytostatic drugs and radiation. In clinical trials using this approach, adenoviral vectors have been employed, in which a TP53 expression cassette replaces a non-essential viral gene.

Trials by resubstitution therapy in humans have been little successful, for several related reasons. The central problem is that essentially only those tumor cells receiving the therapeutic gene can undergo growth arrest or apoptosis. It is difficult to administer sufficiently high amounts of the therapeutic virus, for technical as well as safety reasons. The concentration of the recombinant virus (the '*titer*') that can be produced in cell cultures is limited, and administration of too high titers can elicit an lethal immune reaction in the patient.

Systemic administration of therapeutic viruses, especially of adenoviruses, is also complicated by the ability of the liver to filter and remove viral particles. Up to 90% of all adenoviruses administered are removed during a single pass through the liver. Getting viral particles into the right place is further hampered by mechanical factors due to the disturbed anatomy of solid cancers. As a rule, they have a suboptimal vessel system, which is barely sufficient to provide nutrients, growth factors, and oxygen, and which limits the penetration of therapeutic agents. Even small molecule drugs may not always get optimally distributed into a tumor, least viral particles. The pressure ('*turgor*') within a tumor can be higher than in the surrounding tissue, further impeding the entry of larger particles.

Finally, the repeated administration of therapeutic viruses can lead to immune reactions that decrease efficacy and/or cause adverse immunological reactions in the patient. This effect may limit the applicability of adenoviruses. These are good vectors capable of accomodating quite large genes, infect many human cell types, and are otherwise relatively safe. The unmodified viruses cause at most a light, common cold-like disease when they naturally infect epithelial cells in the airways. Almost everybody has been exposed, and most humans harbor memory B-cells and T-cells directed against adenoviral antigens. These are activated when the viruses are administered as a therapeutic agent and become a more severe problem with each repeated application or upon adminstration of high doses.

For such reasons, the use of recombinant adenoviruses carrying tumor suppressor genes is limited to local administration, for the time being. This could still be useful in those cases, where local tumor growth presents the main problem, but surgery or irradiation are impossible, too risky, or disfiguring. For instance, aggressive brain tumors, glioblastomas, spread within the brain tissue and are often impossible to remove without serious damage to the brain. However, since they metastasize relatively late, local treatment by gene therapy is an option. Similarly, carcinomas recurring in the mouth and throat are often difficult to excise without compromising breathing, swallowing, or speaking. There are thus useful and important applications for this type of gene therapy, but its use in the treatment of systemic disease remains a remote possibility, unless fundamental innovations are made.

Some of these problems are circumvented by a related approach using '*oncolytic viruses*'. Tumor suppressor proteins like RB1 and TP53 not only prevent the carcinogenic effects of tumor viruses, but also impede their replication. Specifically, the replication of DNA viruses, including papovaviruses (SV40), papillomaviruses (HPV), and adenoviruses is inhibited by these tumor suppressor proteins. Therefore, these viruses contain proteins that in turn block the function of RB1 and TP53. In SV40, the large T antigen is responsible for both, while HPV and adenoviruses each contain two separate proteins that inactivate RB1 and TP53, viz. E6 and E7 in HPV, and E1A and E1B in adenoviruses.

The large T protein of SV40 is indispensible because it also functions directly in viral transcription and replication. In contrast, adenoviruses lacking E1B can still replicate and remain cytolytic. However, their replication is blocked in cells that contain functional TP53. Inactivation of TP53 function is common in human cancers, expecially those metastatic carcinomas which represent a major problem in cancer therapy. So, the cells of these tumors ought to allow the replication of adenoviruses that lack the E1B protein directed at the tumor suppressors.

As such viruses remain competent for replication, they are supposed to spread within a cancer, lysing the tumor cells, but they should not be capable of replicating and lysing normal epithelial cells. Since replication-competent viruses are used in this approach, some problems arising in resubstitution therapy are circumvented, viz. the limited efficiency of gene transfer and the requirement for unrealistically high and dangerous virus titers. Other problems remain, such as an eventual immune reaction by the host. However, in this case, there is a chance that the immune reaction might actually be helpful. When it becomes effective some time after administration of the virus, it might be directed not only at the therapeutic virus, but also against the tumor cells in which it replicates. So, this approach could turn out to represent an immunotherapy in disguise.

In clinical trials, however, this elegant concept has not proven as efficacious as one might have hoped, although promising results have been seen. The precise reasons limiting the efficacy of this approach are under investigation. One factor limiting the effect of oncolytic as well as other therapeutic viruses is that cancer cells often express low amounts of receptor proteins used for viral attachment and entry, such as a membrane folate transporter protein (CAR) employed by adenoviruses. Non-viral methods for gene transfer suffer from similar or even worse problems.

Gene therapy strategies that depend on getting a therapeutic gene into each and every cell of a cancer may be generally unrealistic. It appears that a gene therapy strategy aiming at a cure rather than palliation must evoke a '*bystander*' effect, i.e. tumor cells that do not receive the therapeutic gene must also be affected. Eliciting an immune reaction against tumor cells by the replication of a cytolytic virus is one example of a bystander effect. In this case, one hopes that the immune response would be directed at a wider range of antigens, not only those provided by the virus, but also some specific to the tumor cells.

There are more explicit strategies to achieve bystander effects. In one approach employed in several variations, a gene encoding an enzyme that activates a prodrug is introduced into cancer cells. The prodrug is then activated in successfully transfected cancer cells, from which it diffuses to neighboring cells in the tumor. In this fashion, it would kill cancer cells and stromal cells needed for tumor growth, such as endothelial cells. The thymidine kinase of the herpes virus HSV has been used in early trials of this approach. Other than cellular thymidine kinases, this enzyme phosphorylates the nucleoside drug gancyclovir which thereby becomes capable of inhibiting DNA replication. Neighboring cells are affected, if they are linked to the successfully transfected cancer cell by gap junctions which allow the passage of gancyclovir nucleotides. Such cells would most likely be also cancer cells, because gap junctions are typically formed in a homotypic fashion. However, in most cancers, gap junctional communication is down-regulated, which limits the distribution of the active drug. Newer trials therefore employ enzymes that yield better diffusible and more active drugs, e.g. cytidine deaminase, which catalyzes one step in the activation of the prodrug capecitabine to 5-FU.

In this approach, the selectivity of the treatment depends on delivery of the therapeutic toxic gene to the correct cell or on its selective expression there. Again, several strategies are being explored. For instance, the expression of tumor antigens on the cell membrane can be used to target accordingly engineered recombinant viruses. Within a cancer cell, selectivity of expression of a toxic gene can be achieved by using promoters that respond to specific alterations in the tumor ceil or to conditions prevailing in the cancer. For instance, promoters responsive to hypoxia, i.e. to HIF factors, have been designed. These may be particularly useful in clear-cell renal carcinomas in which these factors are constitutively active, but they are certainly not limited to this tumor type.

Other selective promoters exploit the lack of a tumor suppressor that represses them or respond to the oncogenic activation of a cancer pathway in a specific cancer. This is one way to exploit the activation of oncogenes for selectivity in gene therapy. For instance, the activation of β-Catenin in primary hepatocellular carcinomas leads to an increased activity of TCF-dependent promoters. So, such promoters could be employed in gene therapy of liver carcinomas, but also of colon cancers with the same genetic change. Increased promoter activity would also be expected in the large proportion of colorectal cancers in which activation of the WNT pathway is caused by loss of the APC tumor suppressor function rather than oncogenic activation of β-Catenin. A concern in this application is, whether tissue stem cells dependent on WNT signals for their maintenance are also targeted and might become depleted. The promoter of the catalytic subunit of telomerase, hTERT, is also considered, and ought to be applicable in an even wider range of cancers, albeit with the same caveat.

Gene therapy can be targeted at oncogenes and their protein products in a more fashion. For instance, a variety of techniques have become available to down-regulate the expression of specific genes. They are well established in laboratory research and are being developed for suppressing oncogene action in cancer patients. The expression of an oncogenic protein can be blocked at several steps from transcription to translation.

The *MYC* gene, e.g., has been targeted by several methods, although none of them has seriously moved beyond the preclinical stage. It is an attractive target, because it is causally involved in several lymphomas, including Burkitt lymphoma, and at least important, if not essential for the growth of many solid tumors. The *MYC* promoter region contains DNA sequences, e.g. purine-pyrimidine tracts and G-rich regions, which have the potential to form unusual DNA structures such as triplex or quadruplex DNA. So, this gene might be targeted specifically by oligonucleotides designed to stabilize these unusual structures and block *MYC* transcription.

In other genes, where no such unusual structures are available, transcription might be blocked specifically by attaching an intercalating compound like the anthracyclins adriamycin or daunomycin as an obstacle to transcription to an oligonucleotide specific for the oncogene sequence.

Several techniques are available to target the mRNAs of oncogenes by prohibiting their processing or translation, or by promoting their degradation. Antisense oligonucleotides directed against several oncogenes have proceeded to advanced clinical trial stages. They usually contain a modified backbone to protect them from metabolism and increase the stability of the duplex they form with a specific mRNA. Phosphothionates are frequently employed. Nevertheless, huge amounts of oligonucleotides are required to achieve active concentrations in humans, and they have to be highly pure to avoid side effects, especially immune reactions. Thus, their application in humans is not only limited by concerns about their efficacy.

It is hoped that treatment costs may be lower with siRNAs, which are moreover expected to be more efficacious. Antisense oligonucleotides appear to work mainly by blocking the processing and translation of the mRNA to which they bind, although additional effects may contribute. In contrast, siRNAs induce the degradation of their corresponding mRNA. This mechanism increases their efficiency. Furthermore, in theory and indeed in some cells, siRNAs elicit an amplification effect by which a relatively low concentration of siRNA induces an RNase-containing complex that degrades the corresponding mRNAs in the cell. Its activity may be maintained over a period of days to weeks. Thus, less siRNA at larger intervals may be required than in the case of anti-sense oligonucleotides. The concept of using siRNA for gene regulation in mammalian cells, least for therapy in humans, is still very new. It remains to be seen how straightforwardly it can be translated from the laboratory into the clinic.

Anti-sense constructs and siRNA directed at oncogenes are expected to be applied systemically. This raises two critical issues. (1) How can specificity for cancer cells be achieved? (2) Will the down-regulation of one oncogene suffice to inhibit the growth of a cancer? In essence, the answers hinge on how far the '*addiction theory*' discussed previously in this chapter is correct. In other words: There is no doubt that the activation of oncogenes is important in the development of many cancers, but are cancer cells so much more dependent on these proteins than normal cells that there is a useful therapeutic window? And do advanced cancers remain dependent on the activity of oncogenic alterations, or can they evade therapy, e.g., by switching to a different cancer pathway?

In this regard, the example of imatinib use against CML can be interpreted as a pro or as a contra argument. A drug directed at an oncogene thought to be crucial for this cancer indeed induced lasting remissions in the chronic phase of the disease and even transient responses in many patients at the advanced blast crisis stage. This proves that the oncogene product is essential in the chronic phase and remains at least important in some tumor that have progressed. Moreover, the tumor cells recurring after treatment with the drug often harbor genetic changes which alter the structure or expression level of this particular target oncogene protein. However, not all patients respond in the first place, especially among those with advanced disease, and not all cases of drug resistance can be explained by such specific mechanisms.

It seems therefore safe to argue that selection of oncogene targets for antisense and siRNA therapies, too, will require a very thorough understanding of the '*rewiring*' of cancer pathways in a particular malignant tumor.

Future of Cancer Therapy

The first wave of optimism which accompanied the development of novel drugs, immunotherapy and gene therapy for the treatment of human cancers has passed. There is a general feeling that the high hopes pinned on their development have not been fulfilled. A more guarded optimism now prevails and goals are set more realistic (as far as one can tell). In looking back on the 1990's, one realizes how naive some of the novel approaches were. However, this is the benefit of hindsight. After all, human oncogenes and tumor suppressors as such were only discovered during the 1980's and many were identified only in the 1990's. Many of their actions and interactions are not fully understood to this day. So, of course, if one wanted to act at all on the emerging knowledge, it would have to be on an incomplete basis. When dealing with a lethal disease of major importance, it is probably unavoidable that researchers, doctors and companies rush for solutions, once they appear on the horizon. One criticism that may be made with some right is that too often the difficulties ahead have been downplayed and the incompleteness of our understanding has been obfuscated in the rush for success. This may be the reason why now many involved feel that we have been taught a lesson on the complexity and diversity of human cancers which we are to heed in our future efforts at curing this disease.

Some consequences appear to have been drawn. Prevention and early diagnosis are seen as more important than they were in the prime of the enthusiasm associated with the development of novel therapies. Novel therapeutic approaches will be based on a more thorough understanding of the molecular biology of human cancers, acknowledging their diversity and complexity at an earlier stage of the development of therapies. The qualities of the established therapeutic methods, surgery, irradiation and cytostatic drugs, are probably better appreciated, which should faciliate the integration and combination of different types of therapies. For instance, gene therapy with oncolytic viruses has been combined with cytotoxic chemotherapy. Indeed, both '*traditional*' and '*novel*' therapy approaches appear to converge towards the concept of individualized therapy, which aims at taking the properties of each cancer and the constitution and wishes of each patient into account.

The implementation of individualized therapy will constitute new challenges for cancer diagnostics and classification by molecular techniques, as will any extension of cancer prevention and early detection programs. Education of clinicians and scientists will have to evolve to facilitate translational research and its application in the clinic. New options for the therapy, diagnostics and prevention of cancer will have implications for the organization of health systems, in the industrialized Western world as well as in the developing countries of the South. This will require political action and consensus decisions based on public understanding of complex issues. Providing an adequate and solid scientific basis for these developments remains a task that is as challenging as it is important.

5

IMMUNOTHERAPY OF CANCER

Nucleic acid immunization has garnered much attention as a promising approach for cancer therapeutic development. This innovative vaccine strategy uses non live, non replicating, non spreading DNA formulations which utilize the host's cellular machinery for expression of proteins (antigens). Such novel delivered and expressed antigens become recognized by the host immune response and induce specific T and B cell responses against the gene encoded proteins. The foundational basis for DNA vaccines originated from the observation that delivery of gene sequences in vivo could lead to their expression. In the 1950s and 1960s experiments aimed at understanding the fundamental nature of the basis for cancer delivered as either nucleic acid or proteins to animals and followed tumor development. Tumor development segregated with nucleic acids and tumor bearing animals could seroconvert to tumor antigens, establishing the ability of nucleic acid transfer to drive protein expression and activate the immune response. In the 1980s the understanding that the immune response was a nemesis for gene therapy antigen delivery started to impact vector studies. Wolff et al. reported that activity of reporter genes could be detected for up to two months without a delivery system.

Many investigators were focusing on if such proteins implemented for such gene therapy experiments could be employed to express antigens to stimulate the immune system. A study published by Tang et al. utilizing DNA coated gold microprojectiles to transfect cells *in vivo* reported the generation of an antibody response against the DNA encoded proteins. The study utilized a delivery system called a gene gun as this group had doubts that the efficiency of direct injection was likely substantial enough to deliver enough antigen to produce a significant immune response. However, papers appeared from Ulmer and Wang almost coincidently describing different formulations for IM delivery inducing responses against true human pathogens, influenza and HIV, followed rapidly by a paper from Fryan on influenza. These papers demonstrated that not just antibodies could be induced by this technology, but that cellular response as well as cytokine profiles could also be altered. In addition, protection from animal challenge could also be achieved.

Among the most intriguing and yet promising aspect of DNA vaccines is the feasibility of manipulation towards benevolent immune responses, juxtaposed with the remarkable ability to activate both arms of the immune system. These unique attributes are a result of direct transfection of encoding plasmids into cells *in vivo*, whereby direct presentation on MHC Class I can materialize. As will be discussed later, this very principle has been exploited to specifically amplify the cellular arm of the immune response. The other beneficial aspect is its ability to engineer responses robust enough to often break tolerance against nonimmunogenic tumor antigens. This is particularly important when dealing with antigens exhibiting minimal immunogenic properties. In view of these findings, we review the potential utility of applying DNA vaccines as both a therapeutic and prophylactic approach against cancer and other forms of neoplastic growth. The requirement of potent T-cell activation rather than antibody activation as an essential criterion for tumor rejection validates such a use for efficacious treatment for tumor immunotherapy.

Essential Role of Dendritic Cells in Tumor Immunogenicity: Optimizing to Target DC's

In the body's immune system, cells need to process and present antigenic peptides to lymphocytes in order to stimulate antigen specific immune response. Thus, antigen must be processed and presented to T lymphocytes by antigen presenting cells (APCs). Antigen presentation and recognition is a complex biological process that involves many interactions between antigen presenting cells and T cells. There are four primary components that are critical in the professional APCs' ability to present the antigen to T cells and activate them for appropriate immune responses. These components are MHC-antigen complexes, costimulatory molecules (primarily CD80 and CD86), intracellular adhesion molecules, and soluble cytokines. Naive T cells circulate through the body across lymph nodes and secondary lymphoid organs such as the spleen. Their migration is mediated among other factors by intercellular adhesion molecules and cytokines. As the T cells travel, they bind to and dissociate from various *antigen presenting cells* (APCs). Their movement is guided by chemokines but binding to cells is mediated through adhesion molecules. When a naive T cell binds to an APC expressing relevant MHC:peptide complex, the T cell up regulates costimulatory molecules such as CD40L which further activates the APC increasing expression of the T cell costimulatory molecules CD86/CD80. These costimulatory signals bind to CD28 on the T cells inducing increased levels of high affinity IL-2 receptor. Only when this T cell receives a strong enough costimulatory signal through CD80/CD86-CD28 interaction does the T cell make soluble IL-2, which then binds to the receptors and drives the now-armed effector T cell to activate and proliferate.

Much speculation on the immunogenicity of tumor antigens has concentrated on the efficiency of antigen presentation from APCs to T-cells. Specifically, the roles of *Dendritic cells* (DCs) and the essential antigen specific clonal expansion have been thoroughly investigated. When compared with other *"professional" antigen presenting cells* (APCs), dendritic cells are preferentially advantageous due to their exclusive ability to activate naive T-cells within the secondary lymphoid organs. Structurally, dendritic cells express elevated quantities of co-stimulatory molecules including CD80 and CD86, and large amounts of peptide-MHC complexes allowing potent T lymphocyte activation and differentiation.

The role of DC's in regulating tumor antigenicity have been extensively documented. In fact, tumors have developed immune evasive attributes to prevent DC maturation and prevent the eventual antigen specific T-cell generation. For instance, some tumors secrete substantial amounts of Vascular Endothelial Growth Factors (VEGF) which promote not only angiogenesis but also retards the maturation of antigen captured DC's and this effect appears to operate through a direct suppression of NF-κB. Furthermore, continuous infusion of VEGF into mice leads to a dramatic inhibition of dendritic cell development, associated with an increase in the production of B cells and immature Gr-1(+) myeloid cells. In addition to VEGF, some tumor cells secrete IL-10, which directly prevents the maturation of dendritic cells. This effect dramatically diminishes the antigen specific activation of both CD4 and CD8 T cells through the attenuation of DC's, as *ex vivo* generation of bone marrow-derived DC eradicates this effect. These results suggest a paramount theme; tumors suppress the maturation of DC's to impede the functional stimulation of T cells. Unfortunately for the development of anti tumor immunity, this effect is essential for proficient activation of tumor specific T cells.

Essential Role of DCs in DNA-based Immunizations

In addition to anti-tumor immunity, the development of DNA vaccine-based immune responses also requires the activation and and perhaps in part direct transfection of dendritic cells. Condon et al. demonstrated that gene gun delivery of reporter gene plasmids to the skin resulted in expression of the reporter genes in cells exhibiting dendritic cell-like morphology localized within the local draining lymph nodes. Others have proposed that secretion of expressed antigens from somatic cells or their destruction (i.e. muscle cells and keratinocytes) may provide the path for dendritic cells to take up antigen and present through the exogenous MHC class II pathway. In fact purification of APCs from immunized mice will stimulate naive T cells in an antigen specific manner, suggesting that uptake of antigen by APCs is important for DNA immunization based immune activation. Additionally, IM injection of plasmids expressing EGFP results in co-localization of EGFP expressing cells and APC markers CD80 and CD86 in the draining LN's. These results suggest that (1) APC activation and migration to the regional lymph node is essential for immune activation following plasmid immunization, and (2) APCs can take up antigens through direct transfection and/or exogenous phagocytosis. Therefore, vaccine strategies targeting the enhanced uptake of antigens by DCs or increased chemotaxic migration of DCs to the site of antigen expression may provide increased vaccine potency and increased therapeutic potential.

Enhancing DC-directed Antigen Uptake

In addition to powerful signaling, dendritic cells often function as scavenger cells by engulfing and processing apoptotic bodies. Specifically, immature DCs uptake dead cells or apoptotic bodies via surface receptors $\alpha V\beta 5$ integrin and CD36. This uptake promotes a process termed cross-priming whereby exogenous antigens are processed and presented through the endogenous MHC class I pathway. Specifically, the engulfment of these bodies with either tumor or viral antigens by dendritic cells provokes the activation of MHC class I restricted $CD8^+$ CTLs. Both dendritic cells and macrophages have been shown to present apoptotic engulfed antigens but the latter is much less potent at activating naive T-cells, which is a vital step in

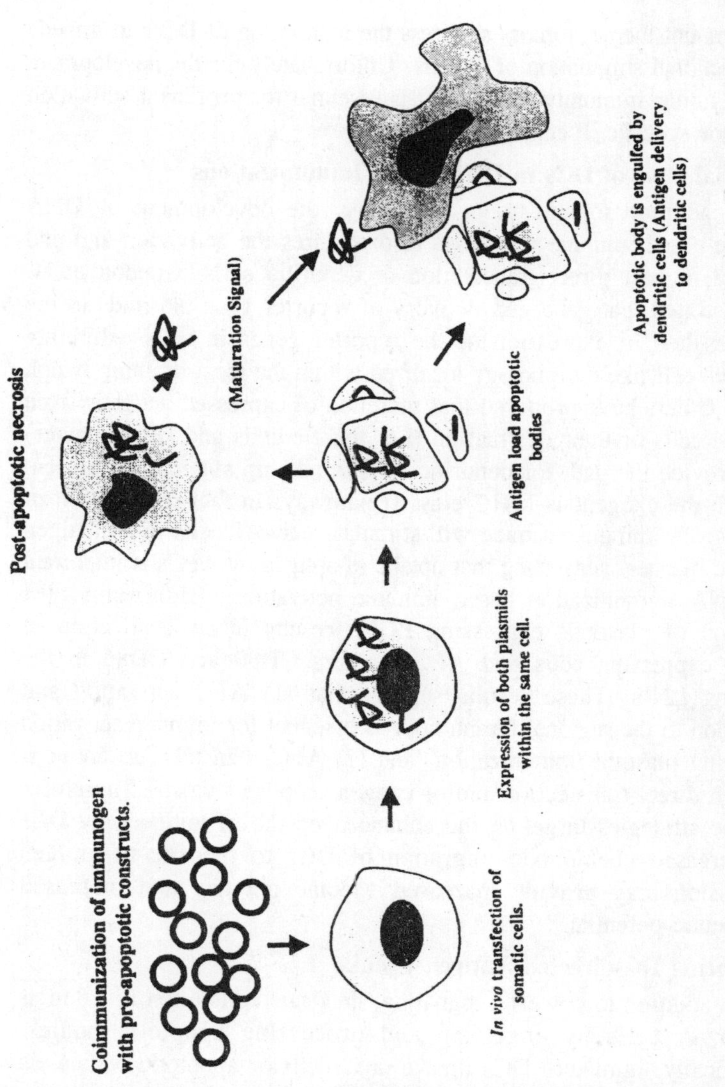

Fig. 5.1. Apoptosis-mediated delivery of DNA vaccine. The following model describes a possible mechanism by which antigen loaded apoptotic bodies deliver and induce maturation of dendritic cells.

the generation of adaptive immunity. Furthermore, several studies also demonstrate that there is a quantitative dependency on apoptotic bodies by dendritic cells in inducing the secretion of pro-inflammatory cytokines TNF-α and IL-1β both *in vitro* and *in vivo*. Accordingly, an optimum strategy to develop potent vaccines would include the activation of dendritic cells and the packaging of immunogens in apoptotic bodies facilitating cross priming and broader cellular immunity. In a recent study, a novel strategy was used whereby immunogen constructs were coimmunized with an apoptosis inducing receptor Fas. This coimmmunization resulted in significant augmentation of antigen specific immune responses as measured by enhanced CTLs and Th1 cytokines including INF-γ and IL-12. There is other evidence to suggest that apoptosis signals that aliquot ample time for immunogen expression will provide adjuvant properties. A more recent study implemented mutant caspases to decrease apoptotic efficiency to increase the time of immunogen expression prior to the apoptotic event, while still delivering apoptosis-mediated antigens to dendritic cells. This specific adjuvant raised both CD4 and CD8 responses, indicating that antigen uptake by DCs presented peptides into both the endogenous and exogenous pathways.

While apoptosis mediated delivery has provided an insight to the possibility of cross priming, others have utilized directly secreted antigens to target dendritic cells. This raises the prospect that exogenous antigens may function in generating MHC Class I-restricted responses by directly entering the cytosol in a DNA vaccine model through the endogenous cross-priming process. It has been previously suggested that antigens can be expressed by transplanted cells, which maintain the ability to induce CTLs through the direct transfer of antigens to host's antigen presenting cells. Various tumor studies directed at ascertaining the precise functions of somatic MHC class I molecules have determined that bone marrow-derived antigen-presenting cells play the dominant role of presenting these somatic-based antigens. Additionally, other exogenous antigens such as bacteria are internalized and processed for presentation by MHC class I molecules.

These reports unequivocally imply extracellular uptake of antigens is a prominent pathway implemented by the immune system to generate CTLs. In this regard, dendritic cells express surface cell receptors for Fc regions of antibodies called FcγR's, which enhances the uptake of antigen-antibody complexes and leads to presentation on MHC class II molecules. These receptors also assist in the activation and maturation of dendritic cells and regulate efficient presentation of exogenous antigens. Hence introduction of exogenous antigens through FcγR-mediated internalization into the cytoplasm may help effectively prime antigens to activate MHC Class I-restricted CTLs. Exogenous antigen endocytosis could then employ the endogenous TAP dependent antigen processing pathway and in theory present peptides on MHC Class I molecules. This strategy was directly tested in a DNA vaccine model by fusing the hepatitis B virus (HBV) e antigen and the Fc portion of an IgG1 antibody. The antigen-Fc immunogen was secreted by somatic cells and taken up effectively by dendritic cells resulting in stimulation of both $CD4^+$ and $CD8^+$ T cells *in vivo*. The adjuvant effectively augmented the secretion of proinflammatory cytokines including INF-γ and IL-2 as well as enhancing CTL and lymphocyte proliferative responses.

Another promising DC targeting immune modulator is the family of chaperones called the *Heat Shock Proteins* (HSPs). The initial experiments that elucidated the immunocapability of HSPs were from purification experiments from antigenically distinct sarcoma cells. In fact, it was later ascertained that this 96 kDa glycoprotein was not itself immunogenic, but became immunogenic in circumstances when it was conjugated with peptides. Overall comparison of immunogenicity with other HSP family members including Hsp70 and Hsp90 suggest that immunogenicity is associated with two vital factors, the associated ATPase activity and the association of HSP with peptides.

The ATPase activity likely determines the ability of the chaperone complex to transfer peptide to acceptor molecules and this association with peptides is the rationale for the autologous nature of these complexes. These chaperones also possess intrinsic inflammatory qualities, including among many properties the maturation and activation of DCs, direct cross-priming abilities, and release of NO from APCs. The endocytosis and eventual presentation of antigens is thought to be a consequence of the universal targeting of all HSPs by its receptor CD91, a natural ligand for alpha 2-macroglobulin. The post uptake processing implements the endogenous pathway, which partially explains the cross-priming effect of these proteins. The significance of HSP in tumor-specific and non-vaccine related circumstances has been examined. Specifically, immunotherapy of cancers with HSPs purified from tumors or reconstituted *in vitro* from tumor cell cultures when administered as vaccines also regressed the growth of tumors.

The copious immunogenic attributes of HSP suggest these complexes may function as useful adjuvants for DNA vaccines. Specifically, the HSP70 of Mycobacterium tuberculosis was fused to the Human HPV-16 E7 antigen generating a chimeric DNA vaccine. The E7-HSP70 DNA vaccine induced significantly enhanced levels of Th1 mediated responses including a ratio of 435:14 (E7-HSP70 to E7) of E7 specific INF-γ spot-forming $CD8^+$ T cells via ELISPOT assays. Additionally, data from this group suggested that the eradication of pre-existing tumors and the resulting immune response was via $CD4^+$ independent mechanisms, implying that cross-priming was crucial for this effect. Where the T cell help for this cross priming event was supplied is unclear.

Another member of the HSP family that has shown to augment the potency of DNA vaccines is calreticulin. The idea of calreticulin as an immune modulator was based on previous findings that calreticulin in conjugation with tumor peptides stimulates potent peptide specific $CD8^+$ T cell responses. Like the other HSP members, calreticulin also implements the CD91-dependent pathway for APC uptake, making cross-priming another presumable immunogenic outcome from use of this molecule. Additionally, calreticulin and its fragment vasostatin also operate as inhibitors of angiogensis. Accordingly, when calreticulin was fused to HPV-16 E7 antigen as a DNA vaccine, a potent, anti-tumor effect was provoked; the resulting response was attributed to both the enhanced immunogenicity against E7 and the generation of anti-angiogenesis.

Amplifying DCs at the Site of Expression

In addition to the enhanced uptake of antigens, an amplification of DC quantity is likely advantageous for enhanced antigen delivery to and presentation within the regional lymph nodes. Compensating for DC paucity can be ameliorated through DNA vaccine-mediated engineering of immune responses. Among various strategies, Flt3 (*Fms-like tyrosine kinase* 3) ligand (FL) has been utilized to stimulate the activation and amplification of dendritic cells. Functionally, FL treatments in mice significantly increase dendritic cell population in many areas including the bone marrow, *gastro-intestinal lymphoid tissue* (GALT), liver, lymph nodes, lung, peripheral blood, peritoneal cavity, spleen, and thymus. FL has revealed tumor suppressive attributes in mice partly by the generation of large number of dendritic cells. Accordingly, recent work indicates enhanced frequency of $CD8^+$ T cells when FL was fused to the human papillomavirus-16 E7 antigen. The response was $CD4^+$ independent and maximum effect was observed when the antigen and FL were fused together. Most importantly, 100% of mice vaccinated with FL-E7 were protected when challenged with TC-1, a tumor cell line derived from C57BL/6 mice cotransformed with HPV-16 E6 and E7 and c-Ha-ras oncogenes.

Other methods have concentrated on the direct chemotatic migration of DCs to the site of injection. One report specifically coimmunized M-CSF and resulted in enhanced levels of $CD8^+$ T cell dependent responses. This effect was in direct correlation with elevated DC migration to the site of injection with an increase in the Beta-Chemokine MIP-1β. Others have reported that coimmunization with GM-CSF augments the migration of immature DCs to the injection site. The maximal migration occurred between days 3–5 post injection and was not positive for CD80 or CD40.

Converting Muscle Cells into APCs

The generation of immune responses via DNA vaccines requires the delivery and/or presentation of immunogens to professional *antigen presenting cells* (APCs). It has been proposed that a significant target for *in vivo* transfection of plasmids are also the muscle cells themselves and their transfer and/or presentation of immunogens may be a vital tool in the development of immune responses. One of the consequences suggested as an issue for muscle delivery of plasmid vectors is that less effective antigen presentation will occur as the muscle cells fail to express the costimulatory molecules (i.e. CD80, CD86, B7RP1) necessary to send a second signal. One approach to this limitation may be to codeliver antigen expressing plasmids with costimulatory molecule expressing plasmids. In theory the coexpression of CD86 on muscles that express a high ratio of MHC class I and can not a highly invasive approach which exploits the host's own immune system to generate intrinsic anti-tumor defenses. In addition, it can be easily combined with other approaches thus is attractive to patients and physicians. Additionally, side effects associated with conventional chemotherapy and radiotherapy are nonexistent with immunotherapies. To this end, several specific TAAs have become targets for DNA vaccine development.

DNA Vaccines Against Melanoma

An imposing barrier for any immune therapy approach is the potential for immune tolerance to tumor antigens. It has been suggested that the unique presentation of tumor specific antigens in the context of DNA vaccines may facilitate breaching of this potential immunological barrier. Among the numerous TAAs that have been identified for melanoma, several have been studied in the context of DNA vaccines. Specifically, an early experiment conducted by Weber et al. targeted the gp75/ tyrosinase-related protein-1 as an antigen in a DNA vaccine model. This specific TAA is well tolerated as a vaccine antigen although it is difficult to develop strong cellular immunity against. However, mice primed with the human gp75 and boosted with murine gp75 appear to be able to break tolerance and developed immunity and tumor protection in a mouse challenge model. This immune response was dependent on both the induction of $CD4^+$ T cells and NK cells.

Another innovative strategy used minigenes as specific targeted immunogenes, by fusing distinct dominant class I epitopes from gp100 and TRP-2 into the vaccine candidate. In addition, the ubiquitin gene was fused on the 5' end of the vaccine and was delivered by oral gavage using an attenuated strain of *Salmonella typhimurium* as carrier. The enhanced effect was concomitant with increased INF-γ production and specific lysis of tumor cells by activated CD8 T cells. The effect is thought to be a consequence of increased processing and targeting of the antigen into the MHC Class I presentation pathway. Several studies have tested plasmid vaccines against different models of melanoma. Some of these studies induced destruction of pigment cells as a possible correlate of destruction of melanoma *in vivo*. However, the early results appear to just be scratching the surface. It is likely that more potent DNA vaccines incorporating molecular adjuvants or in prime boost protocols will be more effective than these early approaches.

DNA Vaccines Against Colon Cancer

Human CEA is a 180-kDa glycoprotein expressed in elevated levels in 90% of gastrointestinal malignancies, including colon, rectal, stomach, and pancreatic tumors, 70% of lung cancers, and 50% of breast cancers. CEA is also found in human fetal digestive organ tissue, hence the name carcinoembryonic antigen. It has been discovered that CEA is expressed in normal adult colon epithelium as well, albeit at far lower levels. Sequencing of CEA shows that it is associated with the human immunoglobulin gene superfamily and that it may be involved in the metastasizing of tumor cells.

The immune response to nucleic acid vaccination using a CEA DNA construct was characterized in amurine model. The CEA insert was cloned into a vector containing the *cytomegalovirus* (CMV) early promoter/enhancer and injected intramuscularly. CEA specific humoral and cellular responses were detected in the immunized mice. These responses were comparable to the immune response generated by rV-CEA. The CEA DNA vaccine was also characterized in a canine model, where sera obtained from dogs injected intramuscularly with the construct demonstrated an increase in antibody levels. Cellular immune responses quantified using the *lymphoblast transformation* (LBT) assay also revealed proliferation of CEA-specific lymphocytes. Therefore a CEA nucleic acid vaccine was able to induce both arms of the immune responses. CEA DNA vaccines are currently being investigated in humans, but as yet there is little data presented for guidance.

DNA Vaccines Against Prostate Cancer

Prostate cancer is the most common form of cancer and the second most common cause of cancer related death in American men. The appearance of prostate cancer is much more common in men over the age of fifty. Three of the most widely used treatments are surgical excision of the prostate and seminal vesicles, external bean irradiation, and androgen deprivation. However, conventional therapies lose their efficacy once the tumor has metastasized, which is the case in more than half of initial diagnoses.

PSA is a serine protease and a human glandular kallikrein gene product of 240 amino acids, which is secreted by both normal and transformed epithelial cells of the prostate gland. Because cancer cells secrete much higher levels of the antigen, PSA level is a particularly reliable and effective diagnostic indicator of the presence of prostate cancer. PSA is also found in normal prostate epithelial tissue and its expression is highly specific.

The immune responses induced by a DNA vaccine encoding for human PSA has been investigated in a murine model. The vaccine construct was constructed by cloning a gene for PSA into expression vectors under control of a CMV promoter. Following the injection of the PSA DNA construct (pCPSA), various assays were performed to measure both the humoral and cellular immune responses of the mice. PSA-specific immune responses induced *in vivo* by immunization were characterized by *enzyme-linked immunosorbent assay* (ELISA), T helper proliferation *cytotoxic T lymphocyte* (CTL), and flow cytometry assays. Strong and persistent antibody responses were observed against PSA for at least 180 days following immunization. In addition, a significant T helper cell proliferation was observed against PSA protein. Immunization with pCPSA also induced MHC Class I $CD8^+$ T cell-restricted cytotoxic T lymphocyte response against tumor cell targets expressing PSA. The induction of PSA-specific humoral and cellular immune responses following injection with pCPSA was also observed in rhesus macaques. These responses were achieved in either female or male animals. As the PSA construct was human in design, and human and rhesus construct are 98% identical these results support that the DNA vaccines could break tolerance in this model. This is a rare demonstration of this ability in a non human primate. In addition to cellular immunity, strong antibody responses were also observed.

Such antibody responses may also be valuable in a clinical setting. Recently, PSMA based DNA vaccines have entered the clinic for initial evaluation. The results of these studies are pending but will likely provide important information about targeting prostate disease using DNA technology.

DNA Vaccines Against Cervical Cancer

Human Papillomavirus (HPV) 16 associated proteins including E6 and E7 are some of the most common proteins in cervical cancers and are ubiquitious expressed within these cells. However, DNA based vaccine targeting these proteins seem to elicit minimal immune responses and may necessitate potent adjuvants to provide efficacious tumor protection. A DNA vaccine based HPV E6 vaccine in mice was able to provide anti-tumor activity when adjuvanted with IL-12 into the skin. This specific study implemented exclusively the amino terminal which of E6, which lacks the transforming property. One of the early E7 vaccines employed mutational variants within the zinc-binding motifs that led to rapid degradation. Ironically, this specific vaccine exhibited stronger E7-specific CTLs. In a similar fashion, several other studies have targeted the processing of HPV vaccines to specific compartments to enhance potency.

An early study by T.C. Wu and colleagues fused the E7 antigen with the *lysosomal-associated membrane protein* (LAMP-1), which directs processing of E7 antigens into the MHC class II pathway for presentation. When compared to the E7 antigen alone, the LAMP-1 mediated targeting enhanced antigen specific $CD4^+$ helper T cells, greater antigen specific E7 CTL activity, and antibody responses. On the contrary, similar manipulation has been implemented to direct proteins into the MHC class I presentation pathway. Specifically, the HSV-1 structural protein VP22, which exhibits an intercellular trafficking property, was directly fused to the E7 antigen to perhaps increase presentation productivity. Incredibly, this specific adjuvant stimulated a 50-fold increase in the overall quantity of E7-specific $CD8^+$ T cells. Similarly, fusion of E7 to gamma-tubulin, a target for the centrosomal compartment which possesses proteasomes, led to a dramatic increase in the quantity of E7-specific $CD8^+$ T cells. This effect was dependent on the proteasome, as mice deficient in TAP-1 failed to develop such an enhancement.

A more recent report within the clinics also suggests that immunization through DNA can also therapeutically attenuate the growth of neoplastic cells in humans. These studies specifically encapsulated DNA plasmids encoding HLA-A2-restricted epitopes of the HPV E7 antigen within biodegradable polymer microparticles. Early work suggests no adverse side effects, while enhancing immune responses when implementing this specific therapy. These results are very exciting as the doses of DNA used in these studies are very low.

In addition to the demonstration of immune response induction these investigators noted a regression in precancerous phenotype in this cervical progression model. While spontaneous regressions are noted in this model, the rate of regression gives hope that this regression was a result of the vaccine. However, strong conformation of these results will await a clinical study that includes a placebo control to firm up these important observations. However, the results remain highly exciting and may mark a turning point in the application of this technology to cancer therapy of Papillomavirus infection.

DNA Vaccines Against Breast Cancer

The *erbB*-2/*neu* proto-oncogene is a member of the EGFR family that dimerizes to activate *trans* phosphorylation to activate signal transduction and is also overexpressed in 15–40% of all human breast cancers. Accordingly, Chen et al. generated DNA constructs expressing the full length *neu*, the extracellular domain, and the extracellular-transmembrane domains. The latter two mutants were created to avoid potential transformation, and all three were immunized and challenged with Tg1-1 cell line, which was garnered from a FVB/N *neu*–transgenic mouse. The authors report protection when challenged with this specific cell line and this effect was augmented with IL-2 as an adjuvant, and was antibody independent. Others have implemented innovative strategies by mutating domains responsible for kinase activity and adding leader sequences to redirect towards antigen processing and have generated similar results.Importantly, the prophylactic attributes of this vaccine was demonstrated when it was shown to prevent spontaneous formation of tumors in FVB/N *neu*-transgenic mice when administered in conjunction with IL-12. One concern for clinical evaluation of this approach is that neu is expressed in many other tissues besides breast cancer, including lining of the brain and in heart tissue, at low levels. The consequences of this expression for DNA immune therapy is at this time unknown but must be considered in clinical trial design.

Concluding Remark

The recent progress of immunotherapy for treatments against cancer can largely be attributed to a greater overall understanding of the immune system. Identification of processing pathways and targeting receptors has allowed the development of novel adjuvants in augmenting the overall potency of these vaccines. In addition, the growing lists of TAAs provide copious targets to develop immunity against tumor formation. Furthermore, therapies can also target factors that are essential for the survival and propagation of tumors. For instance, a recent study targeted the receptor of the angiogenesis factor VEGF. The authors immunized mice against vascular-endothelial growth factor receptor 2 (FLK-1) through an oral vaccine and targeted proliferating endothelial cells in the tumor vasculature. Protection was observed from numerous cell types including melanoma, colon carcinoma, and lung carcinoma.

Accordingly, this combination of basic immunology and TAA isolation is providing an auspicious path for immunotherapies against cancer. All together, these promising results also emphasize the potential of DNA Vaccines as therapies against cancer. The particular advantages of DNA in manufacturing, lack of replication based pathogenesis, specificity for the tumor target, lack of vector immunity allowing for routine reimmunization are all properties of ideal immunization strategies for cancer immune therapies. The challenges as we go forward will be to take these collection of positive attributes and add additional immune potency to the mix. At that time it is likey that DNA vaccines will take their place at the center of programs for tumor immunotherapy.

6

Cellular Immunotherapy of Cancer

In 1909 Paul Ehrlich proposed the idea that immunological defenses provide a normal host with some resistance against malignant cells. Subsequently, Medawar documented that the transfer of immune cells could mediate graft rejection. This seminal finding provided the basis for the work of Mitchinson, and Brncic, Hoecker and Gasic who in the early 1950's documented that the adoptive transfer of lymphoid cells from immunized mice could confer immunity to tumor challenges. In the following Decade investigators began to immunize pigs and rabbits with patient's tumors to obtain immune cells. Subsequently, peripheral blood, lymph node and spleen cells from these animals were adoptively transferred to the peritoneum or pleural cavity of patients with cancer. At the same time, Nadler and Moore immunized pairs of melanoma patients with each other's tumors. Following subcutaneous transplant of malignant cells, patients exchanged white blood cells with reports of clinical improvement in approximately one third of the patients. These studies provided the base on which other investigators, taking advantage of developments in the field of cellular immunology, helped evolve the application of adoptive cellular immunotherapy to where it is today. This chapter will review these developments, provide an overview of the preclinical animal models, their translation into clinical trials and the exciting new strategies that have evolved from an in-depth analyses of basic T cell immunobiology. The focus of this chapter will be on T cells and the "*three-signal*" paradigm for improving efficacy of adoptive immunotherapy. This focus emanates from the appreciation that T cells have the unique capacity to recognize unique or shared determinants on tumor cells, mediate destructive anti-tumor effects, replicate to mobilize additional effector T cells and differentiate into memory cells that can provide long-term anti-tumor immunity.

In 1954, Billingham, Brent and Medawar first used the term "*adoptive immunity*" to describe "an immune state transferred from one animal to another by immunologically activated cells". Today, adoptive T cell immunotherapy of cancer can be defined as the transfer, to the tumor-bearing host, of T cells with anti-tumor properties that can mediate therapeutic effects through direct and/or indirect mechanisms. The earliest studies used fresh isolated immune cells, obtained by repeated immunization of naive animals with irradiated, killed or sub-tumorigenic doses of tumor, or by ligation or excision of a growing tumor. Subsequent developments allowed for the isolation of tumor-specific T cells in a more clinically applicable setting. A key finding of most studies is that adoptive transfer of tumor-specific T cells routinely eliminates micrometastatic disease and provides long-term anti-tumor immunity to treated animals. While results of a recent clinical trial appear to be promising, the majority of clinical studies to date only occasionally report objective responses. Why are objective clinical responses so infrequent and why do the patients which respond, in contrast to their animal counterparts, often relapse? In our opinion it is essential to address a number of fundamental questions before it will be possible to consistently develop effective adoptive cellular immunotherapy for cancer. These questions include: Which T cells mediate tumor regression and what are their properties? Are the same cells responsible for mediating the initial tumor regression and maintaining long-term immunologic memory and preventing recurrence? Are there cells that can suppress or regulate the generation of anti-tumor T cells to be used for adoptive transfer? Can these cells suppress the immediate anti-tumor activity or the development of effective immunological memory following adoptive transfer? How many T cells are required to mediate tumor regression? What can be done to generate more and/or better T cells for adoptive immunotherapy? Following adoptive transfer the majority of transferred T cells die, is it possible to manipulate the environment to expand and maintain the transferred T cells? What is required to promote trafficking of transferred T cells to tumor sites? We will review studies in animal models that address some of these questions, however the importance of these findings ultimately lies in whether their translation into clinical trials improves outcomes.

T Cell-mediated Tumor Regression

The vast majority of preclinical adoptive immunotherapy studies identified $CD8^+$ T cells as the primary mediators of tumor regression and implicated cytolytic activity as the central effector mechanism. Tumor regression could usually be achieved by the adoptive transfer of cytolytic $CD8^+$T cell clones or bulk cultures, in the absence of CD4 help, if IL-2 was administered to the recipient animal. Subsequent studies demonstrated that significant therapeutic activity could be obtained by the adoptive transfer of tumor-specific T cells that lacked cytolytic activity at the time of transfer. However, a subsequent study documented that non-cytolytic $CD8^+$ T cells could acquire cytolytic activity following interaction with tumor in vivo. This highlights a major limitation of studies that attempted to identify the mechanism of effector T cell-mediated tumor destruction in vivo indirectly by characterizing the in vitro phenotype of transferred T cells.

Are Cytotoxic T Cells Responsible for Tumor Regression?

Lymphocyte-mediated cytotoxicity is traditionally defined as the ability of effector T cells to lyse ^{51}Cr-labelled target cells in a 4- to 6-hour in vitro assay. This cytolytic event is mediated by either the perforin-dependent granule exocytosis pathway and/or the Fas ligand (FasL)/ Fas pathway. The development of mice with mutations in the genes encoding either perforin or FasL allowed the first direct examination of whether these pathways were essential for T cell-mediated tumor regression. In both instances, adoptive transfer of tumor-specific T cells generated from perforin or FasL deficient mice were as capable of mediating regression of pulmonary metastases and cure of animals with systemic tumor as wild type (wt) T cells. Since the tumor used in these studies was resistant to killing via the Fas/FasL pathway, the experiments with PKO effector T cells argued against a role for the cytotolytic pathway in T cell-mediated tumor regression. However, cured PKO mice were less resistant to a subsequent s.c. tumor challenge. Consistent with this observation, tumor-specific PKO effector T cells mediated regression of pulmonary or intracaranial tumor and pulmonary metastases, but were ineffective against the same tumor at a subcutaneous site. In this model, regression of subcutaneous MCA-205 sarcomas required the adoptive transfer of effector T cells that expressed perforin. Other studies suggested that perforin was required for regression of EL4 tumor located in the peritoneum. Thus it appears that the mechanisms T cells utilize to mediate tumor regression vary depending on the location of the tumor and are also likely be dependent on the tumor type.

$CD4^+$ T Cells can also Mediate Tumor Regression

The early 1980s saw the accumulation of substantial evidence arguing that $CD4^+$ T cells could also be effective mediators of tumor regression. Fernandez-Cruz and colleagues were the first to show that adoptive transfer of noncytolytic $CD4^+$ T cells could mediate regression of tumors in rats. Subsequent studies by Greenberg and colleagues, confirmed that adoptive transfer of nonlytic $CD4^+$ T cells in combination with cyclophosphamide could mediate regression of the FBL3 leukemia in mice. However, since this tumor was strongly immunogenic, induced by virus and the CD4 response directed against viral genes was therapeutic, there were questions about how translatable this observation was to tumor immunology. Interest in $CD4^+$ effector cells waned in the mid 1980s as cells with a CD8 phenotype and/or cytolytic function were reported to mediate regression of newly-induced "*weakly*" immunogenic tumors. While CD4 T cells played a critical role in priming cultured CD8 effector T cells; tumor regression was mediated by the adoptive transfer of cultured CD8 T cells. These same studies showed that both CD4 and CD8 T cells were required when non-cultured "fresh" immune spleen cells were used for adoptive transfer, but since the clinically applicable cell was one that could be expanded by in vitro culture, most investigators focused on the CD8 T cells. Interest in CD4 T cells was further reduced by evidence that their in vivo depletion did not affect IL-2-induced T cell-mediated regression of large 10-day pulmonary metastases.

Recently, Hu and colleagues, used mice that were congenitally deficient in MHC class II-restricted CD4 T cells (MHCII KO) to reevaluate the role for endogenous CD4 T cell help in tumor regression mediated by adoptive transfer of CD8 effector T cells. Unlike previous studies where animals were transiently depleted of CD4 T cells by mAb, the MHCII KO animals could not recover endogenous help. Similarly to previous reports, adoptive transfer of $CD8^+$ T cells was highly effective at eliminating pulmonary metastases at the time animals were sacrificed, ten days following adoptive transfer. However, when survival studies were performed, $CD8^+$ T cells that were effective at curing established tumor in wt mice failed to cure any tumor-bearing MHCII KO mice. Thus, in this model, where adoptive transfer of CD8 T cells, but not CD4 T cells, is effective at mediating tumor

Immunotherapy			Experimental Pulmonary Metastases		
Effector T cells	IL-2	Recipient mice	day 3	day 14	long term
None	+	wild type		die	
CD8 & CD4	+	wild type			crude/immune
CD8	+	wild type			crude/immune
CD4	+	wild type		die	
CD8	+	wild type			crude/immune
CD8	+	wild type			recurred/die

Fig. 6.1. Tumor-vaccine draining lymph node T cells were activated with anti-CD3 for 2 days and then expanded for 3 days in CM supplemented with 60 IU/ml IL-2 to generate 'effector' T cells.

regression in wt mice, endogenous CD4 T cells are playing a critical role. These results, suggest that CD4 T cells promote the maintenance and/or development of memory CD8 T cells with therapeutic activity and provides a rationale for why the transfer of both CD4 and CD8 T resulted in the dramatic objective responses seen in a recent clinical trial.

One reason for the failure of CD4 T cells to mediate tumor regression in the preceding studies may have been that a greater number of tumor-specific cells were required to mediate the regression of pulmonary metastases than were transferred. However, the detection of tumor-specific class II-restricted CD4 responses is problematic and is less advanced than that for CD8 responses. With the recent identification of class II-restricted tumor-associated antigens, improved culture techniques for expanding and monitoring CD4 T cells and a new appreciation for the role of CD4 T cells in developing and maintaining immunity, there has been a renewed interest in the antitumor effector function of CD4 T cells. Exploiting magnetic bead methods, Kagamu and Shu isolated CD62L^{low} TDLN cells and, after culture, obtained CD4 effector T cells that were highly polarized to a tumor-specific type 1 cytokine profile, secreting greater than 100 fold more IFN-γ than IL-4, and cured mice of intracranial tumor in adoptive transfer studies. A recent report from Mattes and colleagues identified CD4 T cells as mediating the regression of pulmonary and visceral metastases of a CTL-resistant tumor. Together these reports document that the CD4 T cells are capable antitumor effectors that need to be understood and harnessed to improve immunotherapeutic approaches to treat cancer.

Type 1 and Type 2 Cytokine Responses—the Ying and Yang

What mechanisms are non-cytolytic CD8 and CD4 T cells using to mediate tumor regression? An observation of adoptive transfer studies using effector T cells deficient in either perforin or FasL was that the effector T cells released "*inflammatory*" type 1 cytokines (IFN-γ or TNF-α) in response to in vitro stimulation with specific tumor. This is likely an important observation as the immune response is not limited to inflammatory cytokines. In the early 1970s it was suggested that an immune response was a composite of two antagonistic T-cell populations. Today it is generally accepted that these two T-cell populations, composed of both $CD4^+$ T helper (Th) cells and $CD8^+$ T cytotoxic (Tc) cells, can be segregated based on their cytokine release patterns. A type 1 T cell selectively secretes, IFN-γ, TNF-α, TNF-β/LT and/or IL-2, whereas type 2 T cells secrete IL-4, IL-5, IL-6, IL-10, and/or IL-13. This simplistic view of immune regulation has become more complex with the description of Th3 cells, that immunosuppress through the secretion of TGF-β, and the observation that some IL-4 is required to obtain type 1 T cell responses.

The differentiation of T cell subsets along a type 1 or type 2 path depends on the type of antigen, the route and dose of entry of the antigen, the nature of costimulatory signals provided, as well as the genetic background of the host. In addition the most clearly defined factor determining T cell differentiation is the cytokine environment present at the initiation of the immune response. IL-4 is the dominant cytokine influencing type 2 polarization, signaling through the IL-4 receptor and activating Stat-6 and the transcription factors, c-Maf and GATA-3 which commit the T cell to type 2 differentiation. In contrast, IL-12 and IFN-γ are the cytokines that drive type 1 polarization. IL-12 directly influences type 1 polarization by activating Stat-4 in naive T cells. More controversial are the effects of IFN-γ, which likely augment type 1 polarization indirectly by up-regulating expression of IL-12 by macrophages. However, since type 1 responses are not completely abrogated in IL-12 p40 deficient mice and IL-12 poorly induces T-bet, a transcription factor associated with type 1 differentiation, it has been suggested that IFN-γ may also directly influence type 1 polarization. Supporting this reasoning is the observation that T-bet expression is dependent on Stat-1, which is efficiently induced by IFN-γ. Other cytokines, such as IL-18 and IL-1α were thought to act as polarizing signals, but both molecules appear to amplify responses that are already polarized. The antagonistic nature of these T cell populations is evident in that the cytokines that drive polarization of their respective phenotypes inhibit polarization toward the opposing phenotype. The most dominant effect is exerted by IL-4, which induces type 2 polarization and inhibits type 1 polarization. If IL-4 reaches a certain threshold at the beginning of an immune response then a type 2 cytokine profile will dominate that response. One way IL-4 exerts its effect is by down-regulating expression of IL-12Rβ2, thereby blocking the effects of IL-12 on differentiating T cells. IL-4 also inhibits type 1 polarization indirectly by down-regulating IL-12 production of dendritic cells.

Cytokine Profile is Relevant to Disease

The relevance of type 1 or type 2 polarized T cell responses to disease states was first appreciated in infectious disease models. An example is the protection against the parasite, *Leishmania major* (*L. major*), that is associated with a type 1 polarized immune response and this protection is lost in IL-12Rβ2 deficient mice. Mouse strains that are susceptible to *L. major* infection mount predominantly a type 2 immune response. Converting the type 2 immune response toward a type 1 response, in these susceptible mice, provides protection from an infection with *L. major*. The process of promoting a non-therapeutic immune response, as seen in the mouse strains that are susceptible to *L. major*, has been termed '*immune deviation*'. However, it must be noted that all immune pathologies cannot be explained by immune deviation. For example, the cell-mediated disease *experimental autoimmune encephalomyelitis* (EAE) is believed to be mediated by Th1 immune responses that can be ameliorated by Th2 responses. Yet susceptible strains of mice that have the IFN-γ gene disrupted are still susceptible to EAE whereas resistant strains of mice become susceptible to EAE when this gene is disrupted. Whether other type 1 cytokines, such as TNF-α, might be responsible for the pathology observed in EAE is unclear and only underscores the complexity of the immune system. Nonetheless, appreciation of immune deviation has changed the way immunologists look at many disease states. But is this paradigm relevant to cancer?

A Type 1 Cytokine Response is Essential for Tumor Regression

Various studies have implicated the type 1/ type 2 paradigm in the regulation of the host's immune response to cancer however the significance of these two T-cell populations has been controversial. While several reports had made correlations between type 1 responses being therapeutic, Hu and colleagues were the first to show that a poorly immunogenic tumor that failed to prime therapeutic T cells for adoptive immunotherapy, had not ignored the tumor, but had initiated a tumor-specific type 2 response that was non therapeutic. Vaccination with the same tumor that was lipofected with an allogeneic MHC class I gene, primed T cells that exhibited a tumor-specific type 1 cytokine profile and were therapeutic in adoptive transfer studies.

These results suggested that the failure of adoptive immunotherapy, in this model, was not the result of T cells failing to recognize the tumor; rather, it was because the host mounted an ineffective (type 2) immune response. Winter and colleagues examined whether other poorly immunogenic tumors (tumors where vaccination fails to provide protection from a subsequent tumor challenge) stimulated a tumor-specific type 2 cytokine response in the vaccinated host. Examining a panel of tumors, ranging from strongly to poorly immunogenic, they showed that immunogenic tumors primed immune responses that were highly polarized towards a type 1 cytokine response, while a type 2 cytokine response was dominant for poorly immunogenic tumors. Further, To and colleagues, working in the weakly immunogenic MCA-205 tumor model, showed that tumor-specific CD4 T cells polarized to a type 1 response were significantly more therapeutic than $CD4^+$ T cells polarized to a type 2 cytokine profile. In contrast to these findings other groups have suggested that type 2 polarized T cells can mediate tumor regression. However, a careful study using adoptively transferred type 1 or type 2 polarized OT-1 transgenic T cells demonstrated that the type 2 T cells were markedly less therapeutic than T cells from type 1 polarized immune responses.

Additionally, the therapeutic type 2 response was non-therapeutic if the T cells were adoptively transferred into IFN-γ knockout mice. Thus therapeutic type 2 polarized T cells were dependent on the type 1 cytokine, IFN-γ, derived from the recipient, underscoring the importance of a type 1 immune response. Chamoto et al., used the same tumor model system, but transferred non-transgenic T cells and reported that only the adoptive transfer of Th1 cells, but not Th2 cells, induced tumor-specific cytotoxic Tc1 cells in the recipient that led to eradication of the tumor mass *in vivo*. In another study the adoptive transfer of Th2 cells led to tumor eradication; however by inducing necrosis with an infiltration of inflammatory cells into the tumor mass. It is unclear from the design of this last study whether type 1 cytokines played a major role in mediating tumor destruction. Recently, Mattes and colleagues reported that type 2 CD4 T cells mediated, through an eosinophil-dependent process, the regression of pulmonary and visceral metastases of a CTL-resistant tumor. Thus, while the majority of studies support the importance of a type 1 response, there are some examples of type 2 responses mediating tumor regression.

IFN-γ is Critical for in situ Priming but not Effector Function or Protective Memory

In the absence of IFN-γ vaccination fails to provide protective antitumor immunity. In spite of the lack of protection, effector T cells generated from TVDLN of GKO mice exhibited tumor-specific cytotoxicity and adoptive transfer of GKO effector T cells mediated complete regression of pulmonary metastases in both wt and GKO mice. Further, mice cured of experimental pulmonary metastases were resistant to a secondary tumor challenge documenting that IFN-γ is neither required to maintain a protective memory response or to mediate regression of subcutaneous tumor.

These results are generally consistent with an earlier study by Peng et.al. using the MCA-205 sarcoma model. However, this report found that effector T cells from GKO mice were less effective than wt effector T cells, requiring transfer of greater numbers of effector T cells or combination with radiation of the tumor-bearing host. In contrast to these two reports, studies from Prevost-Blondel et. al., using effector T cells from GP33 TCR-tg wt or GKO mice did not see regression of pulmonary metastases when IFN-γ was absent from their system.

However, TCR-Tg effector T cells from GKO mice were able to mediate efficient regression of pulmonary metastases in wt hosts, excluding the possibility that these GKO effector T cells were not efficiently "*primed*". The authors suggest that given the low level of class I on their B16 the lack of therapeutic efficacy may be related to a dependence on IFN-γ to upregulate expression of class I on the tumor in vivo. In the studies of Winter et. al., it is interesting that the effector T cells from GKO mice did not develop a tumor-specific T2 cytokine profile. Subsequent studies showed that effector T cells generated from GKO mice secrete TNF-α in response to stimulation with specific tumor, providing a possible alternative mechanism for these T cells to mediate tumor regression.

Perforin, IFN-γ and TNF—A Triad of Effector Molecules

While the aforementioned studies using gene knock-out or mutant mice deficient in a single effector molecule examined the requirement for that molecule in T cell-mediated tumor regression, they failed to rule-out the likelihood that the immune system of the deficient host would utilize other elements of the immune system to compensate for absence of that molecule. To evaluate whether perforin and IFN-γ were able to compensate for each other when either was absent, T cells from mice deficient in both molecules were evaluated for their ability to mediate tumor regression in the poorly immunogenic B16-BL6-D5 melanoma model. While slightly less effective than T cells from either PKO or GKO mice, effector T cells from perforin-IFN-γ double ko (PKO/GKO) mice could eliminate pulmonary metastases and cure mice of three day established tumor. Analysis of the effector T cells revealed they maintained a type 1 cytokine profile, secreting TNF–α in response to stimulation with specific tumor.

Poehlein and colleagues went on to show that the therapeutic efficacy of these T cells could be blocked by treatment with soluble TNF receptor. These results suggest that a triad of effector molecules exist, any of which may be able to mediate tumor regression. However, strategies that can generate all three responses will likely be the most effective. Consistent with this hypothesis are earlier reports that the administration of type 1 cytokines (IFN-γ, IFN-α, and or TNF-α) together with the adoptive transfer of a cytolytic tumor-specific T cell clone further augmented. therapeutic efficacy. Since the additional cytokines were not expected to support T cell growth better than IL-2, which was administered to all animals, the authors suggested that the IFN-γ, IFN-α or TNF-α worked to augment the susceptibility of the tumor to killing by cytolytic T cells, or that the cytokines mediated antitumor effects independent of CTL.

A Type 1 Immune Response Correlates with Therapeutic Response in Humans

In 1994, Kawakami and colleagues showed a strong correlation with the adoptive transfer of T cells exhibiting tumor-specific IFN-γ secretion and objective clinical response. While a highly selected group of patients, this report supports the link between a type 1 cytokine response and tumor regression. Subsequently, Lowes and colleagues, identified an increase in TNF-β (LT-α) mRNA in melanoma lesions undergoing spontaneous regression and absent in progressing nodules. Since TNF-β is a type 1 cytokine it provides additional support for this paradigm. However, in tumors that are not undergoing regression, elevated levels of type 2 cytokines have been observed. Another study of melanoma and renal cell carcinoma patients reported that T cells from the peripheral blood of patients with no current evidence of disease displayed Th1 responses to the tumor-associated MAGE-6 peptide. Additionally, this report identified that the majority of patients with active disease had a MAGE-6 peptide-specific type 2 immune response, characterized by secretion of IL-5. Other studies have observed tumor-specific type 2 cytokine responses in patients that have progressed following immunotherapy.

Meijer and colleagues detected a mixed tumor-specific type 1 and type 2 cytokine response in the peripheral blood of some patients following adoptive immunotherapy. Mixed type 1 and type 2 responses have also been reported in patients receiving a breast cancer vaccine. While to our knowledge there is no direct evidence that a tumor-specific type 2 response can suppress the therapeutic activity of tumor-specific type 1 effector T cells, it is expected that an established tumor-specific type 2 memory response would interfere with endogenous epitope spreading and the propagation of newly primed tumor-specific type 1 T cells.

Three-Signal Paradigm for Effective Generation of Therapeutic T Cells

Overall the above noted data strongly argue that a type 1 cytokine response is critical for T cell-mediated tumor regression in most models. Further, evidence for immune deviation in additional animal tumor models as well as evidence from clinical studies correlating a type I response with therapeutic effects, spontaneous regression or absence of disease provides additional support for the hypothesis that the development of a tumor-specific type 1 response is critical for effective immunotherapy. These early findings led, in 1999, to the proposition of a three-signal paradigm for the development of effective T cells for adoptive immunotherapy. The first signal is that of specific antigen, presented by MHC to the TCR.

The second is a costimulatory signal(s) and the third are those that polarize the developing immune response to a type 1 cytokine profile and/or block the development of a type 2 cytokine response. This three-signal paradigm provides a basic strategy to induce, augment and maintain the generation of T cells with therapeutic activity. This includes the elimination of factors and/or cells that interfere with these three signals. Combining these strategies with homeostasis-driven

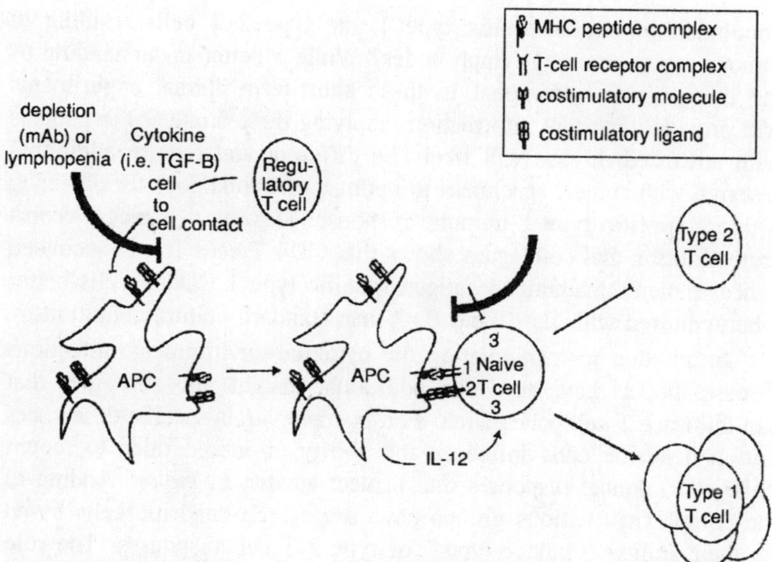

Fig. 6.2. Generation of therapeutic effector T cells requires three signals. This include the well established first "two signals"; including T-cell receptor interaction with MHC-peptide complexes (signal 1) and the interaction of costimulatory molecules with their ligands (signal 2). The third signal (signal 3) polarizes the responding T cell along a type 1 phenotype.

expansion and regulatory T cell depletion provide a basis for a new generation of adoptive cellular immunotherapy trials.

Manipulating the Developing Anti-tumor Immune Response

Since the transfer of T cells with a type 1 polarized tumor-specific cytokine response exhibited enhanced therapeutic efficacy a possible strategy for adoptive immunotherapy is to examine whether type 2 polarized responses could be "*repolarized*" toward a type 1 phenotype. T cells from lymph nodes draining a poorly immunogenic tumor that routinely develop a non-therapeutic tumor-specific type 2 cytokine response could be "*repolarized*" towards a tumor-specific type 1 cytokine response by *in vitro* culture with anti-IL-4 mAb and exogenous IL-12. Coincident with expression of the type 1 cytokine response these T cells exhibited therapeutic efficacy in adoptive transfer studies. The mechanism of this effect is unclear. Did the altered cytokine milieu actually change the cytokine profile of the tumor-specific type 2 cells that were not fully differentiated or did the IL-12 enhance expansion of a small population of tumor-specific type 1 T cells from the mixed population of tumor-specific type 1 and type 2 T cells residing in tumor-vaccine draining lymph nodes? While a better understanding of the mechanisms operational in these short-term animal experiments will provide important information, applying these strategies to patients with advanced disease will likely be different and require additional research with clinical specimens to optimize the conditions for obtaining a tumor-specific type 1 immune response. However, a recent report from Knutson and colleagues shows that CD4 T cells from vaccinated cancer patients maintained antigen-specific type 1 CD4 T cells better when cultured with IL-12 and IL-2 than standard culture conditions.

In addition to manipulating the cytokine environment, infectious disease models have provided additional insight into strategies that can influence T cell polarization. For example, strain-specific differences within dendritic cells influence the ability of inbred mice to mount polarized immune responses that protect against *L. major*. Adding to the complexity, various groups have segregated dendritic cells based on their ability to induce type 1 or type 2 T cell responses. The role of co-stimulation by antigen-presenting cells in skewing immune responses is another potential target for augmenting the generation of tumor-specific T cells for adoptive cellular immunotherapy. CD80 (B7-1) and CD86 (B7-2) have been among the most studied ligands of T cell activation, are critical for priming tumor-specific T cells in vivo and may also affect T cell polarization through a series of interactions; including the strength of signal through the T-cell receptor and differential upregulation of costimulatory molecules. Additionally, constimulation may broaden the repertoire of tumor antigens recognized by the responding T cells, allowing them to respond to subdominant epitopes. This approach, together with polyclonal stimulation with anti-CD3 in vitro, has shown efficacy for improving expansion of effector T cells for adoptive immunotherapy.

While not a polarizing signal, strategies that block the inhibitory signal provided to CD28 through interaction with CTLA4 have already been shown to substantially augment immune responses in preclinical models and clinical trials. CD137 (4-1BB) is a costimulatory molecule expressed on activated T cells that appears to augment type 1 polarization. *In vitro* activation of tumor-vaccine draining lymph node cells with antibodies to CD137, CD3, and CD28 increased tumor-specific IFN-γ secretion more than activation with anti-CD3 and anti-CD28. In adoptive transfer studies T cells activated with all three antibodies were more effective mediators of tumor regression than T cells activated with anti-CD3 and anti-CD28. Another co-stimulatory molecule is CD134 (OX40). This member of the TNF receptor family is expressed on recently activated $CD4^+$ T cells. Ligation of CD134 augments proliferation and cytokine secretion and has been shown to augment the immune response to weakly immunogenic tumors. While some controversy exists, most data suggests that CD134 stimulation augments both type 1 and 2 immune responses. Thus, providing co-stimulation via CD134 will likely have the greatest therapeutic effect when it is administered with a type 1 polarizing signal or in adoptive transfer studies where tumor-specific CD4 T cells are already polarized towards a type 1 cytokine profile.

Costimulation Following Adoptive Immunotherapy

Another way to augment the effectiveness of adoptive immunotherapy is by supplying costimulatory signals to the T cells following adoptive transfer. While a number of investigators have transfected tumors with CD80 for use as vaccines, Bai and colleagues showed that administering an anti-CD28 mAb augmented the therapeutic efficacy of tumor-specific (Tg-TCR) T cells. In conjunction with adoptive immunotherapy, the administration of antibodies against 4-1BB or OX40 also increased therapeutic efficacy of the transferred T cells.

An alternative to providing costimulatory signals is to block inhibitory signals provided by host cells or the tumor. Blocking the inhibitory effect of CTLA-4 is one approach, but as yet we know of no studies that have combined this strategy to promote survival or activity of antitumor effector T cells in adoptive immunotherapy studies. However, given its activity in combination with vaccines, these studies will certainly be performed soon. B7-H1 is a B7 family molecule that provides an inhibitory signal to T cells and is expressed by some tumors. Recently, Strome and colleagues showed that by blocking B7-H1 in vivo at the time of adoptive immunotherapy it was possible to increase therapeutic efficacy against a B7-H1 expressing tumor.

Suppression and Regulatory T Cells

In addition to the inhibitory signals noted above, the immunogenic potential of tumor antigens is dependent on a variety of host immune mechanisms that avoid autoimmunity by ensuring tolerance to self antigens. There is accumulating evidence that immunological tolerance is maintained by T cell-mediated suppression of self-reactive T cells. T cell-mediated regulation is not a new concept as lymphocyte populations that can suppress antigen-specific immune responses were described more than three decades ago. The suppressive lymphocyte population was characterized mainly by function since molecular markers defining this population were unavailable at the time. Subsequent studies demonstrated that $CD4^+$ T cells were responsible for the T cell-mediated suppression. A suppressive lymphocyte population was further characterized as the $CD4^+$ T cell subpopulation expressing the IL-2Rα chain (CD25) that if depleted prior to T cell transfer into athymic nude mice resulted in autoimmune disease.

Other groups demonstrated that elimination of $CD25^+$ T cells resulted in the development of autoimmune diseases such as colitis and diabetes. This $CD25^+CD4^+$ T cell population, which represents 5–10% of peripheral $CD4^+$ T cells in mice, is non-proliferative to antigenic stimulation *in vitro* and potently suppresses the proliferation of other $CD4^+$ or $CD8^+$ T cells. Recently, other markers associated with $CD25^+CD4^+$ regulatory T cells have been described, including GITR, CTLA-4, Foxp3, CD103, $CD45RB^{low}$ and Lag-3 (CD223). Human $CD25^+CD4^+$ regulatory T cells isolated from peripheral blood express $CD45RO^+$, CD62L, and CTLA-4 and can suppress the proliferation of $CD25^-CD4^+$ T cells. It appears that $CD25^+CD4^+$ regulatory T cells require antigen-induced activation to become suppressive, but their suppressive function is antigen independent. They mediate suppression via secretion of immuno-suppressive cytokines, TGF-β and IL-10, but some mechanisms appear to require direct cell-cell contact.

Early on it was postulated that the elimination of "*suppressor*" T cells could enhance effective antitumor immunity in tumor-bearing hosts. Studies from North and Colleagues showed that $CD4^+$ T cells from tumor-bearing mice could inhibit therapeutic adoptive cellular immunotherapy. These results, under appreciated for the past 15 years, correspond closely to what we now appreciate as regulatory T cells. Recent studies have shown that depletion of $CD25^+$ cells augmented both $CD4^+$ and $CD8^+$ T cell responses against tumor. Additionally, *In vivo* depletion of $CD25^+CD4^+$ regulatory T cells using the anti-CD25 mAb, PC61, promoted regression of several leukemias, sarcomas, and a myeloma. Reactivity to the tumor-associated antigen, tyrosinase-related protein-2 (TRP-2), was enhanced in $CD25^+CD4^+$ depleted mice challenged with B16 melanoma and injected with an antibody that blocks CTLA-4. Furthermore, depletion of $CD25^+CD4^+$ regulatory T cells in tumor-vaccinated mice augmented the sensitization of tumor-vaccine draining lymph node cells, which upon adoptive transfer demonstrated augmented antitumor therapy. In support of an important role for IL-2 in the developing anti-tumor immune response, enhanced activity of tumor-vaccine draining lymph nodes did not occur if depletion of $CD25^+CD4^+$ regulatory T cells was performed after tumor vaccination.

The accumulation of data obtained from tumor models has led to a search for $CD25^+CD4^+$ regulatory T cells in humans. Increased percentages of $CD25^+CD4^+$ T cells expressing TGF-β were present in *non-small cell lung cancer* (NSCLC) tumor-infiltrating lymphocytes and ovarian cancer tumor-associated lymphocytes compared to PBMCs from normal patients. $CD25^+CD4^+$ T cells isolated from NSCLC could inhibit proliferation of autologous peripheral blood T cells. Similarly, $CD25^+CD4^+$ T cells from pancreas or breast cancer involved lymph nodes suppressed the proliferation and secretion of IFN-γ of activated $CD8^+$ cells or $CD4^+CD25^-$ cells. Clinical trials designed to deplete $CD25^+CD4^+$ regulatory T cells or block their function will be important steps to determine whether these cells, which play such an important role in preclinical models, are obstacles to effective immunotherapy in humans. One treatment that is already available to delete $CD25^+$ cells is the IL-2-diptheria toxin fusion protein (ONTAK), which could provide a novel strategy for depleting $CD25^+CD4^+$ regulatory T cell population in patients.

When It Comes to Tumor-specific T Cells "More is Better"!

In 1955, Mitchison was the first to demonstrate that the adoptive transfer of greater numbers of tumor-specific T cells increased therapeutic efficacy. This paradigm is now well established in all adoptive transfer models we know of. While obtaining increased numbers of tumor-specific T cells in animal models is often a trivial problem, simply requiring additional mice, obtaining increased numbers of tumor-specific T cells in patients with cancer represents a therapy-limiting obstacle to potentially effective treatment. What limits the expansion of T cells responding to vaccination or following adoptive transfer into a tumor-bearing host? In normal non-lymphopenic hosts homeostatic mechanisms work to maintain a constant level of lymphocytes and the expansion of tumor-reactive T cells is limited. However, in lymphopenic hosts, T cells expand to fill the void. Several hypotheses have been proposed to explain homeostasis-driven T cell proliferation. One of the earliest to be suggested was the "*space*" hypothesis. Here, the creation of space allows responding tumor-specific

T cells to expand, unencumbered by their neighbors and/or inhibitory signals those neighbors may provide. A second is the "*suppressor cell*" hypothesis, which emphasizes the selective elimination of "*suppressor*" or $CD4^+CD25^+$ regulatory T cells by the lymphopenic insult resulting in increased expansion of tumor-reactive T cells. This research has provided solid information on the requirements for T cell expansion in lymphopenic hosts and provides insight into how this information may be exploited to buttress antitumor immunity.

What Controls Homeostatic Proliferation?

The expansion of $CD4^+$ and $CD8^+$ T cells in lymphopenic hosts is dependent primarily on TCR-peptide interactions, with clonal competition for these interactions being a limiting factor for ultimate expansion. However, these interactions are not the sole mechanism for expansion, as an IL-7-mediated component can also drive proliferation independent of TCR signaling and IL-12, which does not play an essential role in T cell expansion, can augment the response. Further, IL-2, costimulation via CD28 or interactions with 4-1BB/4-1BBL and CD40/CD40L are not required for homeostasis-driven proliferation. During expansion naive T cells express a "pseudo" memory phenotype and never revert back to a naive phenotype. Importantly, T cells undergoing homeostasis-driven expansion are hypersensitive to antigen stimulation with a lowered threshold for activation and expression of effector functions.

Augmented Priming of T Cells in Vaccinated Lymphopenic Hosts

Mackall and colleagues were the first to appreciate how exposure to antigen during immune reconstitution of a lymphopenic host could be exploited to skew the T cell response to vaccination. Subsequently Borello and colleagues showed how vaccination, with a GM-CSF transduced B-cell lymphoma, A20, in the post *bone marrow transplant* (BMT) setting could augment therapeutic efficacy more effectively than in a normal host. They also showed how this strategy led to increased expansion of tumor-reactive T cells by reconstitution with trace levels of transgenic TCR T cells reactive with the model antigen expressed by the tumor. Asavaroengchai and colleagues used tumor lysate-pulsed dendritic cells to vaccinate mice post BMT against the MT-901 mammary cancer. This provided effective protection in challenge studies and reduced outgrowth of pulmonary metastases in animals with established tumor prior to BMT and vaccination. Hu and colleagues transfused normal spleen cells into either irradiated or congenitally lymphopenic $Rag1^{-/-}$ mice and vaccinated with a GM-CSF secreting tumor vaccine. Tumor vaccine-draining lymph nodes (TVDLN) harvested from reconstituted lymphopenic mice contained an increased frequency of tumor specific $CD4^+$ and $CD8^+$ T cells and were significantly more effective in adoptive transfer studies. This demonstrated that neither BMT nor the cytokine storm accompanying whole body irradiation were required to obtain the beneficial anti-tumor effects provided by vaccinating a lymphopenic host. Dummer and colleagues reported how lymphopenic animals, either sublethally irradiated or $Rag1^{-/-}$ mice, reconstituted with normal lymph node cells were more resistant to tumor challenge then either control or lymphopenic animals. This response, in non-vaccinated animals, correlated with an increase in tumor-specific cytotoxicity and IFN-γ release. Together, these reports suggest, that by initiating vaccine strategies during periods of lymphopenia-driven T cell expansion it is possible to skew the T cell repertoire towards tumor antigens, resulting in a dramatic expansion of tumor-specific T cells. Since adoptive immunotherapy has been limited to tumors where it is possible to generate substantial numbers of tumor-specific T cells, this maneuver could be used to obtain tumor-specific T cells in malignancies where it has previously been impossible to do so.

Adoptive Immunotherapy in Lymphopenic Hosts Augments Therapeutic Activity

Homeostasis-driven proliferation can also have a tremendous impact when exploited at the efferent stage of immunotherapy. The adoptive transfer of antigen-specific lymphocytes into a lymphopenic host, has been shown to augment the effector activity of the transferred cells. This was first shown by Harris and colleagues, who in 1954 reconstituted irradiated rabbits with immune lymph node cells and documented substantial increases in antibody production. Over the intervening decades the observation that immunosuppression prior to adoptive transfer improves therapeutic efficacy has remained consistent. While the creation of space, elimination of suppressor cells or a direct anti-tumor effect were frequently used to explain the advantage conferred by immunosuppression, in some models it is likely that all three mechanisms played a role in the augmented antitumor effect. Based on the preponderance of preclinical data supporting its use, many clinical studies used immunomodulatory doses of cyclophosphamide prior to infusion of transferred cells even though there was little clinical evidence to support its use. The recent success of stem cell transplant strategies in renal cell cancer prompted Rosenberg and colleagues to reevaluate the degree of immunosuppression employed prior to adoptive transfer. Their success in adoptive cellular immunotherapy in melanoma patients receiving a mix of tumor-specific T cell clones and bulk $CD4^+$ and $CD8^+$ TIL following a non-myeloablative conditioning regimen has created a great deal of enthusiasm in the field of adoptive immunotherapy. The unparalleled expansion and persistence of tumor-specific T cells, greater than 70% of circulating $CD8^+$ T cells in some patients, will undoubtably lead to additional trials of this approach in melanoma and other malignancies.

While trials exploiting homeostasis-driven proliferation at the afferent limb (priming) or the efferent limb (transfer of effector cells) are underway or have recently been reported. Given the strong preclinical and recent clinical data it is only a matter of time before studies will be instituted that exploit the advantages of homeostasis-driven proliferation at both the afferent and efferent stages of the immune response. In the following sections we will review clinical trials of adoptive cellular immunotherapy, in some cases discussing preclinical studies that were relevant to the clinical trial.

Adoptive Cellular Therapy Using Non-specific Cells

Macrophages

Macrophages play an important role as antigen presenting cells and as effector cells in humoral and cellular immunity; however, their role in mediating anti-tumor effects is not well established. The infiltration of macrophages and monocytes into many different tumors, e.g. *colon carcinoma*, *mammary carcinoma* and *melanoma*, has been shown, although the degree of infiltration can vary greatly even in tumors of the same histology. Preclinical adoptive transfer experiments with in vitro activated macrophages revealed their potential to inhibit pulmonary metastases and to induce regression of transplanted human melanoma cells in SCID mice. Although activated macrophages were effective at inhibiting the formation of metastases, they were generally ineffective at mediating regression of established tumors. Additionally, strategies that activated macrophages in vivo, using lymphokines or synthetic analogs of muramyl dipeptide, had limited success mediating tumor regression. Further, macrophages can release growth factors that promote angiogenesis and support tumor growth complicating their application to treat cancer.

However, these preclinical studies were sufficiently encouraging that clinical trials employing adoptive transfer of macrophages were performed. To increase the number of macrophages in the peripheral blood prior to leukapheresis, patients were pretreated for 7 days with GM-CSF. Harvested macrophages were stimulated in vitro with IFN-γ and LPS and adoptively transferred. Macrophages accumulated at sites of tumor metastases, but no objective responses were observed in the treatment of 22 colorectal cancer patients, 10 melanoma patients and 11 non small cell lung cancer patients (NSCLC). A recent study repeatedly administered, intravesicularly, IFN-γ activated macrophages to 17 patients with superficial bladder cancer following trans-urethral tumor resection. 15 patients received 6 or more infusions of 0.9 to 2.5×10^8 activated macrophages. Urinary IL-8 and GM-CSF were markedly increased and the recurrence rate in the 12 months following initiation of therapy was significantly less than the year preceding the first adoptive transfer. Future studies will be needed to confirm these promising findings. Another possible strategy to improve the efficacy of this approach would be to combine adoptive transfer of macrophages with bi-specific antibodies that exploit FcγR or FcαR expression of macrophages to target these effector cells to antigens expressed on cancers.

Phytohemagglutinin-Activated Killer Cells (PAK)

Phytohemaglutinin (PHA) is a plant lectin that is mitogenic for T cells. PHA-activated peripheral blood lymphocytes mediate cytolytic activity against fresh autologous and allogeneic tumor targets, but not normal cells, through lectin-dependent cellular cytotoxicity. While the adoptive transfer of PHA-activated killer cells (PAK) directly into the tumor or intravascularly had little therapeutic success, the later was an important step as it proved the feasibility of expanding large numbers autologous lymphocytes and adoptively transferring them back to cancer patients.

Lymphokine—Activated Killer Cells (LAK)

The discovery that it was possible to generate *lymphokine-activated killer* (LAK) cells, that could lyse fresh "*non-cultured*" tumor cells, simply by culturing lymphocytes for three days with a high concentration of IL-2 created a good deal of excitement in the 1980's. The earliest studies used lectin-stimulated lymphocytes to generate *T cell growth factor* (TCGF) that was used as the source of IL-2. The availability of recombinant IL-2 rapidly expanded the number of investigators studying LAK cells. Initially controversy existed over whether LAK activity was derived from T cells or NK cells. The earliest studies using TCGF characterized LAK cells as being T cells while later studies identified them as being NK cells. Subsequently it was shown that the variations in LAK precursor phenotype were due to whether TCGF or recombinant IL-2 were used to generate LAK; TCGF induced both T cells and NK cells to generate LAK activity while IL-2 worked predominantly on NK cells.

The first clinical trial of "LAK" cells adoptively transferred TCGF cultured PBMC, that exhibited lysis of autologous tumor, into three patients. There were no clinical responses, but relatively few cells were given and patients did not receive systemic IL-2. The failure of this approach would subsequently be predicted from animal models which showed that therapeutic efficacy of LAK cells was optimal when maximal numbers of cells were transferred and the maximal tolerated dose of exogenous IL-2 was administered. Translation of these observations to the clinic required that patients first be treated with IL-2 alone. The first clinical studies administered Jurkat cell-derived, or recombinant IL-2 alone at different doses, routes and schedules to 39 cancer patients. No therapeutic effect was observed in these trials but the toxicity of IL-2, particularly the increased vascular permeability was identified. The knowledge that IL-2 could be administered safely paved the way for trials that combined adoptive cellular therapy with IL-2 support. A prospective randomized trial of high dose IL-2 alone or in conjunction with LAK cells in patients with melanoma, renal cancer, colorectal cancer, non Hodgkin lymphoma and other tumors revealed no significant difference between the two groups with 10 CR and 4 PR among 85 patients treated with IL-2 and LAK versus 4 CR and 12 PR among 79 patients treated with IL-2 alone. These findings were similar to those of the cytokine working group.

One explanation for the failure of adoptively transferred LAK cells to mediate tumor regression is the possibility that they are not able to traffic in large numbers to the tumor site. To overcome this roadblock, local administration of LAK cells was studied in patients with peritoneal disease. One study treated patients with ovarian cancer and reported 1 PR for 10 patients treated. A second study reported 2 PR for 10 ovarian cancer patients and 5 PR for 12 colon cancer patients treated by intra-peritoneal administration of LAK cells and IL-2. Both studies identified ascites, abdominal pain and intraperitoneal fibrosis as limitations to this approach.

Another explanation for the limited success of adoptive immunotherapy is that patients treated on these trials generally have advanced disease that is more difficult to treat. Since preclinical models predict that adoptive immunotherapy would be more effective against minimal residual disease some have sought to combine adoptive immunotherapy in the adjuvant setting. Kimura and colleagues performed a prospective, controlled study that randomized stage IIIA NSCLC patients, following curative resection of locally advanced primary lung cancer, to either no adjuvant therapy, chemotherapy alone or chemotherapy and adoptive immunotherapy with LAK cells and IL-2. Patients receiving chemo-immunotherapy had a significantly better 5-year survival rates (53.4%, n = 25) versus chemotherapy alone (33.4%, n = 26), or no additional adjuvant therapy (15.3%, n = 13). These encouraging results may be due to applying immunotherapy in the adjuvant setting and/or to the combination of adoptive immunotherapy under conditions that support homeostasis-driven proliferation of adoptively transferred cells. Future studies will address both components.

Enriching for the subset of LAK cells that mediate anti-tumor effects is another approach to increase the efficacy of adoptive immunotherapy. IL-2-activated NK cells selected by their adherence to plastic surfaces (adherent NK cells, ANK) were shown to have increased anti-tumor activity in vitro and in animal models. However, initial clinical trials with adoptively transferred ANK have had little success.

Anti-CD3 Activated PBL

In 1989 Anderson and colleagues reported that anti-CD3 activated spleen cells exhibited cytolytic activity against NK-resistant tumor targets and mediated regression of 5 day established pulmonary metastases. An advantage of this approach compared to LAK cells was a substantially increased yield of activated killer cells. A clinical trial of this approach adoptively transferred PBMC that had been activated by an overnight in vitro culture with anti-CD3. Subsequently, all patients received systemic administration of IL-2 to support in vivo expansion of the transferred T cells. In this trial all patients received low dose cyclophosphamide for the purpose of reducing "*suppressor*" cell activity. There was one PR in 24 treated patients. Additional preclinical studies using anti-CD3 stimulation of naive spleen cells demonstrated that the dominant mediator of therapeutic activity was a $CD4^+$ T cell. In this model, transfer of anti-CD3 activated CD4 T cells was more effective than the transfer of anti-CD3-activated CD8 or bulk unseparated spleen cells. Based on this and other in vitro human studies supporting this concept, Curti and colleagues performed a second clinical trial using CD4 T cells obtained by negative selection of leukapheresis product. Isolated CD4 T cells were activated with anti-CD3 and expanded in IL-2 (90 IU/ml) for 4 days prior to being adoptively transferred with all patients receiving systemic IL-2. An interesting component of this trial was that PBMC were obtained from patients following cyclophosphamide treatment at a time when their WBC count was dropping towards its nadir or as the WBC was recovering from its nadir. Recovery of CD4 T cells was greatest when leukapheresis was performed when the WBC was dropping following cyclophosphamide administration. Most patients were treated with CD4 T cells obtained in this way. There was 1 CR and 2 PRs for 31 treated patients, but 8 of 17 patients with the greatest CD4 expansion exhibited some anti-tumor effects.

Adoptive Cellular Therapy Using Tunor-specific T Cells

Tumor-Infiltrating Lymphocytes

Reports of tumor-specific T cells in the peripheral blood of melanoma patients encouraged the idea that the immune system might be exploited to treat melanoma. However, the inability to regularly isolate these tumor-specific T cells or obtain them in large numbers was one limitation to their application in adoptive transfer studies. This changed when it was discovered that by culturing freshly isolated tumor preparations with high doses of IL-2, it was possible to routinely generate cultures of Tumor-infiltrating lymphocytes (TIL). In preclinical studies the TIL exhibited tumor "*specificity*" and were 50 to 100 times more effective at reducing established pulmonary metastases than LAK cells. Consistent with preclinical reports, TIL generated from some melanoma patients could lyse autologous tumor targets specifically. The initial clinical trial of TIL administered with IL-2 and cyclophosphamide (25 mg/kg), showed 11 partial responses in the 20 patients treated. A subsequent study of 86 melanoma patients reported an objective response rate of 34% with 5 CR and 24 PR. In this study approximately 2/3rds of the patients were pretreated with cyclophosphamide (25 mg/kg) 36 hours prior to adoptive transfer. However the overall response rate was not different: 31% for TIL + IL-2 and 35% for cyclophosphamide, TIL + IL-2.

A general disadvantage faced by immunotherapists, is that most patients treated on adoptive immunotherapy trials have advanced and bulky disease that is difficult to treat. Recently, there have been two reports using adoptive immunotherapy with TIL as adjuvant therapy for resected stage III-IV melanoma, i.e. patients with minimal residual disease. In one trial, lymph node metastases from stage III patients, rendered disease free by surgery, were randomly assigned to receive either TIL plus interleukin-2 (IL-2) for 2 months, or IL-2 only. Eighty-eight patients entered the trial with 44 in each group. While there was no difference in overall survival for the 2 groups, subset analysis suggested a significantly increased survival for that group of patients with only a single invaded lymph node that received TIL and IL-2. Labarriere and colleagues further analyzed the in vitro properties of TIL generated from 40 patients where autologous melanoma cell lines were available and showed that patients receiving TIL specific for autologous tumor, measured by intracellular staining for IFN-γ, had a longer relapse free interval than patients receiving TIL that were not specific. The second trial treated 25 stage III and IV patients with TIL and IL-2. Eight of 22 stage IIIC (>3 lymph nodes involved) patients that received between 0.27-to 85 $\times$ 10^{10} TIL were disease free at a median follow-up of 5 years.

The initial success in treating melanoma patients encouraged investigators to consider other malignancies. Kradin and colleagues, generated TIL and treated 7 patients with adenocarcinoma of the lung, but saw no responses where there was greater than 50% reduction at all sites. Bukowski and colleagues treated 18 renal cell carcinoma patients with TIL alone or supported with escalating doses of IL-2 and saw no objective clinical responses and were unable to generate TIL from 7 patients. While TIL from most patients exhibited non-specific cytotoxicity, TIL from one patient exhibited tumor-specific cytolytic function. A subsequent trial from Belldegrun and colleagues pretreated patients with IFN-α prior to radical nephrectomy for TIL generation. TIL were then adoptively transferred and patients received IL-2 and IFN-α. TIL were generated in 11 of 11 patients attempted and there were 2 CR and one surgical CR. Subsequently, a large multi-center trial of CD8 TIL for renal cancer enrolled 178 patients, randomizing 160 to either TIL + IL-2 (n = 81) or IL-2 alone (n = 79). Of the 81 patients enrolled to TIL + IL-2 only 72 were eligible for TIL therapy and sufficient numbers of T cells could be grown on only 39 patients. Intent-to-treat analysis demonstrated objective response rates of 9.9% (8/81) and 11.4%, which was not different for the two groups. Notable differences between this trial and the 86 patients treated by Rosenberg and colleagues were the requirement to transport tumor specimens to a central facility, the isolation of only $CD8^+$ TIL for expansion and infusion, the relatively low number of T cells infused in some patients and the selection of patients with renal cancer.

Why didn't more renal cancer patients respond? In concert with some clinical trials, investigators looked for surrogate markers of therapeutic effector T cells. The first report of a correlation was provided by Aebersold et al., who showed that tumor-specific cytolytic activity of TIL was associated with clinical responses in melanoma patients. Another study of selected melanoma patients observed a significant correlation between the adoptive transfer of gp100-specific, IFN-γ secreting T cells and tumor regression. However, of the renal cancer studies listed above, only one reported functional analysis of TIL cultures and only a single patient was noted to express autologous tumor-specific cytolytic activity.

More extensive characterization of TIL in vitro function might have provided additional insights about why the response rate is so low. However, immunological monitoring in renal cancer patients has been somewhat limited by the absence of defined renal cancer-specific/associated antigens. Recently, determinants have been identified that appear to represent common renal cancer tumor antigens; brightening the prospects for immunological monitoring in this disease. However, since the generation of renal cancer-specific T cells from TIL is a rare event, better ways of generating renal cancer-specific T cells are needed before increased response rates are likely to be seen for this disease.

Tumor Vaccine-Draining Lymph Node T Cells—in vitro Sensitization

While tumor-specific T cells can be grown from TIL of most melanoma patients, it is not possible to reliably generate autologous tumor-specific T cells for adoptive transfer from most other tumors. One potential problem with TIL is that the T cells present at the tumor site may be suppressed by association with tumor factors and/or T reg cells and be ineffective at mediating tumor regression. Simultaneous with the identification of TIL, Shu and colleagues, showed that T cells from the lymph nodes draining a progressively growing tumor were a good source of anti-tumor T cells. These tumor-draining lymph node (TDLN) T cells, following in vitro sensitization (IVS) with tumor cells and IL-2, exhibited tumor-specific cytolytic activity in vitro and were highly therapeutic in adoptive transfer studies. It was speculated that this approach, utilizing in vitro activated tumor vaccine-draining lymph node T cells (TVDLN) or vaccine primed lymph nodes (VPL) might circumvent some of the obstacles associated with TIL. The clinical application of IVS-TVDLN cells was studied in 17 melanoma patients and 3 renal cell cancer patients. In these studies irradiated autologous tumor cells were combined with *Bacillus Calmette Guerin* (BCG) and used as the vaccine. TVDLN were harvested 10 to 14 days later, stimulated with cryopreserved autologous tumor and expanded in media containing 600 IU/ml of IL-2 and subsequently transferred to the patient in combination with IL-2. One patient receiving adoptively transferred T cells developed a partial response compared to none in the IL-2 control cohort. An interesting observation from this study was that T cell transfer conferred DTH reactivity to autologous tumor while vaccination and IL-2 treatment alone did not. A serious limitation of this strategy was the requirement for large numbers of tumor cells to perform IVS.

Tumor Vaccine-Draining Lymph Node T Cells—Anti-CD3 Activation

Frustrated by the limitation of the prior trial, Shu and colleagues investigated alternatives to using tumor to drive in-vitro expansion of T cells with therapeutic efficacy. They found that stimulating TVDLN cells with anti-CD3 appeared to mimic antigen-specific stimulation, supporting the maturation of T cells that were specific for the tumor used in the vaccine. In animal models anti-CD3-activated TVDLN cells mediated regression of tumors in the brain, skin and lung. In a clinical trial 11 melanoma and 12 renal cell cancer patients were vaccinated with autologous tumor cells and BCG. The TVDLN were activated with anti-CD3 and IL-2 and adoptively transferred in combination with IL-2. A 33% response rate was achieved in RCC patients (2 PR and 2 CR), while only one PR was observed in melanoma patients. A subsequent Phase II trial of 39 stage IV renal cell cancer patients reported 4 CRs and 5 PRs for an overall response rate of 27%.

An interesting observation of this report was the correlation of clinical response with the transfer of T cells that exhibited a high IFN-γ: IL-10 ratio for tumor-specific cytokine release. Chang and colleagues applied this same approach to 6 patients with advanced head and neck cancers. Patients were vaccinated with autologous tumor and BCG, TVDLN were harvested, expanded with anti-CD3 and IL-2, and infused into patients who received 15 doses of IL-2. Analysis of infused TIL for 4 of 5 patients identified tumor-specific secretion of IFN-γ and GM-CSF but no IL-4 or IL-10 (3 of 3 patients reported).

No objective clinical responses were observed. A similar approach vaccinated 21 NSCLC patients with autologous tumor cells and GM-CSF. After 2 vaccinations lymphocytes were activated with anti-CD3, expanded in IL-2 and patients received T cells numbering between 0.5- to 6.1×10^{10}, with 18 patients receiving more than 1.6×10^{10} T cells. Median survival of all 21 patients was 18.6 months, with a 1-year survival of 51.6%.

Tumor Vaccine-Draining Lymph Node T Cells—Superantigen Activation

The staphylococcal enterotoxins also known as microbial superantigens are small proteins that can cross link distinct Vβ subunits of the TCR with MHC Class II molecules and lead to selective expansion of T cells, which express the appropriate Vβ TCR. Preclinical studies demonstrated that staphylococcal enterotoxin C or staphylococcal enterotoxin B two potent microbial superantigens, exhibited to specific IFN-γ release and were therapeutic in the treatment of murine pulmonary and intracranial metastases. In humans, *staphylococcal enterotoxin A* (SEA) is the most potent mitogen, and activates greater than 80% of human T cells. There have been four clinical trials performed by Shu and colleagues where SEA-activated TVDLN were expanded in low dose IL-2 in vitro and adoptively transferred to patients with advanced disease. A major difference between these four studies and most other adoptive cellular immunotherapy trials is that they did not provide systemic IL-2 to support in vivo survival of transferred T cells. This strategy was undertaken based upon this group's preclinical data showing that adoptive immunotherapy with activated TVDLN was more effective against intracaranial and subcutaneous tumor when systemic IL-2 was not provided.

In the first clinical trial, ten patients with malignant glioma were vaccinated with irradiated autologous tumor cells and received GM-CSF. The TVDLN cells were stimulated ex vivo with SEA, expanded in IL-2 and then expanded a second time with anti-CD3 and IL-2 in order to generate high numbers of T cells. Patients were administered 10 mg/kg cyclophosphamide and 24 to 48 hrs later had their T cells infused. Three patients experienced a PR lasting 6, 7 and >13 months. A subsequent trial was performed with newly diagnosed gliomas. Patients were vaccinated with autologous tumor and GM-CSF. In this study harvested TVDLN cells were activated once with SEA, expanded in low dose IL-2 for 6–8 days and adoptively transferred to patients pretreated with cyclophosphamide. Four patients experienced a PR lasting 11, 14, 17 and >29 months. A third clinical trial repeated this strategy in patients with metastatic renal cell carcinoma. Patients were vaccinated with autologous tumor mixed with GM-CSF and TVDLN were activated by culture with SEA, expanded in IL-2 and adoptively transferred. All patients pretreated with cyclophosphamide and no systemic IL-2 was administered. There was 1 PR reported for 20 patients treated (318). The fourth trial was undertaken in patients with unresectable squamous cell carcinoma of the head and neck (SCCHN). Patients were treated as noted above and sufficient T cells were obtained to treat 15 of 17 patients enrolled. There were no objective clinical responses in this trial. Overall this approach had the greatest success in Glioma where there were 7 PRs for 22 patients treated.

Tumor Vaccine-Draining Lymph Node T Cells—Gene Modified Vaccines

Although murine models show that vaccination with poorly immunogenic tumors fails to sensitize therapeutic T cells, genetic modification of these ineffective vaccines can convert them to effective inducers of effective T cells for adoptive immunotherapy. Modification with an allogeneic MHC class I gene or a construct encoding GM-CSF are two approaches that are effective in preclinical models. The first to enter clinical trials was modification of alloantigen-modified autologous tumor. Patients received unmodified autologous tumor cells and BCG in one extremity and HLA-B7-lipofected autologous tumor in an alternate extremity. Ten to 14 days later TVDLN draining both vaccine sites were isolated and expanded independently so that possible differences in vaccine effectiveness could be evaluated by in vitro assays.

For adoptive cellular therapy anti-CD3 activated TVDLN draining both vaccine sites were combined and administered together with systemic IL-2. This report failed to observe any responses in 9 melanoma and 11 renal cancer patients treated. In contrast to preclinical studies that saw lipofected vaccines shifting the tumor-specific T cell response towards a type 1 cytokine profile, here the HLA-B7-modified vaccine promoted a tumor-specific IL-5 response that was higher than that observed for the TVDLN draining autologous tumor and BCG. Given this and other findings of tumor-antigen specific IL-5 in patients with progressive disease, future investigations will need to explore whether tumor-specific IL-5 responses might interfere with therapeutic efficacy or be a marker of other type 2 cytokines that have that ability.

Chang and colleagues used a similar trial design to study the effectiveness of a GM-CSF-transduced autologous tumor vaccine to prime tumor-specific T cells for adoptive immunotherapy. Five melanoma patients were vaccinated with autologous tumor transduced with a vector encoding GM-CSF in one extremity and unmodified tumor cells alone at a different site. TVDLN were harvested 7 days later, activated and expanded separately so that immunological comparisons could be made and the two populations of T cells were combined for adoptive transfer. Four patients received T cells and IL-2 with one patient undergoing a CR.

Tumor-specific immunological monitoring was possible on 2 patients, but did not include the patient with the CR. While there were no consistent differences between tumor-specific T cells primed by either vaccine, the yield of TVDLN cells was consistently greater in the LN-draining the GM-CSF-modified vaccine. While this report of Chang and colleagues is preliminary, the application of GM-CSF secreting autologous tumor vaccines is an approach that is already showing promising results in NSCLC. The combination of a GM-CSF transduced-tumor vaccine with other strategies (eg. Non-myeloablative conditioning and/or $CD25^{+}$ T cell depletion) and adoptive cellular immunotherapy will certainly be tested in clinical trials in the near future.

Selected Tumor-Specific T Cells

An underlying tenant of adoptive immunotherapy is that if you could select and transfer only tumor-specific T cells with therapeutic activity you could improve the response rate of treated patients. Thus strategies that identify the tumor-specific T cells maybe crucial to the success of adoptive immunotherapy. Recently, Kagamu and colleagues developed an approach to select the subset of T cells that have been specifically sensitized to tumor during vaccination. T cells that expressed a low level of L-Selectin (L-selectin^{Lo}), a well-established marker for recently activated and memory T cells, were isolated using magnetic bead technology, expanded in vitro and studied for their ability to mediate regression of the weakly immunogenic MCA-205. Consistent with its ability to mark recently activated "*responding*" T cells, the L-selectin^{Lo} TVDLN T cells contained all of the therapeutic activity. Others have repeated this observation using therapeutic vaccine strategies in different tumor models with similar success.

But is this strategy translatable to cancer patients? Currently efforts are underway to characterize the in vitro anti-tumor properties of L-selectin^{Lo} TVDLN T cells from cancer patients. Combining this approach with the polarizing signals suggested above (three-signal paradigm) this approach might improve not only the therapeutic efficacy but also help to reduce the high costs of expanding large numbers of cells for AIT.

Tumor-Specific T Cell Clones and Lines

In review of the proceeding clinical trials, one limiting factor has been the requirement to generate large numbers of tumor-specific T cells. For many cancers, there is still a paucity of evidence that this feat can be routinely accomplished. However, for melanoma and EBV associated malignancies, while technically challenging, it is a therapy, which can be attained by experienced laboratories. Proof of the feasibility and efficacy of this approach was provided by Walter and colleagues, who reconstituted cellular immunity against *cytomegalovirus* (CMV) in patients following bone marrow transplant. While the development of anti-virals limited the application of this technology for CMV, it paved the way for its application in cancer. Stimulated with tumor cells or APC and T cells are cloned or cultured in bulk to generate CTL lines. Rooney and colleagues have used adoptive immunotherapy with EBV-specific CTL lines to either prevent or treat EBV-induced lymphoma in allogeneic transplant recipients. In their prevention study they successfully generated CTL lines for 69 of 70 patients attempted. None of 39 evaluable patients developed EBV lymphoma, contrasting with an incidence of 11.5% in a control population from the same institution. This same group also reported CTL transfer was effective at treating lymphoma in two patients who received CTL transfer following onset of disease.

Unfortunately, the efficacy of Tumor-specific CD8^{+} T cell clones has been disappointing. In 2001 Dudley reported on 13 patients treated with CD8^{+} T cell clones reactive with gp100 epitope. The first 12 patients received T cell clones alone with no evidence of clinical response. Eleven of these patients and one previously untreated patient went on to infusions of T cell clones and either subcutaneous or intravenous IL-2. There was one minor response in a patient receiving T cells and intravenous IL-2. Subsequently, Yee and colleagues transferred T cell clones generated by in vitro culture with autologous dendritic cells pulsed with an HLA-A2-restricted peptide for either MART1/MelanA or gp100. Clones were selected for their ability to lyse antigen positive tumor targets in ^{51}Cr-release assays. They reported 2 minor responses but no PR or CR in 10 patients treated with 4 cycles of CTL infused at two-week intervals. An interesting component of their study was an internally controlled comparison of how T cell survival was affected by IL-2 administration. The median T cell survival following the initial infusion of CTL, when no IL-2 was administered, was 6.68 days. This compared to a median T cell survival of 16.92 days.

Mitchell and colleagues obtained T cells by leukapheresis and used tyrosinase peptide-pulsed Drosophila cells transduced with HLA-A2.1, CD80, and CD54 to prime/expand T cells in IVS. T cells were adoptively transferred and patients immunized with peptide. One PR was seen in 10 patients treated with adoptive transfer of 108 cells.

Tumor-Specific T Cell in Non-Myelo Ablated Patients

Dudley and colleagues reported on a similar trial that transferred Tumor-specific $CD8^+$ T cell clones into patients who first received a non-myeloablative regimen of cyclophosphamide and fludarabine. The first 6 patients received no systemic IL-2 treatment following T cell infusion. The next three received 15 doses of 72,000 IU/Kg and the remaining six received 720,000 IU/Kg every 8 hours till tolerance (mean 11 doses). There were no clinical responses for the 15 patients enrolled. One reason for the disappointing result of these studies could be the use of T cells directed against a single antigenic epitope. A recent report using a human MART-1-specific T cell clone for the adoptive immunotherapy of human melanoma in SCID mice showed that this treatment leads to immunoselection of MART-1 antigen-loss variants and treatment failure.

Rosenberg and colleagues performed a subsequent trial where patients received the same non-myeloablative chemotherapy regimen and high dose IL-2 but instead of receiving Tumor-specific $CD8^+$ T cells alone, received a mixture of $CD4^+$ and $CD8^+$ T cells. In striking contrast to previous trials where $CD8^+$ T cell clones or lines rapidly disappeared from circulation, some patients on this trial had T cells expand and persist at frequencies as high as 75% of $CD8^+$ T cells for 120–140 days. The most striking finding of this report was that 6 of 13 patients had objective clinical responses. These observations raised several important questions. First, why did a high percentage of patients respond? Is it solely a result of transferring $CD4^+$ T cells that may contain some HLA-DR-restricted tumor-specific cells? One supposition is that it is likely a combination of creating "*space*" in the lymphopenic host and deleting $CD4^+$ T reg cells that promotes the expansion and persistence of transferred T cells. A second supposition is that the expansion and persistence of the transferred T cells relies on the presence of some tumor-specific $CD4^+$ T cells. There is some evidence from preclinical models that $CD4^+$ T cells play a valuable role in maintaining anti-tumor immunity long-term.

Approaches to Expand Tumor-Specific T Cells

The encouraging results seen in trials combining CD4 and CD8 T cells with nonmyelo ablation will lead to additional trials of this approach. As noted above, a three signal paradigm has been proposed to generate T cells with therapeutic efficacy. However, methods are still needed for the large-scale expansion of antigen-specific T cells. Artificial APC is one approach that is being explored. Maus and colleagues developed used a cell line that expressed ligands for the TCR, CD28 and 4-1BB and have used it to expand functional CD8 T cells. Others have used beads coated with either anti-CD3 and anti-CD28. This approach can rapidly expand T cells and has already seen application in a clinical trial. A similar approach generated a bead with a soluble class I molecule and anti-CD28. An advantage to this approach is that it can be loaded with specific peptides. Multiple expansions with this approach triggered expansion of T cells that retained antigen-specific function. A similar approach provided TCR signaling to CD 4 T cells with good results.

Concluding Remark

From our perspective a great deal has changed in the past few years. We now appreciate that tumor-specific T cells have at least a triad of properties (perforin, IFN-γ, and TNF) that they can utilize to mediate tumor regression. We also have a basic understanding of in vitro methods to polarize primed T cells towards a "*therapeutic*" type 1 cytokine profile (IFN-γ and TNF). Additionally, combining vaccination at a time when host T cells are undergoing homeostasis-driven proliferation has been shown to dramatically increase the frequency of tumor-specific T cells generated by the host. The discovery of $CD25^+CD4^+$ regulatory T cells at tumor sites and the success of combining adoptive transfer of CD4 and $CD8^+$ TIL with a non myeloablative conditioning regimen that includes fludarabine, a drug that preferentially decimates $CD4^+$ T cells, are likely to be related. The availability of antibodies or ligands that block negative signals (CTLA4) or provide costimulatory signals (4-1BB, OX40) will be extended or initiated soon. The next several years should prove particularly informative as trials incorporating combinations of strategies make their way to the clinic.

7

Peptide Vaccines

Multiple vaccine modalities have been explored in the search for an effective immunotherapy for cancer, but to date, only limited success with any one of these has been reported. Each has potential advantages and disadvantages. Peptide vaccines have turned out to be the most successful approach so far for melanoma, using either free peptides or peptides coated on dendritic cells. They have the feature of focusing the immune response on specific epitopes, of particular advantage for the many tumor antigens that are self antigens. This approach has been shown to facilitate the breaking of tolerance to self, for example in the case of Her-2/neu. In the case of mutant molecules unique to the tumor, peptides also have the advantage of targeting only the mutant epitope that identifies the tumor cells, and avoiding other parts of the antigen that would be present in normal cells. Peptides are also relatively easy to modify, so that panels of variants can be studied to increase affinity for the relevant *Major Histocompatibility Complex* (MHC) molecules, to make the peptides more immunogenic, a process we have termed epitope enhancement. Likewise, the peptide sequence can be modified also to increase the affinity of the peptide-MHC complex for the T cell receptor. Here we will review how these peptide vaccine approaches have been used to target a variety of tumor antigens in both animal models, human *in vitro* studies, and human clinical trials.

Vaccine Strategies Using Peptide Vaccines

Several approaches have been developed to immunize with peptides, as single free CTL epitope peptides are not inherently as immunogenic as larger constructs or live viral vectors.

Table 7.1. Strategies to increase peptide vaccine efficacy

Approach	*Mechanism*
Inclusion of helper T cell epitopes	Induce helper T cells to activate/mature antigen presenting cells and secrete cytokines (It is not necessary to use a peptide from the same antigen as the CTL epitope.)
Incorporation of immunostimulatory molecules	Recruit professional antigen presenting cells (dendritic cells) to the site of antigen administration and skew T cells to the Th1 and CTL phenotypes
Blockade of negative regulators	Blocking negative regulatory cytokines and receptors to relieve mechanisms that dampen the response to the vaccine
Delivery of peptide on dendritic cells	Directly use professional antigen presenting cells which express high levels of co-stimulatory molecules to serve as a natural adjuvant; also to bypass the factors from the tumor that inhibit dendritic cell maturation
Epitope enhancement	Enhance binding ability of peptides to MHC without changing T cell interaction or increase affinity for T cell receptor without changing binding affinity for MHC

Requirement for Attached or Intrinsic T Helper Epitopes

First, for induction of a CTL response, a helper epitope is necessary in addition to the CTL epitope to obtain an optimal CTL response. We originally found that for non-emulsion adjuvants, covalent linkage of helper epitope and CTL epitope is critical, whereas when the two peptides are physically associated in an emulsion adjuvant or other physical linkage, covalent linkage is not necessary. It is likely that this association is needed to get both epitopes into the same antigen presenting cell, so that the helper T cell can activate this presenting cell to "*license*" it to activate the CTL precursor. When a helper epitope is intrinsic to the peptide containing the CTL epitope, no additional helper epitope is needed. Even priming with just a helper epitope led to a protective CTL response against an MHC class II negative tumor. Accordingly, it was recently found that a longer peptide from human papillomavirus E7 protein containing both a helper and a

CTL epitope was more effective at inducing a CTL response and treating an established E7-expressing tumor than the free CTL epitope, in a murine tumor model. For these reasons, peptide vaccines should optimally be designed to contain both helper and CTL epitopes.

Incorporation of Cytokines, Chemokines, and Costimulatory Molecules

Second, incorporation of cytokines, chemokines, costimulatory molecules, or immunostimulatory DNA sequences (CpG oligonucleotides) can enhance the response to a peptide vaccine. An emulsion adjuvant such as incomplete Freund's or the human grade equivalent, Montanide ISA-51, is conducive to incorporation of such agents, because they can be emulsified together with the antigen so that they are present in the same slow release depot and drain to the same draining lymph nodes. The most widely used are cytokines, such as GM-CSF, which we showed increased antigen presenting cells and function in the draining lymph node. We and others also found synergy between GM-CSF and IL-12, which act by different mechanisms.

In addition, we reasoned that if GM-CSF recruited dendritic cells, CD40L might mature them, and indeed, we found that the combination of GM-CSF and CD40L is synergistic. Costimulatory molecules can also increase the magnitude of the CTL response, as well as select for higher avidity CTL that are more effective at clearing virus or killing tumor cells. IL-15 as an adjuvant in a vaccine has also been found to select for CTL with a long-lived memory phenotype that remains responsive to IL-15-induced homeostatic proliferation for at least 14 months, more than half a mouse lifetime. Some of these cytokines have been tested in human clinical trials. Chemokines have also served as successful adjuvants, attracting T cells to the site of the vaccine. Finally, CpG-containing immunostimulatory oligonucleotides can be used to steer the response toward Th1 cyokine production and CTL, and can even be covalently linked to the antigen to induce an even stronger CTL response.

Blockade of Negative Regulatory Pathways and Signals

Third, one can also block negative regulatory pathways that dampen the immune response. For example, IL-13 made by regulatory NKT cells dampens or partially inhibits natural tumor immunosurveillance mediated by CTL, and blockade of IL-13 with a soluble receptor construct, IL-13Rα2-Fc, or elimination of the CD4$^+$ NKT cell mediating the suppression can enhance immunsurveillance and prevent tumor recurrence or increase the efficacy of vaccines aimed at eliciting CTL.

Similarly, one can block IL-10 or TGF-β made by $CD25^+$ and other immunoregulatory cells or eliminate such $CD25^+$ suppressive cells. Likewise, CTLA-4, a costimulatory receptor that paradoxically delivers an inhibitory signal to the T cell, can be blocked to increase CTL responses to tumors. Indeed, blockade of CTLA-4 and elimination of $CD25^+$ suppressor cells was synergistic in a murine tumor model.

Peptide Presentation on Dendritic Cells

Fourth, peptides can be coated or pulsed onto *dendritic cells* (DC) or other antigen presenting cells, and these used as an autologous cellular vaccine. This approach has the advantage that dendritic cells are the professional antigen presenting cells that most effectively activate naive T cells, and that serve as "*nature's adjuvant*". Dendritic cells as purified from bone marrow, spleen, or peripheral blood, or as differentiated in vitro from monocytes, tend to be immature, better at antigen uptake and processing than at antigen presentation. However, these cells are low in costimulatory molecules, and negative or dull for CD83 in the human, and relatively poor at presenting antigen. When matured by various agents, the dendritic cells express CD83, lose their facility at antigen uptake, but upregulate costimulatory molecules and become much more effective at stimulating T cells. Indeed, different methods for maturing dendritic cells can affect their potency as vaccines when pulsed with antigen.

The most effective agent for maturing dendritic cells is CD40L, which corresponds to the natural molecule on helper T cells that matures the dendritic cell when it binds to CD40 on the cell. There is some evidence that immature dendritic cells, which are low in costimulatory molecules, can actually be tolerogenic, as found in a human clinical trial. Therefore, most clinical protocols using dendritic cells as antigen presenting cells now employ matured DC. Furthermore, use of autologous dendritic cells matured in vitro bypasses the problem that *vascular endothelial growth factor* (VEGF) and perhaps other factors made by tumors can inhibit the maturation of dendritic cells in tumor-bearing animals and patients. Thus, peptides have the advantage that they can be easily coated onto dendritic cells *ex vivo*, circumventing this impass to induction of vaccine responses in cancer patients.

Epitope Enhancement

Finally, the epitopes incorporated into peptide vaccines can be improved by sequence modification, a process we call epitope enhancement. Natural epitopes from cancer cells may not be optimal for binding to MHC molecules, because tumors probably lose the most immunogenic epitopes to become malignant. Many tumor antigens are self proteins, and self-tolerance is likely to delete the high avidity T cells specific for the most dominant epitopes. Thus, subdominant epitopes, to which there is less tolerance, may turn out to be the most effective tumor antigens. However, such subdominant epitopes may have suboptimal affinity for the MHC molecule, and therefore suboptimal immunogenicity.

To improve immunogenicity, the sequence can be modified by epitope enhancement to increase the affinity for the MHC molecule. The idea is to alter only residues interacting with the MHC molecule, so that the surface of the peptide-MHC complex recognized by the T cell receptor is unchanged, in order to induce T cells that still respond to the natural sequence present in the tumor (or virus). In practice, some alterations may affect both MHC and T cell receptor binding, so care must be taken to achieve the right balance between increased MHC affinity and T cell cross-reactivity. This approach has been applied to viral vaccines, as well as to tumor antigens, such as gp100, a melanocyte differentiation antigen, and to p53, a tumor suppressor protein.

An alternative related approach is to modify the amino acid residues interacting with the T-cell receptor, rather than with the MHC molecule. By this approach, one can generate peptide MHC complexes with higher affinity for a particular T cell receptor. If this receptor or ones like it predominate in the response to that epitope, then one can create a more immunogenic peptide to use as a vaccine, including epitopes from tumor antigens *carcinoembryonic antigen* (CEA) and p53.

Tumor Antigen Targets of Peptide Vaccines

Mutant Oncogene or Tumor Suppressor Gene Products

p53

The tumor suppressor gene p53 is mutated almost 50% of cancers of many common types, and the mutant protein is usually overexpressed in the cancer cells. These two features make p53 a potential target for vaccine immunotherapy, since the mutation is a unique marker for the cancer cells, and the overexpression may also distinguish cancer cells from normal cells. One caveat to the latter concept is that the overexpression appears to be due to reduced degradation, rather than increased production, and as such, might decrease the amount of mutant epitope processed and presented, rather than increase it. Nevertheless, T cells specific for wild-type p53 sequences have been found to preferentially kill tumors with mutant p53 that is overexpressed, so the overexpression can favor CTL recognition of tumor. Mutations in p53 have been shown to create neoantigenic epitopes in p53 which allow killing of cancer cells without harming normal cells. Also, mutant p53 peptides given with cytokines such as IL-12 or pulsed onto dendritic cells have been able to induce anti-tumor immunity and even treat established tumors in mice. Such murine CTL to mutant p53 can also lyse human tumor cells expressing the p53 mutation.

The disadvantage of focusing the immune response on the mutation is that there are so many different p53 mutations found that each vaccine would have to be custom-made for each tumor, and not all mutations would be in amino acid sequences that could bind to and be presented by the HLA molecules of the patient. Therefore, investigators have searched for common sequences that might be more immunogenic in cancer cells. A few of these that are presented by HLA-A2 have been described and some have been improved by epitope enhancement. Indeed, in one case the wild type epitope was not presented by HLA-A2 in individuals with a mutation one residue downstream of the epitope, presumably because of a processing problem, but surprisingly, it was possible to reverse the defect by compensatory amino acid substitutions within the epitope itself. CTL to wild-type p53 epitopes have also been found to recognize peptides presented by other HLA molecules, including HLA-A24, HLA-B51, HLA-B46, and others in patients with bladder cancer and head and neck cancer, colon cancer, and breast cancer. Human CTL raised in vitro by stimulation with peptide-pulsed dendritic cells have been found to lyse human tumor cells overexpressing p53.

Although most of the work on p53 as a tumor antigen have focused on $CD8^+$ CTL responses, p53-specific $CD4^+$ T cell responses have also been described and been shown to be important for induction of CTL as well as potentially for their own effector function in the anti-tumor immune response. Overall, as either a custom peptide to uniquely target a cancer expressing a p53 mutation, or as a broader vaccine focused on overexpressed wild-type p53 sequences, p53 remains an attractive target molecule for the immunotherapy of cancer.

Ras

Ras is mutated in a number of human cancers, including about a third of colorectal cancers and a larger fraction of pancreatic cancer.

Unlike p53, only a handful of mutations occur commonly, mostly in codon 12, in which a glycine residue is replaced by a valine, aspartic acid, alanine, cysteine, or arginine. Some mutations occur less commonly in codon 13 or codon 61. Codon 12 and 13 were found to fall within a 10-residue sequence that has a binding motif for the most common class I HLA molecule, HLA-A2.1.

The mutations actually increase the ability of the epitope to be presented compared to the wild type ras sequence, but the affinity is still relatively low. Much work has been done showing efficacy of CTL raised against mutant ras in mouse tumor models, reviewed previously. Cheever's group pioneered the idea of targeting ras as a tumor antigen in mice, defining $CD4^+$ T cell responses to the Arg 12 mutant ras and the Leu 61 mutant form. Skipper and Stauss first identified murine $CD8^+$ T cell responses to mutant ras targeting a codon 61 mutation (Lys 61), and Peace et al. mapped residues 59–67 as the best binder able to elicit specific CTL. Fenton et al. then showed that a recombinant mutant ras protein with the Arg-12 mutation was able to elicit CTL and protect mice against challenge with tumors expressing this mutation.

Human $CD4^+$ T cell responses have also been reported to ras codon 12 and 61 mutations. Indeed, promiscuous $CD4^+$ T cell epitopes were found encompassing codon 12 and codon 61 mutations. However, a clinical trial of peptide-pulsed PBMC induced T cell proliferative but not clinical responses in pancreatic cancer patients.

Also, human CTL have been raised *in vitro* against some of the common codon 12 or 13 mutant peptides, from blood of patients either unimmunized or immunized with mutant ras peptides, and have been shown to lyse human tumors. On the other hand, several attempts to raise CTL to such mutant ras peptides resulted in CTL that would kill only targets pulsed with peptide, not tumor cells expressing mutant ras. Several clinical trials have been carried out to immunize against mutant ras in cancer patients, including use of 13-residue peptides in adjuvant and 10-residue or 17-residue peptides pulsed onto antigen presenting cells, either peripheral blood mononuclear cells or enriched dendritic cells.

Although no clinical responses were seen in these studies, a correlation between specific cytokine response and survival was observed. In another study of ras peptide intradermal immunization of pancreatic cancer patients using GM-CSF as adjuvant, some clinical responses were seen, and median survival was longer in those achieving an immune response to the vaccine. A clinical trial of peptide-pulsed autologous CD40L-matured dendritic cells with codon 12 and codon 13 mutant ras peptides in colorectal cancer patients is underway in the National Cancer Institute. Thus, mutant ras peptides remain a promising target for therapy of a number of types of cancer.

VHL

The *von Hippel Lindau* (VHL) protein was originally found to be mutated in this syndrome involving hereditary renal cell cancer, and then was also found to be mutated in sporadic renal cell carcinoma. The mutations occur at many positions, more like the case of p53 than that of ras. However, a number of them fall within sequences predicted to bind to HLA-A2.1, so a clinical trial is underway to examine whether peptides spanning these mutations can induce a CTL response and/or a clinical remission in HLA-A2^{+} patients with renal cell cancer.

Chromosomal Translocations

A number of types of malignancy are associated with chromosomal translocations, especially sarcomas, and *chronic myelogenous leukemia* (CML). In general, these chromosomal translocations have been found to contribute to the malignant phenotype by creating fusion genes at the junction of the two chromosomes that produce a new oncogene. Usually these involve genes that regulate other genes, such as transcription factors. For example, the DNA binding domain of one transcription factor may be joined to the activation domain of another transcription factor, resulting in aberrant transcription.

However, the fusion protein created by the chromosomal translocation, which is responsible for the malignancy, may also be its Achilles heel. At the breakpoint junction within the fusion protein, there is a new amino acid sequence for every peptide that spans the breakpoint, that does not occur in either of the normal proteins that are the parents of the fusion. These new peptides may serve as neoantigenic determinants that can flag the tumor for recognition by the immune system, since these amino acid sequences are absent in non-malignant cells. Furthermore, the tumor cannot afford to lose or turn off production of the fusion gene product, because this product is also serving as an oncogene to maintain the malignant phenotype.

Bcr-Abl is a the classic example of a fusion protein, in this case formed by the t(9;22) chromosomal translocation associated with the Philadelphia chromosome of CML (95% of cases) as well as 10% of childhood and 25% of adult *acute lymphocytic leukemia* (ALL). The tyrosine kinase activity of the fusion protein is increased compared to the normal C-Abl tyrosine kinase and the fusion protein has transforming activity, so it is likely the tumor cells cannot lose it without losing their malignant state. Cheever's group first targeted the BCR-ABL fusion protein in mice, inducing $CD4^+$ T cell responses, and similar responses have been seen in human $CD4^+$ T cells. Murine CTL to the fusion protein were not able to lyse tumor cells expressing the fusion protein, but subsequent studies of an epitope presented by HLA-A3 showed that human CTL could lyse tumor cells, supporting the use of BCR-ABL as a tumor vaccine antigen. Recent clinical trials of BCR-ABL breakpoint peptides as vaccines in CML patients have induced cellular immune responses but not yet achieved clinical remissions.

PAX3-FKHR, EWS-FLI1, SSX-SYT are all examples of fusion proteins created by translocations in pediatric sarcomas, such as alveolar rhabdomyosarcoma, Ewing's sarcoma, and synovial sarcoma, respectively. Murine CTL raised to a peptide spanning the breakpoint of the PAX3-FKHR fusion protein were able to lyse adenocarcinoma cells transfected with the full-length PAX3-FKHR DNA. Some of the peptides spanning the breakpoints have been found to bind to common HLA molecules, such as HLA-A3, A1 or B7. In such cases, it has been possible to raise human CTL to these peptides that can recognize and kill human tumor cells expressing the fusion protein, for example in the case of an SSX-SYT fusion peptide of synovial sarcoma presented by HLA-B7. Some of these are currently in clinical trials as therapeutic vaccines in patients.

Her-2/neu

Her-2/neu is a 185 Kd transmembrane protein in the epidermal growth factor receptor family of tyrosine kinase receptors. Her-2/neu is overexpressed in about 30% of breast carcinomas in humans, and so has been considered a target for immunotherapy of breast cancer. Its value as a target is underlined by the success of trastuxumab (Herceptin), a monoclonal antibody to Her-2/neu licensed to treat breast cancer. As a vaccine target, both antibodies and T cell immunity have been sought. With regard to antibodies, a peptide vaccine consisting of B cell epitopes joined to a promiscuous helper T cell epitope induced antibodies in rabbits that inhibited human breast cancer cells in vitro, and substantially protected 83% of Her-2 transgenic mice from development of spontaneous breast cancers. With regard to T cells, Cheever, Disis and colleagues found that it was easier to break tolerance to murine Her-2 in mice with short peptides as vaccines than with the whole protein. Thus, this may be an ideal case for a peptide vaccine. Clinical trials of Her-2 peptides in humans were successful in inducing $CD4^+$ T cell proliferative responses that correlated with *delayed type hypersensitivity* (DTH) responses.

A later study using peptides that contained both helper epitopes and CTL epitopes presented by HLA-A2, with GM-CSF as an adjuvant, induced both $CD4^+$ T cell proliferative responses and $CD8^+$ HLA-A2-restricted CTL in patients previously treated for breast, ovarian, or lung cancer that overexpressed Her-2, with no evident or minimal residual disease. T cells induced by the vaccine lysed human tumor cells expressing Her-2 and persisted for more than a year in some patients. However, some CTL induced by peptides from Her-2 have been found not to recognize Her-2-expressing tumors. Also, short peptides are less likely to induce antibodies that may have clinical benefit like that of trastuxumab. Nevertheless, Her-2/neu remains a promising target for cancer vaccines.

MUC1

MUC1 is a mucin-family glycoprotein that is overexpressed as well as under-glycosylated on many types of cancers of epithelial origin compared to normal epithelial cells. It contains multiple copies of a 20-residue repeat sequence. Early studies of human CTL responses to MUC1 revealed a surprising lack of HLA restriction that was thought to be related to the multivalency of the repeat structure. In addition, conventional HLA-restricted epitopes have been found. MUC1 peptides pulsed on dendritic cells were more effective than the same peptides in adjuvant at eliciting CTL and inducing tumor rejection in both wild-type mice and mice transgenic for MUC1, indicating an ability to break tolerance. Several clinical trials of peptide vaccines have succeeded in eliciting $CD4^+$ or $CD8^+$ T cell responses and specific antibodies, and antibodies raised to MUC1 peptides conjugated to *keyhole limpet hemocyanin* (KLH) as carrier in patients can mediate antibody-dependent cellular cytotoxicity against tumor cells in vitro, but so far no consistent clinical responses except for stabilization of disease has been observed.

CEA

Carcinoembryonic antigen (CEA) is an embryonic antigen not normally expressed substantially in the adult, but overexpressed in most colorectal, gastric, breast, pancreatic, and non-small cell lung cancers. An immunodominant CTL epitope has been identified presented by HLA-A2.1, called CAP-1, and by application of epitope enhancement, an improved epitope has been shown to have higher affinity to the most frequently used T cell receptors. Several early clinical trials used the CAP-1 peptide as a vaccine either in adjuvant (Detox) or pulsed onto autologous dendritic cells. T cell responses have been observed, but no consistent clinical responses were seen, although there was one case of a partial remission in a thyroid carcinoma patient treated with peptide-pulsed dendritic cells.

However, a more recent clinical trial of the epitope-enhanced CAP-1 peptide CEA605-613 pulsed onto dendritic cells that had been expanded with Flt3 ligand produced clear tumor regressions in two colorectal cancer patients, of 12 HLA-A2$^+$ patients with colorectal or non-small-cell lung cancer studied. Another CEA peptide presented by HLA-A2 (CEA691) has been improved by epitope enhancement, and immunzation with autologous dendritic cells pulsed with an HLA-A24-presented peptide of CEA (CEA652) has been associated with stable disease in two of ten patients. Also, a promiscuous T helper epitope of CEA (residues 653–667), presented by HLA-DR4, DR7, and DR9, has been identified, overlapping the latter HLA-A24-presented CTL epitope. Therefore, much recent progress has been made toward developing peptide vaccines against CEA that can impact the clinical course of cancers expressing this antigen.

Melanocyte Differentiation Antigens

As melanoma is one of the tumors most associated with spontaneous remissions thought to be immune-mediated, it has been a major focus of cancer vaccines and immunotherapy. Using tumor infiltrating lymphocytes as probes, several shared tumor antigens have been identified, many of which turned out to be melanocyte differentiation antigens, such as Mart-1/Melan A, gp100, tyrosinase, and tyrosinase-related protein (TRP)-2. Patients treated with vaccines or adoptively transferred T cells specific for these antigens often develop vitiligo, or depigmentation in patches of skin, confirming the cross-reactivity of the T cells for normal melanocytes and melanoma cells.

Indeed, there is a correlation between vitiligo and clinical remissions, in that cases of vitiligo have been seen only in patients showing some clinical response to the therapy. This side effect, largely cosmetic, has been considered an acceptable trade-off if one can successfully treat a largely fatal malignancy. One of the most effective vaccine approaches has been found to be synthetic peptides corresponding to HLA-A2-binding segments of these antigens. In a phase I trial of

MART-1 peptide in incomplete Freund's adjuvant, 10 of 22 patients developed interferon-γ responses specific for the peptide and these responses correlated with prolonged relapse-free survival. A modification of this peptide has been described to increase stability in plasma.

Epitope enhancement has been applied to make a more effective vaccine of gp100 peptide 209–217, by substituting a methionine at position 2 in the peptide sequence. In a clinical trial comparing the wild type and enhanced peptide, the enhanced peptide was much more effective at eliciting a $CD8^+$ T cell response. When given with IL-2, this peptide was also the most effective at producing clinical remissions, significantly more than in the case of treatment with IL-2 alone. This promising finding has led to a phase III clinical trial in progress.

Interestingly, however, the use of IL-2 that increased clinical responses reduced the CTL activity detectable in peripheral blood, suggesting sequestering at the tumor site. In that regard, it was found that when melanoma patients were vaccinated with a mixture of four peptides from gp100 and tyrosinase restricted by HLA-A1, A2, and A3, with GM-CSF in Montanide ISA-51 adjuvant, CTL could be detected in 5/5 patients in lymph nodes draining the immunization site, but in only 2/5 patients in the peripheral blood. In addition, a MART-1 peptide vaccine in two types of emulsion adjuvants increased the number of antigen-specific T cells ex vivo, but did not convert them to an active effector state seen after virus infection, suggesting the need for additional vaccine components to activate the T cells induced.

In this regard, responses to the gp100-209-217 (2M) peptide could be increased by immunization of melanoma patients with the peptide in Montanide ISA-51 adjuvant when recombinant human IL-12 was administered at the same sites. In a trial of $CD34^+$ progenitor cell derived dendritic cells pulsed with 4 different melanoma peptides presented by HLA-A2.1, response to more than two of these peptides correlated with lack of disease progression. Thus, melanocyte differentiation antigen peptides remain one of the most promising types of tumor antigen for vaccine therapy.

Tumor-Testis Antigens (MAGE, etc.)

Some of the first T-cell tumor antigens mapped were found by cloning genes using T lymphocytes as a probe. The first one, MAGE, found in melanoma, turned out to be the prototype of a class of tumor antigens called *tumor-testis antigens* because they were found primarily in tumors, but also in one normal tissue, testis. These proteins contain segments presented by HLA-A1 or A2 and peptides from these antigens binding HLA molecules have been used in cancer vaccine clinical trials for melanoma, either in adjuvant or pulsed on dendritic cells, resulting in some clinical tumor regressions and/or lack of progression. Peptides pulsed on to dendritic cells have also induced $CD4^+$ Th1 cell responses to MAGE peptides in melanoma patients.

Viral Tumor Antigens: HPV 16-E6 and E7

The most foreign tumor antigens are ones that are actually encoded by a viral genome rather than the human genome. Although several virally-induced tumors are known, such as B cell lymphomas related to *Epstein-Barr virus* (EBV) and adult T-cell leukemia/lymphoma associated with HTLV-I, the best characterized antigenically is cervical carcinoma associated with *human papillomavirus* (HPV). Over 95% of human cervical cancer is now believed to be caused by human papillomavirus, primarily types 16 and 18. The premalignant dysplastic cells and carcinoma in situ, as well as invasive cancer, all express two oncogene products encoded by the virus, E6 and E7. E6 contributes to the malignancy by binding to and facilitating the degradation of the tumor suppressor protein p53, while E7 contributes by binding and inactivating another tumor suppressor protein, Rb. Together they have been shown to be sufficient to transform cells, and so they must be retained to maintain the malignant phenotype.

Much work has been done to target these with vaccines, but they have not proven to be the most immunogenic proteins. Nevertheless, a dominant epitope of E7 presented by a murine class I MHC molecule has been shown to be an effective vaccine against murine tumors expressing E7. Epitopes binding to human HLA-A2 and other HLA molecules have been mapped, and human CTL raised. These have been the subject of a number of clinical trials of peptide vaccines.

Initial clinical trials with HPV-16 E7 peptide vaccines were not very successful at inducing CTL or clinical responses, but a more recent one using two peptides from E7 (residues 12–20 and 86-93) showed increased CTL activity to E7 in 62% of individuals tested and some viral clearance from cervical scrapings in two thirds. It is not clear why such a foreign tumor antigen as a viral antigen should be so weakly immunogenic. Nevertheless, if these problems can be overcome, E6 and E7 remain strong choices for cancer vaccines because they are so completely foreign that at least tolerance does not need to be broken, and no autoreactivity should be induced.

Concluding Remark

Much recent progress has been made in the identification of new tumor antigens and their epitopes that may serve as potential cancer vaccines. Many of these have been studied as synthetic peptide vaccines corresponding to epitopes identified as presented by particular common human class I HLA molecules, especially HLAA2.1, the most common human class I molecule. Although a number of strategies for immunization against cancer have been investigated, no strategy targeting a specific antigen has yet proven consistently more clinically effective than synthetic peptides.

Peptides have the advantage that they can be easily modified by epitope enhancement to improve binding to the MHC molecule or the T cell receptor, and they can be combined with cytokines, chemokines, and costimulatory molecules to increase vaccine potency and steer the responses toward a desired phenotype, such as CTL or Th1 cells. Peptides can also be coated onto dendritic cells, the ultimate professional antigen presenting cell, to bypass any defect in antigen-presenting cell function or maturation related to the presence of the cancer. Thus, as both research tools and as potential clinical vaccines, synthetic peptides remain at the forefront of research in the vaccine immunotherapy of cancer.

8

OPTIMIZING PEPTIDE VACCINE

Methodological progress at the end of last century in the identification of tumor associated antigens specifically recognized by *cytolytic T lymphocytes* (CTL) made possible the characterization of numerous peptides (p) presented by class I *Major Histocompatibility Complexes* (MHC). These p-MHC complexes are the ligands for clonotypically distributed *T cell receptors* (TCR). The latter are heterodimers of α and β chains bearing structural homology with immunoglobulins. As such, they are composed of constant and variable segments. Three hypervariable regions can be identified, of which the Complementary Determining Region 3 (CDR3) is both the most variable and involved in the interactions with the peptide amino acid residues in the p-MHC complex.

The tumor associated antigenic peptides identified thus far are derived from a large variety of cellular polypeptides. These may include regular proteins from different cellular compartments, isoforms encoded by alternatively spliced genes, the products from alternative open reading frames, mutated genes or frameshifts and may even result from the transcription of the antisense strand of DNA. In one case, the antigenic peptide was shown to be generated by a protein splicing mechanism, thus far unknown in the eukaryotic world. Thus, the variety of cell biological mechanisms uncovered so far as giving rise to antigenic peptides reveal the highly opportunistic nature of tumor recognition by CD8 T lymphocytes. This is the result of two concurrent mechanisms leading to antigen recognition by T lymphocytes. On one hand, the process of antigen recognition involves a sophisticated molecular apparatus able to discriminate as few as 1–10 p-MHC complexes on the surface of the antigen presenting cell that normally display up to 10^4–10^5 p-MHC complexes. Thus, the system has evolved to attain an exquisite sensitivity and is endowed with powerful discrimination and amplification properties. On the other hand, the repertoire of αβ T cells is shaped by positive and negative selection processes during thymic development. As a result the majority, up to 95% of immature thymocytes that successfully rearrange TCRs, are eliminated from the mature repertoire. The coupling of these two thymic selection forces ensures that the TCRs expressed by T cells exported for immunesurveillance in the periphery possess sufficient affinity for interaction with self MHC molecules but are depleted of potentially dangerous TCRs with high affinity for self p-MHC complexes. As a result self tolerance is firmly established. However, this does not mean absence of autoreactive T cells. In fact, these cells exist in the peripheral T cell repertoire but possess a low to intermediate avidity for a high number of self antigens. Thus, despite the considerable diversity of tumor associated peptides, many of those identified thus far are derived from conventional polypeptides that are expressed by both normal and tumor cells.

Practical issues in specific therapy of cancer favour the use of those antigens that are expressed in the maximum number of patients with a given type of tumor. In this regard, most of the antigenic peptides from mutated gene products are poor candidates for widely applicable vaccines because their expression is limited to individual tumors. Consequently, the best candidates for vaccine development in terms of cancer population coverage are those derived from self antigens. Thus, an expected limitation of these generic cancer vaccines is the existence of self tolerance. Such constraints have been clearly demonstrated in studies conducted in experimental mouse models. For instance, large differences in TCR avidity for a p53-derived class I restricted T cell epitope can be measured when comparing the TCR repertoires of wild type mice and p53-genetically deficient counterparts. Similar findings were reported in a transgenic mouse model system for CTL recognizing a dominant viral antigen. Another elegant illustration of this phenomenon comes from the comparative analysis of the HLA-A2 restricted CD8 T cell repertoire for a tyrosinase-derived melanoma associated antigen in strains of mice expressing or not the *tyrosinase* gene product.

Attempts to vaccinate patients with such peptides result in the selection of a specific CTL response. Moreover, appropriate immunization may elicit a tumor protective response mediated by the low avidity CD8 T cell repertoire in a mouse model. Interestingly, it has been shown in well defined animal models that similar or even more efficient CTL responses can be obtained by immunization with peptides modified at key residues. These studies clearly demonstrate that this class of peptide analogues have the ability to mobilize the intermediate/low avidity T cell repertoire and induce protective anti-tumor CTL responses. Here we review the sequence and structural basis of p-MHC complexes formation and show how antigenic peptide modifications can improve the peptide's immunogenicity.

Peptide Binding to MHC

Sequence Analysis

To fulfil their immunological functions, MHC Class I molecules have evolved to bind with sufficient affinity a large number of peptides with widely divergent amino acid sequences. Sequence analysis of the peptide population obtained by elution of immunoaffinity purified MHC class I molecules revealed the presence of allele-specific binding motifs. For instance, *HLA-A*0201* encoded molecules selectively bind peptides with L, M or I at the second position of the peptide, or P2, and V or L at PΩ, i.e. the residue occupying the carboxyl terminal position of the peptide. In contrast, P2 needs to be a Y or F and PΩ an I or an L in peptides binding to the mouse K^d molecule as well as in those binding to the human HLA-A24 molecule. Nearly identical results were obtained by a completely functional approach using substituted peptides as competitors of antigenic peptides to inhibit lysis of chromium labelled targets by H2 K^d restricted CTL clones. These results suggested that there are distinct amino acid residues in the peptide that are directly involved in MHC binding, while the remaining peptide residues are relatively unconstrained at the sequence level.

Since this pioneering work, large amounts of data have been collected on the nature of peptide sequences restricted to different MHC allelic products. For instance, the MHC-PEP database has been regularly updated and contains information on peptide binding for several MHC together with experimentally determined affinity constants for MHC. There are currently over 2500 peptide sequences known to bind HLA-A2, allowing statistics to be made, though care should be taken since the peptide population is subject to certain bias. Table 8.1 shows the occurrence of each of the twenty naturally occurring amino acids at specific peptide positions for the panel of peptides known to be naturally associated with HLA-A2 in somatic cells. The first number is computed for the entire database, and the second one for high affinity peptides only (246 sequences). The main anchor residues described above are clearly still predominant and the Table provides information on which alternate residues are allowed.

Table 8.1. Anchor residues specificity for the different pockets of HLA-A2.

Amino acid	*P1*	*P2*	*P3*	*P(Ω-3)*	*P(Ω-2)*	*P(Ω)*
A	13/6	4/3	10/5	9/3	13/10	5/4
C	0/1	0/0	1/0	2/0	1/1	0/0
D	0/0	0/0	6/2	1/1	2/0	0/0
E	2/0	0/0	2/1	1/0	2/0	0/0
F	10/13	0/0	5/10	9/13	13/25	0/0
G	11/23	1/0	7/8	5/7	4/7	1/1
H	1/0	0/0	2/1	1/0	3/2	0/0
I	6/5	13/15	4/4	7/6	5/3	10/6
K	9/8	0/1	2/3	2/1	1/2	0/0
L	7/11	60/64	17/25	9/7	11/8	28/30
M	2/1	7/6	1/2	1/1	0/0	1/1
N	1/1	0/0	5/3	1/1	2/2	0/0
P	1/0	0/0	7/9	8/7	8/14	0/0
Q	2/1	0/0	1/0	2/3	2/1	0/0
R	3/4	0/0	1/0	1/0	1/0	0/0
S	6/5	0/0	5/5	5/7	3/3	0/0
T	2/2	4/3	2/1	5/4	3/2	3/2
V	4/3	3/1	5/4	15/24	9/7	42/52
W	1/2	0/0	4/4	0/0	2/2	0/0
Y	5/6	0/0	3/4	2/4	2/1	0/0

Due to the strong selectivity at positions P2 and PΩ, these two residues are referred to as *main* or *primary* anchor residues and those occupying the less selective positions P1, P3 and PΩ-3, PΩ-2 to as *secondary* anchor residues. An additional regular feature of MHC class I binding peptides is their defined length of 9–10 residues. Indeed, despite the identification of occasional T cell epitopes whose optimal length is clearly at variance with this rule, the large majority of known T cell epitopes as well as sequenced MHC class I-associated peptides are nona or decapeptides. Thus, relatively simple sequence motifs can be defined for sets of peptides binding to well defined class

I MHC molecules, both from murine and human origin. These motifs can be defined by three components. The first, the primary anchor residues. The second, the secondary anchor residues and the third component is a defined peptide length.

The sequence motifs described here find their explanation in the specific p-MHC architecture in three dimensions. An immediate application of these insights has been the design of computer algorithms to identify candidate peptides in proteins of known sequence that would bind a given MHC class I molecule. Two such computer programs have gained wide recognition: the bioinformatics and molecular analysis section (BIMAS) algorithm and the one based on the SYFPEITHI database. Another algorithm with the same purpose has been reported recently.

Numerous studies have been performed leading to the identification of potential T cell epitopes in proteins of interest for immunotherapy of infectious or autoimmune diseases and cancer. Such an approach has been dubbed "*reverse immunology*" to emphasize the fact that, in contrast to the initial methods leading to CTL-defined antigen identification, the starting "*reagent*" is the bioinformatic tool and the end-product the isolation of the peptide-specific T cell.

Structural Analysis

A major step in the understanding of peptide binding to MHC molecules was the elucidation, by X-ray crystallography, of the three dimensional structure of the p-MHC complex. It allowed to derive general rules on the strategy of peptide binding by MHC. So far, the structures of around 60 different p-MHC complexes have been solved by X-ray crystallography.

Non-Natural Peptide Antigen Analogues Resistant to Biodegradation

The efficient use of antigenic peptides as therapeutic agents may be limited by the high sensitivity of peptides to degradation by peptidases present in biological fluids. Initial *in vitro* studies showed that peptide degradation by proteases in serum could decrease the presentation of exogenous antigenic peptide by MHC on the surface of presenting cells. In addition, the degradation of the antigenic peptide *in vitro* was correlated with a diminution of their persistence *in vivo*.

Further studies indicated that local persistence of the antigenic peptide could be associated with the induction of an optimal immune response. Together, these factors could limit the immunogenicity of the antigenic peptide as tumor vaccine. Thus, rendering antigenic peptides resistant to degradation by peptidases could have important implications in the design of efficient peptide based vaccines for immunotherapeutic treatment of cancer.

To this end, an effective approach consists in introducing structural modifications to the antigenic peptide. This has been showed for both MHC class-I or class-II restricted antigenic peptides. The structural changes in the antigenic peptide involve either a variety of chemical modifications of the peptide bond or substitutions with non-natural amino acids. A drawback, however, was the simultaneous appearance of dramatic negative effects on the MHC binding properties of the antigen and/or on the recognition by antigen specific T lymphocytes. Such detrimental effects must be minimised in order to use such peptidase resistant pseudopeptides as efficient therapeutic compounds. To preserve the antigenicity and immunogenicity of the antigenic peptides, a more rational approach was taken to introduce minimal modifications of the peptide structure. In this approach, the knowledge of the degradation mechanism of the antigenic peptide guides the choice of structural modifications targeted to the appropriate position in the peptide's structure, the one(s) susceptible to proteolytic attack.

The detailed mechanism of tumor antigenic peptide degradation was initially determined by the analysis using an on-line HPLC mass spectrometry (HPLC/ESIMS) method of the degradation fragments generated after incubation of the antigenic peptide in human serum for various periods of time. In line with the findings of this study, the analysis of the degradation of the MelanA/MART-1 related peptide $MelanA_{26-35}$ A27L indicates the involvement of aminopeptidases and di-peptidylcarboxy peptidases. Interestingly, the degradation of the antigenic peptides from their amino- and the carboxy-terminal ends was found to be sequential and no endopeptidase activity was involved. The kinetics of amino- and carboxy-terminal degradation can be different from one peptide to another leading to slightly different degradation profiles. The analysis of the degradation of Melan-A/MART-1 nona- and decapeptide related peptides suggest that the nature of the amino-terminal residues has a direct or indirect effect on both amino- and carboxy-peptidase enzymatic activities.

The degradation model of the peptide $MelanA_{26-35}$ A27L predicts that the peptidase sensitive bonds are the first (Glu^1-Leu^2) and the eighth (Leu^8-Thr^9). Within the $MelanA_{26-35}$ A27L sequence, the peptidase sensitive peptide bonds were targeted for the introduction of a variety of structural modifications. Protection of the N-terminal and C-terminal

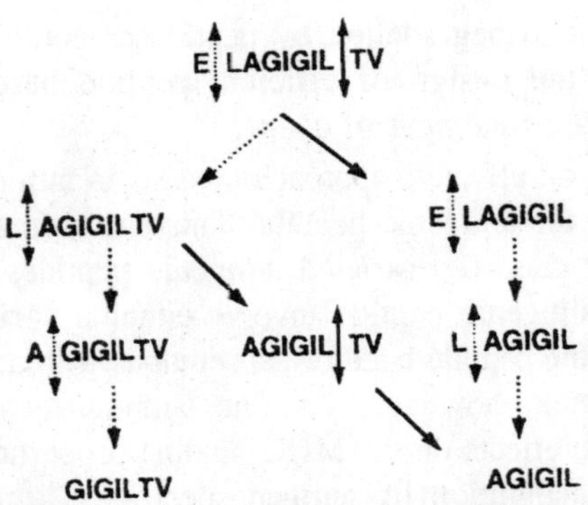

Fig. 8.1. Degradation model of Melan-A$_{26\text{-}35}$ A27L antigenic peptide.

ends of the peptide was explored by acetylation and amidation, respectively. Peptides with backbone modifications such as reduced or retro-inverso peptide bonds were also synthesised. Finally, substitutions of peptide residues by non-natural amino acids such as the D series amino acids, β-amino acids, cyclic amino acids, N-hdroxylated amino acids or methylated amino acids (NMe-amino acids or αMe amino acids) were also investigated.

Although the introduction of one structural modification in only one of the sensitive peptide bonds does not significantly improve the half-life of the peptide in human serum, most of the structural modifications were efficient to locally protect the peptide against peptidase. The short half-life of the mono-protected analogues was related to the degradation of the non-protected end of the peptide. We have shown that only the analogues carrying both amino- and carboxy-terminal modifications of the peptide were fully protected against degradation and display a remarkable stability in the serum with a half-life superior to 24 hours, compared to 2 minutes for the natural peptide. Not all the structural modifications were efficient to locally protect the peptide against peptidase activities. We have found that the amidation of the carboxy terminal end of the peptide were not fully protective against the degradation. The doubly protected analogues with amidated C-terminal ends display a half-life between 11 to 20 hours. This result confirms previous observations showing that the Angiotensin Converting Enzyme (ACE), the most abundant di-peptidylcarboxy peptidase in the serum, was able to cleave peptide with amidated carboxy-terminal ends.

Structural modifications of antigenic peptide could have a negative impact on its immunological properties. The first important biological property affected by structural modifications of the antigenic peptide is its binding to MHC molecules. We have shown that most of the structural modifications of MelanA$_{26-35}$ A27L have a negative effect on the MHC binding properties of the antigen. Not surprisingly, this could occur even when the MHC non-anchor residues are modified. In case of the amino- and carboxy-modified analogues, the negative effects of the modifications are always additive. Structural modifications could modify the peptide ability to fit properly the MHC peptide-binding groove. For example, methylated or cyclic residues could increase the steric hindrance. Other studies indicate that the peptide backbone flexibility could be reduced by the introduction of retro-inverso or reduced peptide bonds.

Molecular modeling of the non-natural analogues in the MHC binding groove indicates that the hydrogen bond network between MHC residues and the peptide backbone or the peptide ends could be disturbed. In rare cases, structural modifications of the peptide could have a positive impact on MHC binding. Indeed, non-natural antigenic peptides including structural modifications such as β-amino acid or N-hydroxylation have been shown to display a better affinity for the MHC compared to the unmodified peptide. In our study, the introduction of β-amino acid or N-hydroxylation within the first peptide bond of the MelanA$_{26-35}$ A27L peptide did not significantly change binding to HLA-A*0201. We have also shown that other structural modifications such as α-, or N-methylation of appropriate residues in the peptide sequence have minimal effects on the MHC binding properties of the non-natural analogues. We have identified MelanA$_{26-35}$ A27L non-natural analogues bearing both amino- and carboxy-terminal structural modifications with MHC binding properties very similar to the unmodified peptide. In addition to the MHC binding affinity, the peptide-MHC complex stability could also be considered to determine if the non-natural analogues could be efficiently presented by the MHC.

The second aspect of the antigenicity that could be impaired by structural modification of antigenic peptides is the efficiency of recognition by specific T cells. After normalizing the efficiency of T cell recognition to the change in binding to MHC, non-natural analogues could be recognised in very different ways by the T cell receptor. Previous studies, including ours, reported that non-natural antigens with reduced peptide bond, although showing similar or improved binding to MHC, were poorly recognised by antigen specific T cell clones. Other studies have shown that recognition of the non-natural analogues could be clone specific depending on the region of the peptide recognised by each clone, illustrating how the peptide backbone and structural modifications of nonanchor residues could modify the shape adopted by the peptide in the MHC binding groove and ultimately affect the recognition by the specific T cell receptor.

Fortunately, in some cases, structurally modified antigenic peptides can be recognised efficiently by antigen specific T cells. In our studies, we have identified amino and carboxy-modified analogues of $MelanA_{26-35}$ A27L that were efficiently recognised by a Melan-A specific T cell line. We have shown that the non-natural peptides bearing α-methylation, N-hydroxylation or β-amino acid were recognised by the Melan-A specific T cells within a concentration range similar to that of the non-modified peptide in cytolytic assay. Thus a stepwise approach to design the non-natural analogues of $MelanA_{26-35}$ A27L allows the identification of fully protected peptides against peptidases with a binding to the MHC and a recognition by the Melan-A specific T cells similar to the non-modified peptide.

However, even when they are efficiently recognised by antigen specific T cells, the non-natural analogues can yet trigger T cell effector functions different from those triggered by the native antigenic peptide. Thus, structural modification of the antigenic peptide could have profound effects on the functional properties of the antigen, and the effector functions of the antigen specific T cells recognising the non-natural analogue must be carefully checked.

An essential requirement for their use as therapeutic agents is that the non-natural peptide analogues must be able to induce an efficient antigen specific immunity after vaccination mediating recognition and elimination of tumor cells expressing the antigen. The immunogenicity of the non-natural analogues resistant to peptidase degradation was initially tested *in vitro*. Using the ELISpot method, a previous study described the cross-reactivity of T cells induced by $Melan\text{-}A_{27-35}$ non-natural analogues with the non-modified peptide. In our study, we used HLA-A*0201/$MelanA_{26-35}$ A27L tetramers to quantify the number of Melan-A specific cells induced after *in vitro* stimulation of PBMC from healthy donors with the structurally modified analogues. We showed that amino- and carboxy-modified analogues, efficiently presented by the MHC and recognised by the antigen specific T cells, were able to induce the expansion of Melan-A specific cells from PBMC of healthy individuals. Three $MelanA_{26-35}$ A27L protease resistant analogues induced a higher number of Melan-A specific cells than the non-modified peptide, indicating that protection against proteolysis could significantly enhance the *in vitro* immunogenicity of the antigenic peptide.

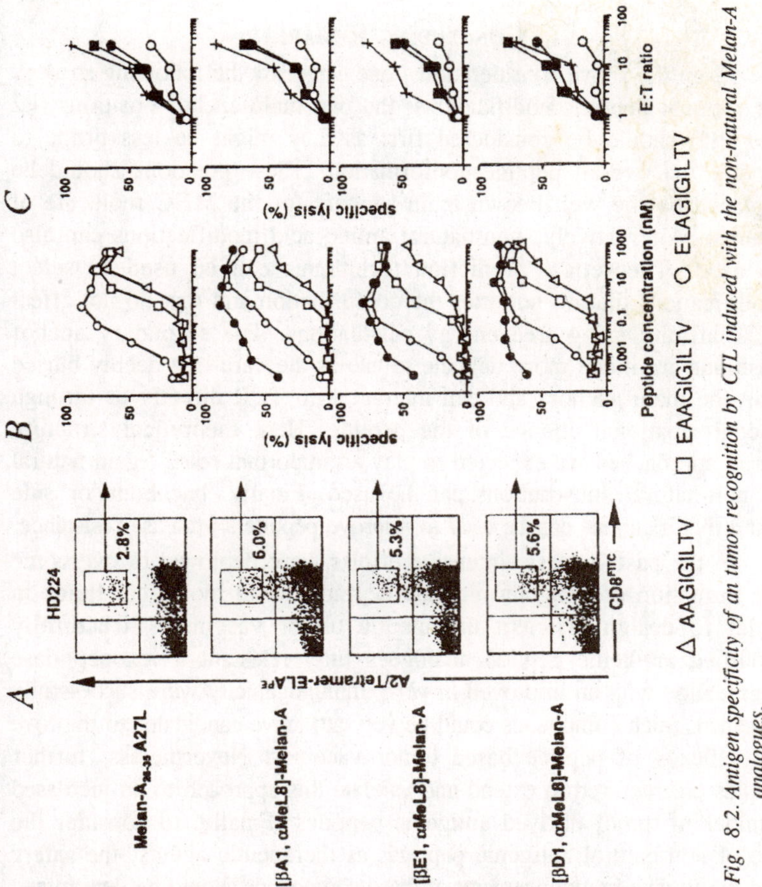

Fig. 8.2. Antigen specificity of an tumor recognition by CTL induced with the non-natural Melan-A analogues.

More importantly, the Melan-A specific $CD8^+$ T cells induced by stimulation with some of the protease resistant Melan-A peptide analogues were also able to recognise not only the unmodified $MelanA_{26-35}$ A27L peptide, but also $MelanA_{26-35}$ or $MelanA_{27-35}$ native peptides. Finally, the Melan-A specific T cells induced by the non-natural Melan-A analogues showed robust cytolytic activity against Melan-A expressing melanoma tumor cell lines, indicating their ability to recognise the Melan-A antigen naturally processed and expressed by tumor cells. The immunogenicity of structurally modified antigenic peptides has been also shown *in vivo*. Indeed, immunization of mice with antigenic pseudopeptides with reduced bonds induced a native antigen-specific immune response and conferred a better resistance against lethal challenge with tumor cells expressing the target antigen.

Concluding Remark

From the above considerations, one can draw the following strategy for rational peptide modifications; the two main anchor positions (P2 and PΩ) should be considered first as they might be less prone to modify the overall peptide conformation. These positions should be replaced by the well known main anchors for the MHC molecule of interest. Alternatively, non-natural amino acid modifications can also be used. Theoretical prediction techniques can be used to select modifications that do not alter the conformation and that do not affect TCR affinity using free energy calculations. The secondary anchor positions are much more delicate to use as they are less deeply buried than the main anchors and can interact with TCR directly or through a conformational change of the peptide. Here theoretical structure based approaches are expected to play an important role. Again natural or non-natural substitutions can be used. Finally, backbone or side chain modifications can be used to improve peptide's protease resistance.

In the past 7 years, intensive efforts were deployed to overcome the limitation of antigenic peptide degradation in biological fluids in order to design efficient therapeutic tumor vaccines. Structurally modified antigenic peptide analogues fully resistant to exopeptidase degradation with an improved *in vitro* immunogenicity were successfully designed. Such compounds could be very attractive candidates to improve the efficacy of peptide based tumor vaccines. Nevertheless, further studies are required to extend and validate this approach to an increased number of tumor derived antigenic peptides. Finally, to consider the use of non-natural antigenic peptides as therapeutic agents, the safety and the *in vivo* immunogenicity of these compounds should be determined more precisely in clinical studies. It can be anticipated that such stable peptides should be carefully confined in such way that they selectively reach mature professional antigen presenting cells. The risks of inducing tolerance when delivery of immunogenic peptides allows prolonged systemic persistence has been demonstrated in an animal model. In summary, any peptide modification should be followed by both MHC binding assays and analysis of the CTL fine specificity of recognition for a large panel of clones. Some modifications might abrogate recognition by some of the TCR but not by others as the affected part of the epitope might be more or less important for each individual TCR. Tinkering with nature offers many opportunities but it should be carefully monitored and the many variants of natural peptides should undergo a rigorous, experimentally driven selection process.

9

MULTIMODALITY THERAPY

There has been a long-standing interest in manipulating the immune system for cancer treatment. Our evolving understanding of the fundamental principles of tumor immunology has accelerated the clinical development of cancer vaccines. A number of small cancer vaccine trials documented the induction of tumor-specific T cells in some patients, with some promising evidence of clinical response. Despite these encouraging early results, larger clinical trials testing cancer vaccines as a single intervention in patients with advanced cancers have been generally disappointing. Furthermore, while few trials have incorporated cancer vaccines directly into or in sequence with combined modality therapy, current data suggest that standard chemotherapy regimens can significantly curtail the vaccine-mediated induction of antitumor immunity. Here we review the development of *granulocyte-macrophage colony-stimulating factor* (GM-CSF)-secreting cell-based cancer vaccines in the context of these observations. Integrating these vaccines into standard cancer treatments should minimize the deleterious impact of tumor burden, and the negative influences of both pre-existing tumor-specific immune tolerance and the combined modality treatment regimens themselves. Moreover, carefully elucidating the pharmacodynamic interactions between traditional cancer treatment modalities and cancer vaccines in clinically relevant, preclinical models can identify novel combinatorial strategies with the potential for augmenting vaccine-activated, tumor-specific immunity. The scientific rationale underlying the development of future clinical trials should be based on both preclinical and clinical data in order to maximize the information gained, and to facilitate the development of the most effective vaccination regimens for incorporation into clinical practice.

A significant focus of therapeutic cancer research over the last twenty years has been to develop the optimal combination of the traditional cancer treatment modalities, including surgery, radiation therapy, and drug-based therapies. Although optimal combined modality treatment can cure a significant percentage of leukemias and lymphomas, it is generally less effective against the solid tumors. The efficacy of combined modality therapy in solid malignancies is generally regarded to be primarily limited by a therapeutic drug resistance inherent to the tumor cell, and to a lesser extent by the collateral damage to normal tissues conferred by the imprecise specificity of radiation therapy and cytotoxic chemotherapy. This has led to increasing enthusiasm for the development of highly targeted treatment approaches that either disrupt the regulatory pathways that promote transformation and metastasis, or specifically deliver a therapeutic hit by targeting the drug to a structural phenotype specific to the cancer cell. Immunotherapy represents a unique biologically targeted treatment approach potentially capable of circumventing mechanisms of intrinsic therapeutic resistance by marshalling the patient's own immune system to reject the tumor. Intensive research both in applied biotechnology and molecular immunology has converged to facilitate the development of cancer vaccines as the fourth major cancer treatment modality, and a number of initial Phase II and III trials have suggested the promise of active immunization for cancer treatment. When combined with the three historical treatment strategies, tumor vaccines offer the added value of exquisite tumor specificity, minimal systemic toxicity, and a persistent and durable antitumor effect by virtue of immunologic memory. Despite these advantages, the efficacy of tumor vaccines is also potentially limited by the magnitude of the tumor burden, vigorous pre-established mechanisms of tumor-specific immune tolerance, and the potential antigenic plasticity of the tumor cells themselves. Here we focus on the development of GM-CSF-secreting cellular cancer vaccines, and review approaches for integrating these vaccines with the traditional treatment modalities of surgery, radiation, and drug-based therapies in additive or synergistic treatment regimens that maximize the efficacy and minimize the limitations of each individual therapeutic approach.

Genetically Modified GM-CSF-Secreting Tumor Cell Vaccines

Genetically modified granulocyte-macrophage colony-stimulating factor (GM-CSF)-secreting tumor vaccines represent an innovative cell-based cancer vaccine platform capable of activating immunity specific for solid tumors historically considered to be inherently non-immunogenic. An early systematic analysis compared the ability of a variety of cytokines (including IL1, IL2, IL4, IL5, IL6, GM-CSF, IFNγ, and TNFα) delivered to poorly immunogenic B16F10 melanoma cells by retroviral transduction to effect tumor rejection. GM-CSF clearly stood out as the most potent inducer of an antitumor immune response capable of mediating tumor rejection in animals with small burdens of pre-established tumors. GM-CSF secretion at the vaccine inoculation site recruits and activates dendritic cells to take up and process antigen delivered by the tumor vaccine cells, cross-priming an effective antigen-specific immune response dependent on $CD4^+$ T helper type 1 and 2 cells as well as $CD8^+$ cytotoxic T cells.

Dose-finding studies have suggested that increasing the number of tumor cells delivered, and thus the quantity of tumor antigen, augments the induction of antitumor immunity. The concentration of GM-CSF in relation to tumor cells is also important, with a minimum of 35 ng of GM-CSF/10^6 cells/24 hours for 4 to 5 days after inoculation *in vivo* required for the effective induction of antitumor immunity. The paracrine secretion of GM-CSF induces cellular infiltrates at the inoculation site that consist of predominantly macrophages, dendritic cells, and eosinophils up to three days after vaccination, evolving to mature lymphocytes and eosinophils at day seven. These latter three observations thus establish the base-line parameters for designing and evaluating clinical trials testing GM-CSF secreting cancer vaccines alone and combined with other cancer treatment modalities.

Promising results in preclinical studies prompted the clinical testing of both autologous and allogeneic GM-CSF-secreting tumor vaccines as a single therapeutic intervention in patients with metastatic renal cell carcinoma, metastatic melanoma, metastatic prostate carcinoma, and early or advanced non-small cell carcinoma of the lung. These initial trials established the safety of the vaccination strategy, and provided clinical validation of the relevance of antigen dose, level of GM-CSF secretion, and the cellular infiltrates at the vaccination site. The most recent clinical trials of GM-CSF-secreting cancer vaccines have tested treatment regimens that integrate these tumor vaccines into standard treatment modalities. The first reported clinical trial of GM-CSF-secreting tumor vaccines integrated with combined modality therapy for the treatment of pancreatic cancer was conducted by Jaffee and colleagues. They conducted a dose escalation trial testing a mixture of two allogeneic pancreatic carcinoma cell lines secreting GM-CSF at levels of 220 ng/10^6 cells/24 hours in patients with Stage II or Stage III pancreatic cancer after pancreaticoduodenectomy. Patients were initially vaccinated immediately after surgery and just prior to adjuvant chemoradiation. Those who remained disease-free after six months of aggressive adjuvant chemoradiation were eligible to receive an additional three monthly vaccinations. This study identified 5×10^8 vaccine cells (the highest dose tested) as a safe and bioactive vaccine cell dose for testing in future trials. Four of five patients who received this dose developed serum levels of GM-CSF that recapitulated the pharmacokinetics observed in preclinical models. No patient treated at lower vaccine dose levels developed detectable levels of serum GM-CSF.

Clinically significant *delayed type hypersensitivity* (DTH) responses (≥ 1.0 cm) to dissociated autologous pancreatic tumor cells developed after the first vaccination in 1 of 3 and 2 of 4 patients who received 1×10^8 and 5×10^8 vaccine cells respectively. These 3 patients remained free of disease for over 2 years, suggesting a potential survival benefit. A Phase II trial of similar design to evaluate the efficacy of the integrated treatment regimen is now in active accrual. In the aggregate, these trials have demonstrated the safety of GM-CSF-secreting vaccines, with side effects limited primarily to local erythema and induration at the inoculation sites.

While they have provided encouraging preliminary evidence of bioactivity, they have also more clearly defined the challenges facing the effective clinical development of cancer vaccines. These include the hurdle posed by established tumor burdens, the barrier of pre-existing tumor-specific immune tolerance, the potential plasticity of the antigenic profile displayed by the tumor as it continues to evolve, and the impact of standard cancer therapy on vaccine-activated immunity. As discussed below, integrating tumor vaccines appropriately with traditional treatment modalities can potentially surmount each of these obstacles to the efficacy of tumor immunotherapy, thereby maximizing the antitumor immune response.

Challenges in Cancer Vaccine Development

The magnitude of the tumor burden is the first significant influence on the development of antitumor immunity. When tumors are small, they grow without accessing peripheral lymphoid tissues and are essentially ignored by the immune system. The tumor thus "*sneaks through*" immune surveillance at its earliest stages. Once it has reached sufficient size, the tumor invades local lymphoid tissue. This initiates an interaction with the immune system relatively late in tumor development. At this stage immune-mediated tumor rejection is determined by the relative balance between the growth kinetics and physical burden of the tumor cells compared to the intensity and diversity of the induced effector T cell response. Superimposed on this imbalance, tumor cells employ several strategies to evade the developing immune response. Tumor cells can elaborate inhibitory cytokines (interleukin 10, transforming growth factor-β(TGF-β), and prostaglandin E_2) that inhibit the function of tumor infiltrating T lymphocytes (TIL). They can also express surface fasL (CD95L), thus inducing the apoptosis of TIL engaged by the tumor cells.

Tumor-specific immune tolerance represents the second major barrier to the effectiveness of cancer vaccines. Vaccination for the prevention of infectious diseases sets the stage for a vigorous antigen-specific immune response capable of rejecting an exogenous infectious challenge. In contrast, tumor cells arise endogenously. Thus, with the exception of *de novo* genetic mutations, most tumor antigens are recognized as self. This typically results in either the central thymic deletion of those components of the T cell repertoire with the highest affinity for tumor-specific antigens, or their peripheral deletion by *activation-induced cell death* (AICD) in the setting of widely disseminated tumor. However, the process of thymic selection is imperfect, and allows the emigration of T cells that recognize self antigen with low avidity or by virtue of specificity for a cryptic antigenic epitope not commonly seen by the immune system.

This latent population of T cells may be activated under the appropriate conditions to exert potent antigen-specific immunity. Additionally, tumor cells do not evolve to present antigen effectively, and are typically detected by the immune system in the absence of an associated inflammatory response. These two factors lead to the presentation of tumor antigens in the absence of the costimulatory signals critical for immune activation, thereby rendering potentially responsive T cells unresponsive or anergic. Further, the compartmentalization of tumor antigens away from the immune system either by expression restricted to embryologic development or immunologically privileged sites, or by extremely low levels of antigen expression, can result in the peaceful coexistence of tumor and tumor-specific T cells that simply fail to see their target. If T cells are activated, a phenotypically skewed cytokine/chemokine receptor profile can render them functionally impotent by virtue of cytokine deviation and aberrant trafficking. Finally, novel subsets of dendritic cells and regulatory T cells have recently been characterized. These can down-regulate the antigen-specific immune response, resulting in immune tolerance rather than immune activation. Thoroughly dissecting the impact of these diverse mechanisms of immune tolerance on the tumor-specific T cell repertoire available for therapeutic manipulation should facilitate the development of innovative combinatorial vaccination strategies for overcoming them.

The third challenge for effective tumor immunotherapy is the diversity and plasticity of the antigen expression profile of tumors themselves. Tumors can down-regulate the expression of tumor antigens targeted by an antigen-specific vaccine or therapeutic antibody, resulting in the outgrowth of antigen loss variants resistant to the therapeutic intervention. The use of highly defined antigen-specific cancer vaccines is further limited by the fact that only a few tumor antigens are likely to represent true tumor rejection targets. Tumor rejection antigens are defined as antigens preferentially associated with a cancer cell that elicit an effective immune response capable of causing clinically meaningful tumor regression.

The distinction between tumor antigens capable of eliciting an immune response and those that elicit an immune response that translates into a clinical response are well illustrated by studies of the natural and vaccine-induced immune responses in melanoma patients. Many patients have significant numbers of functional cytotoxic effector T cells specific for the melanoma antigens MART-1/Melan-A or gp100, but their disease continues to progress. Moreover, the numbers of antigen-specific T cells in these patients can be augmented with targeted vaccines, but this does not influence the immunodynamics of the antitumor response in a clinically meaningful way. Adding further complexity to the host-tumor interaction, tumors can also down-regulate multiple components of the antigen-processing machinery, including MHC Class I and Class II molecules, different proteosome subunits, and the TAP transporter. Importantly, these altered antigen-processing phenotypes have been found to correlate with poor clinical outcome.

These fundamental principles of tumor immunology can be combined with the lessons of traditional drug development to guide both the preclinical and clinical development of cancer vaccines. It is clear from the principles discussed above and the results of clinical cancer vaccine trials to date that cancer vaccines as a single treatment modality are not likely to have the potency required to overcome immune tolerance and surmount the tumor burden present in patients with established disease. Moreover, traditional drug development typically calls for early clinical testing in heavily pretreated patients with extensive disease. Both a greater number of prior chemotherapy regimens and close proximity to a prior chemotherapy treatment was recently demonstrated to limit the induction of carcinoembryonic antigen (CEA)-specific T cell prescursors in patients with advanced colorectal carcinoma treated with the canary pox vaccine ALVAC-CEA. Additionally, the serial ELISPOT analysis of post-vaccination, antigen-specific $CD8^+$ T cell responses of patients treated on the Phase I trial testing the integration of a GM-CSF-secreting pancreatic cancer vaccine with adjuvant chemoradiation also demonstrated the detrimental effect of close proximity to a prior chemotherapy treatment on vaccine-induced immune responses.

The mismatch between tumor growth kinetics and the intensity of the vaccine-induced antitumor response achievable with current vaccination regimens is a strong argument for testing vaccine therapy in patients with minimal or undetectable disease after standard therapy. However, our own experience and the results of the ALVAC-CEA trial suggest that the potential negative impact of some standard treatment modalities on the potency of cancer vaccines must also be considered. The scientifically based sequencing of tumor vaccines with surgery, radiation therapy, chemotherapy, and biologically targeted therapy is thus a critical aspect of clinical cancer vaccine development that should be determined in relevant preclinical models when possible.

Immunomodulatory Effects of Chemotherapy

In cancer treatment, chemotherapy agents have been historically used for their direct cytotoxic activity on tumor cells. However, novel approaches to the use of chemotherapy have revealed that some drugs also have dose- and sequence-specific antiangiogenic or immunomodulatory effects. The frequent administration of Cyclophosphamide, Paclitaxel, Doxorubicin, or Vinblastine at very low doses (so-called metronomic administration) preferentially targets the tumor vasculature compared to tumor cells. Additionally, many chemotherapeutic agents (including Cyclophosphamide, the taxanes (Paclitaxel and Docetaxel), Doxorubicin, Melphalan, Gemcitabine and 5'-aza-2'-Deoxycytidine) can either potentiate or antagonize an antigen-specific immune response depending on the drug dose and timing in relation to an antigen exposure. Here we review the immunomodulatory activities of these drugs in the framework of their impact on the antigen-specific immune response, existing mechanisms of tumor-specific immune tolerance, the tumor microenvironment, and tumor antigen expression profile of the tumor itself.

Chemotherapy and the Adaptive Immune Response

At standard doses, many chemotherapeutic drugs clearly suppress cellular immune responses; these include Cyclophosphamide, Paclitaxel, Gemcitabine, and Doxorubicin. Cyclophosphamide in particular has been widely used for its immunosuppressive effects in the treatment of autoimmune disease. Importantly, the timing of administration in relation to drug exposure is a critical determinant of the ensuing immune response. The humoral response to an antigenic challenge is markedly enhanced if Cyclophosphamide is given one to three days prior to antigen exposure. Similarly, treatment of animals with Doxorubicin three to five days prior to antigen exposure enhances the induction of adaptive cell-mediated immunity, likely by modulating cells of the monocyte/macrophage lineage. In contrast, administering Cyclophosphamide at the time of antigen exposure abrogates the primary antigen-specific humoral immune response in guinea pigs exposed to ovalbumin. Re-challenge of these same animals three months later again failed to induce an antigen-specific antibody response, although the animals did develop significant antibody titers to an unrelated antigen. This observation suggests that the simultaneous administration of Cyclophosphamide with antigen induces antigen-specific immune tolerance. Cyclophosphamide has a similar impact on the induction of contact hypersensitivity, a manifestation of cellular immunity.

In addition to modulating the induction of immunity to new antigens, Cyclophosphamide can also break both natural and acquired immune tolerance. For example, animals challenged with either syngeneic or autologous testicular cells develop significant *delayed type hypersensitivity* (DTH) reactions consistent with adaptive cellular immunity only if the challenge is preceded by Cyclophosphamide administration. Similarly, the treatment of mice with palpable MOPC-315 plasmacytomas initiates immune-mediated tumor rejection in 92% of animals, with cured mice retaining the ability to reject a subsequent MOPC-315 tumor challenge. The effect of Cyclophosphamide was abrogated by prior immunosuppression, and markedly diminished in mice with nonpalpable tumor burdens (a tumor rejection rate of 10%), arguing for the importance of pre-existing antitumor immunity in tumor rejection. Cyclophosphamide, Paclitaxel, and Melphalan can also promote a therapeutic balance between T helper type 1 and T helper type 2 lymphocytes. As discussed below, we have found that both Cyclophosphamide and Paclitaxel treatment one day prior to an antigen-specific vaccination can reverse immunologic skew, favoring the development of antigen-specific T helper type 1 antitumor immunity capable of orchestrating the delay of tumor outgrowth in a tolerogenic murine model of breast cancer. Cyclophosphamide has also been reported to upregulate type I interferons, an observation that has been associated with the development of T helper type 1 immunity and ultimately correlated with an augmented production of $CD44^{high}$ memory T lymphocytes in the treated mice. Cyclophosphamide is also thought to abrogate regulatory T cell activity, although most of this data was generated prior to the resurgence of interest in suppressor T cell populations as they are currently defined.

The impact of Gemcitabine on adaptive immune responses is perhaps the least studied. Importantly, it has been reported to abrogate the humoral antigen-specific immune response. The administration of five doses of gemcitabine (120 μg/g every three days) to hemagglutinin (HA) T cell receptor transgenic mice completely abrogates HA-specific IgG responses in the context of a minimal to moderate augmentation of HA-specific T cell proliferation. We have found that Gemcitabine potently inhibits vaccine-induced T cell immunity. Gemcitabine may thus be a chemotherapeutic agent to avoid in combinatorial cancer vaccination regimens.

In summary, multiple chemotherapeutic agents significantly impact the adaptive immune response. Whether the influence is positive or negative depends largely on the agent under consideration, the dose given, and the timing of administration of the drug in relation to antigen exposure. These observations taken together argue for the careful pharmacodynamic analysis of cancer vaccines and chemotherapeutic agents in clinically relevant preclinical models rather than the simple addition of a vaccine to a treatment regimen considered to be the standard of care.

Chemotherapy and the Tumor Microenvironment

Chemotherapy can also modulate the tumor microenvironment, either discouraging or promoting the development of an effective antitumor immune response. The preferential antiangiogenic effect of metronomic chemotherapy could physically disrupt access to the tumor by the immune system, thus abrogating the efficacy of existing tumor-specific immunity. Furthermore, when integrated directly with active, specific immunotherapy, the metronomic scheduling is likely to inhibit the induction of antitumor immunity due to sequencing effects. Alternatively, chemotherapy can augment tumor-specific immune responses by inhibiting the secretion of immunosuppressive cytokines by the tumor, or by upregulating tumor cell expression of costimulatory molecules for effective antigen presentation. For example, Bleomycin has been shown to inhibit the production of tumor-derived TGF-β, thus partially abrogating the negative effect of the tumor cells themselves in the developing immune response.

Melphalan can induce the secretion of tumor necrosis factor-α (TNF-α) by tumor cells, thereby facilitating the development of a cytotoxic $CD8^+$ T cell response. The mechanism of TNF-α upregulation was more recently characterized, and was found to be dependent on the early production of interferon-β. This is reminiscent of the influence of Cyclophosphamide on the type I interferons discussed above. It is potentially important given the promotion of the T helper type I cytokine response by the type I interferons that is known to be critical for an effective antitumor response. Melphalan also upregulates the expression of both B7-1 and B7-2 in MOPC-315 tumor cells and host cells; a similar effect was demonstrated in P815 plasmacytoma cells. Importantly, both Mitomycin C and γ-irradiation can also upregulate B7-1. This suggests that some chemotherapeutic agents and/or radiation therapy could potentiate the induction of antitumor immunity by upregulating critical costimulatory molecules, thereby rendering the tumor cells themselves more effective antigen presenting cells.

Other cytotoxic drugs (Doxorubicin, 5-Fluorouracil, Gemcitabine, and Paclitaxel) and γ-irradiation can modify the tumor microenvironment by inducing tumor cell apoptosis, potentially enhancing antigen presentation. Importantly, several groups have successfully combined apoptosis-inducing chemotherapy or γ-irradiation with intratumoral dendritic cell administration to induce effective antitumor immunity. Paclitaxel, which is known to upregulate proapoptotic molecules and phosphorylate bcl-2, is of particular interest. Clinically, the degree of induction of apoptosis and mitotic arrest after one cycle of neoadjuvant Paclitaxel treatment was demonstrated to predict therapeutic response in women with locally advanced breast cancer. Further, the first dose apoptotic response correlated with the development of TIL in 67% of patients with clinical complete responses and pathologic residual disease. In contrast, only 25% of patients with a clinical partial response developed TIL. In addition to its potent apoptotic effects, Paclitaxel also has a variety of immunomodulatory activities. Paclitaxel is known to efficiently mobilize peripheral blood stem cells, likely through inducing GM-CSF secretion by macrophages and B cells. Thus, Paclitaxel may increase antigen presenting cells and cytotoxic T cells for participation in the induction of antitumor immunity, while simultaneously creating a potent source of tumor antigen in the form of apoptotic bodies produced due to the cytotoxic effect of the drug. Importantly, vigorous apoptosis itself can induce dendritic cell maturation. This process could be further facilitated by the lipopolysaccharide-mimetic effect of Paclitaxel, which results in the secretion of the pro-inflammatory factors interleukin 1β (IL1β), GM-CSF, TNFα, *nitric oxide* (NO), and interleukin 12 (IL12).

The demethylating agents represent a novel class of chemotherapeutic drugs that exert an antitumor effect by promoting cellular differentiation. The drugs function by facilitating the re-expression of genes under active transcriptional repression as the result of methylation of important transcriptional regulatory regions. Importantly, restoring the expression of MHC Class I and cancer testis antigens by pretreating tumor cells with the demethylating agent 5'-aza-2'-Deoxycytidine *in vitro* can restore melanoma- and renal cell carcinoma-specific CTL activity. These results suggest that treatment of tumors *in vivo* with demethylating agents could circumvent the development of MHC Class I and antigen loss variants that sometimes underlie the failure of antigen-specific immunotherapy.

GM-CSF-Secreting Cancer Vaccines and Multimodality Therapy

Given the cytoreductive and immunomodulatory potential of many anticancer drugs, the integration of these agents and GM-CSF-secreting vaccines for the treatment of locally advanced or metastatic cancer holds great appeal. Chemotherapeutic agents are commonly used for their cytotoxic effects, and are clearly immunosuppressive at standard doses. However, some can also either augment or reduce antigen-specific immune responses, depending on the drug dose and timing of administration in relation to the antigen exposure. Furthermore, emerging data suggests that therapeutic monoclonal antibodies could synergize with active vaccination by recruiting innate immune effectors. Two areas that clearly warrant further investigation are thus the integration of GM-CSF-secreting vaccines with traditional chemotherapy, and the integration of these vaccines with therapeutic, monoclonal antibody-based therapy.

Chemotherapy as a Vaccine Adjuvant for GM-CSF-secreting Vaccines

The sequencing of chemotherapy and GM-CSF-secreting tumor vaccines can be considered in the context of chemotherapy as a vaccine adjuvant, or in the context of the altered host environment created by autologous or allogeneic bone marrow transplantation and other types of lymphoablative therapy. The use of low to standard dose chemotherapy as a vaccine adjuvant has been examined in two preclinical models. In the first, a variety of chemotherapeutic agents was tested in sequence with a GM-CSF-secreting CT26 colon carcinoma whole cell vaccine in BALB/c mice.

In this nontolerogenic system, Cyclophosphamide (50–250 mg/kg) given one or two weeks prior to vaccination failed to increase the induction of CT26-specific $CD8^+$ cytotoxic T cells, whereas the drug given at the time of or subsequent to vaccination abrogated vaccine activity. Conversely, Doxorubicin (2–6 mg/kg) given one week prior to vaccine prevented immune induction, whereas similar doses given at the time of or subsequent to vaccination augmented CT26-specific $CD8^+$ T cell immunity. Vaccination followed by Doxorubicin treatment protected mice from a lethal CT26 tumor challenge, and cured 40% of mice with established tumor burdens. Doxorubicin alone cured 10% of such mice, whereas Cyclophosphamide plus vaccination or vaccination alone cured between 30–35% of tumor-bearing mice. Other chemotherapeutic agents tested in this system, including Vincristine, Vinblastine, Etoposide, Methotrexate, 5-Fluorouracil, Cytarabine, Cisplatinum, and Dexamethasone clearly reduced vaccine efficacy.

Because the CT26 model system is not characterized by antigen-specific immune tolerance, we extended these studies to the *neu* transgenic mouse. These mice are one of the most clinically relevant preclinical models for evaluating combinatorial immunotherapy regimens. Due to MMTV-driven expression of the protooncogene *neu*, the mice spontaneously develop *neu*-expressing breast cancers histologically similar to those of patients, and have a pre-established *neu*-specific immune tolerance. The impact of *neu*-specific immune tolerance on vaccine-activated immunity is profound. Whereas parental FVB/N mice vigorously reject *neu*-expressing tumors in response to *neu*-targeted, GM-CSF-secreting vaccination, *neu* transgenic mice have at best a tepid antitumor response to the vaccine. In fact, tumor outgrowth rates are similar in *neu* mice who receive a mock vaccine and those who receive a *neu*-targeted, GM-CSF-secreting vaccine. Importantly, giving the vaccine in sequence with some chemotherapeutic drugs can partially overcome tolerance, and enhance vaccine efficacy in *neu* mice. Both parental FVB/N mice and tolerized *neu* transgenic mice demonstrate a more robust tumor rejection response to a *neu*-targeted, GM-CSF-secreting cellular vaccine preceded by either Cyclophosphamide (100 mg/kg) or Paclitaxel (20 mg/kg) one day prior to vaccination compared to vaccine alone. Similar to observations in the CT26 system, sequencing the vaccine with Doxorubicin (5–8 mg/kg) seven days later also resulted in an enhanced antitumor response, but only in the *neu* mice. Underscoring the importance of drug dose, the positive interaction between drug and vaccine diminished with nadiring T cell counts.

Recapitulating previous observations, reversing the order of Cyclophosphamide, Paclitaxel, or Doxorubicin inhibited vaccine activity. Cisplatinum was not observed to have a positive interaction with the vaccine in *neu* transgenic mice. The activity of the drugs as a vaccine adjuvant was suggested by their ability to enhance the rejection of a subsequent tumor challenge, and confirmed by the documentation of augmented *neu*-specific T helper type 1 cellular responses by ELISPOT with combinatorial therapy compared with vaccine alone. A combination chemoimmunotherapy regimen including specifically timed Cyclophosphamide, vaccine, and Doxorubicin demonstrated the greatest potency, curing pre-existing tumor burdens in up to 30% of tolerized mice. A Phase I clinical trial testing timed sequential therapy with Cyclophosphamide, Doxorubicin, and a GM-CSF-secreting allogeneic cell-based breast cancer vaccine will explore the safety and bioactivity of this approach in patients with metastatic breast cancer. Additional trials testing GM-CSF-secreting vaccines preceded by Cyclophosphamide in patients with metastatic pancreatic cancer or metastatic non-small cell lung cancer are also planned.

GM-CSF-Secreting Vaccines and the Lymphocyte-Depleted Host

Lymphopenia-induced homeostatic T cell proliferation is a recently described mechanism for restoring the memory T cell compartment. Manipulating the T cell repertoire with cancer vaccines during immune reconstitution after lymphoablative treatments might skew the immune system toward a desired antitumor specificity. Consistent with this concept, the selective induction and expansion of functional melanoma-specific T cells was documented in Rag-1-deficient, lymphopenic, tumor-bearing mice in response to a GM-CSF-secreting melanoma vaccine. The presence of this altered T cell repertoire correlated with significant tumor regression. Highlighting the potential clinical relevance of this phenomenon, several preclinical studies have demonstrated that vaccine-induced antitumor immunity can be enhanced by vaccinating tumor-bearing mice with GM-CSF-secreting tumor vaccines during early engraftment after syngeneic or allogeneic T cell-depleted bone marrow transplantation. Furthermore, altering the host microenvironment prior to the transfer of syngeneic tumor-specific T cells with sublethal irradiation in mice can result in an effective antitumor immune response as measured by CTL activity, IFN-γ secretion, and the persistence of memory T cells. The most recent study reported the efficacy of combined modality chemoimmunotherapy in the chemotherapy–resistant 4T1 model of metastatic breast cancer.

Tumor-bearing animals underwent surgical resection, then treatment with a nonmyeloablative allogeneic stem cell transplantation where the conditioning regimen included irradiation and Cyclophosphamide. Subsequent treatment of animals with post-transplant *donor lymphocyte infusions* (DLI) and a tumor vaccine comprised of autologous tumor cells admixed with GM-CSF-secreting bystander cells resulted in potent systemic antitumor immunity capable of curing mice of metastatic mammary tumors. Similar results have been observed with the adoptive transfer of melanoma-specific TIL to patients with metastatic melanoma pretreated with a nonmyeloablative chemotherapy regimen consisting of Cyclophosphamide and Fludarabine.

While the phenomenon of homeostatic proliferation has not yet been rigorously demonstrated in patients, this study suggests that it could be clinically relevant. Since many standard cancer therapies result in lymphopenia, carefully delineating the influence of radiation therapy and/or chemotherapy on the kinetics, persistence, and functional quality of antigen-specific immune reconstitution will be required for the effective application of cancer vaccines to the lymphopenic setting. Clinical trials evaluating the bioactivity of GM-CSF-secreting vaccines administered in the context of autologous or allogeneic bone marrow transplantation in multiple myeloma and acute myelogenous leukemia are currently underway.

GM-CSF-Secreting Vaccines and Therapeutic Monoclonal Antibodies

Combining GM-CSF-secreting vaccines with monoclonal antibody therapy is another promising area for research. Trastuzumab and Rituximab are two monoclonal antibodies that play clear roles in the management of breast cancers and B cell lymphomas, respectively; a number of additional therapeutic monoclonal antibodies are currently in active clinical development. There is emerging data to suggest that humoral immunity may play an important role in antitumor immunity that has not been previously appreciated. For example, we demonstrated that the passive transfer of HER-2/*neu*-specific antibody and HER-2/*neu*-specific CTL results in a more robust antitumor effect than the passive transfer of either alone in the tolerogenic *neu* mouse model of breast cancer. Furthermore, we have also demonstrated that the combination of HER-2/*neu*-specific monoclonal antibodies and a GM-CSF-secreting HER-2/*neu*-targeted vaccine is more effective than either vaccine or monoclonal antibody alone in *neu* transgenic mice. Consistent with these observations, others have shown that humoral and cellular immunity can synergize to mediate the rejection of established lymphomas through a process dependent on $CD8^+$ T cells and $CD11b^+$, Fc-γ receptor-expressing macrophages.

A number of mechanisms for synergism between humoral and cellular immune mediators have been suggested. Trastuzumab can exert an antitumor effect by inhibiting growth-promoting signaling pathways, and could render the tumor cell more sensitive to apoptosis. Like Rituximab, it can also recruit innate immune effectors by functioning as a nidus for the initiation of *antibody-dependent cellular cytotoxicity* (ADCC). Furthermore, Trastuzumab has been recently demonstrated to enhance the lytic activity of MHC Class I restricted, HER-2/*neu*-specific CTL against HER-2-overexpressing breast and ovarian tumor cells. It was proposed that degradation of internalized HER-2/*neu* protein could increase the amount of HER-2/*neu* peptide epitopes available for loading onto MHC Class I molecules, thereby augmenting antigen presentation. Although not directly proven, support for this mechanism is provided by observations that Trastuzumab promotes the ubiquitination and degradation of HER-2/*neu*.

Geldanamycin, an ansamycin antibiotic that also induces the ubiquitination and degradation of HER-2/*neu,* was demonstrated to augment the presentation of HER-2/*neu*-specific peptide epitopes by ovarian carcinoma cells, thereby enhancing the activity of antigen-specific CTL against treated HER-2/*neu*-over-expressing ovarian carcinoma targets. While recruiting innate immune effectors and augmenting antigen presentation are at least two potential mechanisms for the positive interplay between therapeutic monoclonal antibodies and cancer vaccines, potential also exists for antagonism. Rituximab can inhibit the induction of primary and secondary humoral immunity, and can also abrogate the manifestation of antibody-mediated diseases by eliminating both normal and malignant B cells responsible for antibody production. Thus, the integration of cancer vaccines with Rituximab might not be optimal when humoral immunity is thought to play an important role in tumor rejection. Regardless, these observations together demonstrate that integrating cancer vaccines with therapeutic monoclonal antibodies is an area that clearly warrants further research.

CONCLUDING REMARK

Improvements in our understanding of tumor immunology have facilitated significant progress in the development of cancer vaccines. Early clinical trials have generated evidence for the safety of tumor vaccines, and have provided a suggestion of clinically significant bioactivity. They have also highlighted the challenges of cancer vaccine development. These include developing strategies for overcoming immune tolerance, and approaches for identifying the most active tumor rejection antigens for cancer vaccine formulation. Furthermore, these early studies highlight the importance of identifying important pharmacodynamic interactions between standard cancer treatment modalities and tumor vaccines.

Surgical debulking is one approach for minimizing the impact of tumor burden, and patients with minimal residual disease are likely to be the most ideal candidates for vaccine therapy. The impact of chemotherapy on vaccine activity is a developing area of clinical research, with regard to both its positive and negative impact on the development of antigen-specific immunity.

The impact of ionizing radiation on the immune response to cancer vaccines is an underdeveloped area that also warrants further investigation. Finally, the advent of biologically targeted therapies such as the monoclonal antibodies Trastuzumab and Rituximab offer new opportunities for combining cancer vaccines with novel drugs in combinatorial treatment strategies with the potential for significant synergism. It is clear that the careful preclinical and clinical investigation of these issues will guide the most effective clinical testing of cancer vaccines, and facilitate their ultimate incorporation into standard clinical practice.

10

Dendritic Cell-based Vaccine

Dendritic cells (DCs) were initially described in 1973 by Ralph Steinman, who observed in mouse spleen a subpopulation of cells with a striking dendritic morphology. DCs originate from the bone marrow, and their precursors migrate via the bloodstream to almost all organs of the body, where they reside as immature cells with high phagocytic capacity. They *acquire antigens* (Ag) in peripheral tissues and migrate to lymphoid organs where they present processed peptides to naive T cells and initiate the immune response. During this process, DCs lose their Ag-capturing/processing capacity as they differentiate into mature, fully stimulatory, antigen-presenting cells. In addition, DCs interact with B lymphocytes to enhance B cell expansion and antibody production, as well as with *natural killer* (NK) cells to augment cytolytic activity and interferon-γ (IFN-γ) production.

The past 20 years have witnessed a dramatic expansion in the understanding of the relationship between DCs and the cellular immune response. DCs appear to be central to the regulation, maturation, and maintenance of a cellular immune response to cancer. Encouraging results from vaccination studies in animal models and the development of protocols to generate sufficient numbers of human DCs for clinical application have led to the first early-phase clinical trials of DCs for the treatment of cancer in patients. These studies have established the safety and feasibility of this approach and have produced some encouraging evidence of therapeutic efficacy.

This chapter will focus on mouse and human DCs, their generation, as well as selected strategies being pursued to harness their potent antigen-stimulating activity for their use in clinical trials and murine experimental models, and finally highlighting issues for future trial design.

EXPERIMENTAL ANIMAL MODELS

Generation of Murine DCs

Although monocyte-derived DCs are the most commonly used type of human DCs, they are only rarely prepared from mice largely because the yield is small (1×10^5/mouse), and there are other easier methods available to produce murine DCs.

Mouse bone marrow is a major source of DCs when cultivated with *granulocyte-macrophage colony-stimulating factor* (GM-CSF) and interleukin (IL)-4. Most published reports of mouse DCs use cells derived from BALB/c or C57Bl/6 mice. However, there is no reason not to use mice of other genetic backgrounds for certain applications. In general, mice 8–12 weeks old yield sufficient numbers of DCs, precursor and progenitor cells to be easily manipulated. The technique described by Inaba et al. has been modified over the years. Once generated, DCs are collected on day 5 or 6, and enriched by 14.5% (w/v) metrizamide density gradient separation. Further purification can be achieved by FACS sort on CD11b and CD11c, or by using CD11c-coated paramagnetic beads. Typical DC yields are approximately 5×10^6 cells/mouse. Further maturation of DCs can be achieved by LPS or TNF-α treatment.

Progenitor $CD34^+$ cells obtained from mouse bone marrow will differentiate into DCs when cultured with GM-CSF plus the ligand for the receptor tyrosine kinase fms-like tyrosine kinase 3 (Flt-3L). $CD34^+$ cells may be obtained from mouse marrow by depletion of lineage+, nonadherent cells followed by sorting. These cells will differentiate into $CD11c^+CD11b^+$ and $CD11b^-$/dull$CD11c^+$ subsets upon culture with GM-CSF, TNF-α and CSF, which may be sorted by FACS on day 6 for independent culture. Addition of *stem cell factor* (SCF) or Flt-3L to bone marrow cultures increase the yield of DCs ultimately derived, especially when used in combination.

DC-Based Vaccination in Animal Tumor Models

A growing number of studies have reported the successful use of DCs for inducing antitumor immune responses in animals. Most of these experiments have involved in vitro isolation of DCs, followed by pulsing of DCs with different forms of tumor antigen and injection of the antigen-loaded DCs into syngeneic animals as a cancer vaccine. Tumor development was induced by injection of established tumor cell lines of various tissue origins. Following interaction with tumor cells or selected tumor Ags, DCs were effective as prophylactic tumor vaccines against subsequent challenge with the same tumor. Initial approaches using DCs loaded with tumor lysates, tumor antigen-derived peptides, soluble protein tumor antigen expressed by a B cell lymphoma, synthetic class I-MHC-restricted peptides, RNA, DNA and whole protein have all been demonstrated to generate tumor-specific immune responses and antitumor activity against subsequent tumor challenges, and even therapeutic efficacy was reported, leading to the induction of regression of preexisting tumors. Such immunologic and anti-tumor effects depend on additional critical factors, e.g., the route of DC administration. Using vaccination with tyrosinase-related protein-2-derived peptide-loaded, Indium-111-labeled DC vaccination in a fully syngeneic B16 melanoma tumor model, Eggert et al. observed a delay in tumor growth, improved survival, as well as increased antitumor cytotoxic T-cell reactivity after s.c. delivery compared to i.v. delivery. In contrast, a pilot clinical trial, performed by Fong et al., using Ag-pulsed DCs as a tumor vaccine in patients with metastatic prostate cancer suggest that activated DCs can prime T cell immunity regardless of route of administration. However, these investigators reported that the "*quality*" of this response and induction of Ag-specific Abs might be affected by the route of administration.

With these studies providing the "*proof-of-principle*" for Ag-pulsed DC vaccination against cancer with respect to route of administration, recent investigations have focused on discovering more effective methods of delivering tumor Ags to DCs. One strategy has been to use recombinant viruses as a highly efficient means of introducing genes into DCs. Mouse tumor models have extensively been used to test the in vivo therapeutic efficacy of DCs transduced with viral vectors that encode different cytokine cDNAs such as GM-CSF, IL-12, or Flt-3L, immunomodulatory molecules like B7-1, ICAM-1, or LFA-3, or cDNAs encoding for model antigens or TAAs. Studies have addressed the question whether DCs genetically engineered are capable of eliciting antitumor immunity in vivo. Adenovirus-mediated gene delivery into DCs has been studied extensively in murine models since 1997. A number of reports have shown DCs to possess enhanced antitumor properties after adenoviral transfer of therapeutic transgenes. For example, mice immunized with Trp2 gene-transduced DCs were capable of inducing protection against mouse melanoma-induced lung metastasis. Another report showed that DCs infected with adenoviral vectors encoding endogenous TAA expressed by the murine melanoma line B16 could elicit antitumor immunity in this poorly immunogenic tumor model. DCs overexpressing IL-12 as a result of adenoviral-mediated IL-12 gene transfer have been found to induce antitumor immunity when injected directly into tumors. Because of the emerging evidence that chemokines play an important role in the priming of naive T cells by DCs, introduction of chemokine genes into DCs are now being reported as well. For example, a recent study showed that immunization with DCs adenovirally co-transfected with gp100 and lymphotactin, a C chemokine that specifically regulates the migration of T cells and NK cells, could enhance protective and therapeutic antitumor response more effectively in a B16 melanoma model. Our group has studied direct administration of DCs genetically modified to express *secondary lymphoid tissue* chemokine (SLC) into growing B16 melanoma. SLC, a CC chemokine found in high endothelial venules and within the T-cell zones of both spleen and lymph nodes, is capable of recruiting both DCs and naive T cells via the CCR7 receptor found on both cell types. We reported that intratumoral injections of SLC-expressing DCs could result in tumor growth inhibition with a substantial, sustained influx of T cells within the mass.

A long-puzzling phenomenon was the improved efficacy of DNA vaccines containing unmethylated *cytidine-phosphate-guanosine* (CpG) dinucleotide (CpG-ODN) motifs that are common in bacterial DNA but not in mammalian DNA. Synthetic oligodeoxynucleotides containing CpG-ODN in specific sequence contexts mimic the immunostimulatory qualities of bacterial DNA. These agents can activate an "*innate*" immune response by activating monocytes, NK cells, DCs, and B-cells in an independent manner. The effects of CpG on DCs include increased DC migration to lymph nodes, enhanced activation of $CD8^+$ T cells, and protective CTL responses against both viral and tumor antigens. In vivo, CpG act also as an effective adjuvant for a tumor vaccine consisting of DCs cocultured with irradiated tumor cells, which provide a substantial increase in both prophylactic and therapeutic activity in several murine tumor models. Clinical vaccination trials that use CpG-ODN as immunologic adjuvants are currently underway.

Utilization of exosomes, small vesicles of endosomal origin, might be another attractive approach in cancer immunotherapy, combining the anti-tumor activity of DCs with the advantages of a cell-free vehicle. Both DCs and tumor can secrete exosomes constitutively. Tumor-derived exosomes contain whole native cytosolic and/or endosomal tumor antigens and constitutive *heat shock proteins* (hsps). Exosomes transfer tumor antigen to DCs and induce peptide-specific, MHC class I-restricted cross presentation to T cell clones and, in vitro, tumor-specific CTL responses in patient's lymphocytes. Exosomes produced by DCs, display a discrete set of proteins involved in antigen presentation, in particular MHC class I and II molecules, but also costimulatory molecules (CD86), and are selectively enriched in molecules potentially involved in effector cell targeting, such CD11b, lactadherin, and CD9 molecules. Isolation of exosomes is usually carried out by differential centrifugation, followed by floatation on sucrose density gradients to collect the exosomes. Zitvogel at al. have shown that not only do DCs trigger T cell responses through direct cell-cell contacts, but exosomes secreted by DCs can also stimulate T cells. In this study, exosomes secreted by bone marrow-derived DCs (BM-DCs), which were challenged with tumor-derived peptides, activated CTLs, causing the eradication of established tumors.

The mechanism of action of exosomes in vivo is poorly understood. Exosomes could stimulate T cells directly, through the MHC-peptide complexes they harbor, or they could be captured by other professional APC, which could then use peptide-loaded MHC molecules, Ags, or peptides present in exosomes to stimulate T cells. When compared with the tumor peptide-loaded DCs, DC-derived exosomes showed higher efficiency in eliciting tumor regression of the established p815 mastocytoma and TS/A mammary adenocarcinoma. Moreover, in several mouse tumor models, Wolfers et al. showed that immunization of mice with DCs loaded with tumor-derived exosomes resulted in tumor prevention as well as the regression of established lesions. The antitumor immunity was mediated by $CD8^+$ T cells, because their depletion in vivo inhibited the anti-tumor effect of exosomes. These results suggest that exosomes derived from tumor cells or DCs provide another promising avenue for the development of DC-based cancer vaccines. A clinical trial has recently been launched, aimed at vaccinating patients with metastatic melanoma and inoperable lung cancer with autologous DC-derived exosomes pulsed with MAGE-3 MHC class I- and II-associated peptides.

Fusion of tumor cells with DCs is a powerful new technology to increase tumor vaccine immunogenicity, and as been explored as a means to potentially endow DCs with the full complement of TAAs expressed by the tumor cell. In this strategy, DCs can be loaded with tumor antigens by simply fusing them to tumor cells. These cell-fusion studies have shown effective responses against both primary tumors and secondary metastases, and stimulation of both $CD4^+$ and $CD8^+$ T cells as well as NK cell anti-tumor responses. The commonly used procedure for the preparation of DC-tumor fusion cells has used *polyethylene-glycol* (PEG), a classical fusogenic agent that is widely used to produce B or T cell hybridomas. This procedure can be time and labor intensive because after fusion, 7–14 days of culture are usually required for selection and expansion. Among a number of means for achieving cell-cell fusion, electro-fusion seems to be particularly attractive. A recent study has compared the therapeutic efficiency of PEG versus electric pulse-mediated fusion protocols in a poorly immunogenic and it demonstrated metastatic murine mammary carcinoma cell line, and it demonstrated that electro-fusion is as efficient as PEG mediated fusion in generating an immunogen capable of inducing protective anti-tumor immunity. Therefore, both techniques seem to be promising for clinical application. However, in a more recent study, the further optimization of the electro-fusion parameters resulted in superior activity compared to chemical fusion.

Another approach that may supersede the need for ex vivo expansion and manipulation of DCs, is the administration of the cytokine Flt-3L. Treatment of mice bearing certain immunologic tumors with Flt-3L has been shown to result in tumor regression. In an *acute myelogenous leukemia* (AML) model, Pawlowski et al. have also shown that a significant protection against AML challenge in naive or bone marrow-transplanted mice was provided by either in vitro tumor-lysate pulsed DCs or in vivo Flt-3L-generated DCs, but only when initiated prior to AML challenge.

Despite the immunologically privileged status of the brain, numerous pre-clinical studies of DC-based immunotherapy for malignant brain tumors since 1997 have demonstrated that immunotherapy may be feasible and efficacious in both protection and treatment models for intracranial models of glioma and melanoma. Numerous strategies of loading DCs with tumor antigens have been investigated including pulsing with tumor lysate, acid-eluted peptides, synthetic or virally transfected peptides, whole tumor cDNA, DC-tumor fusions, RNA, apoptotic tumor, and irradiated tumor cells. While all utilized immature, bone-marrow derived DCs, the number and characterization of the DCs used, the frequency and technique of vaccination, and *in vitro* and *in vivo* assays utilized were highly variable. The multiplicity of techniques and tumor models makes meaningful comparisons impossible. Nonetheless, nearly all demonstrated efficacy in the models studied. Several also implicated the importance of $CD8^+$ T cells, $CD4^+$ T cells, and NK cells in anti-tumor efficacy. The single negative study was that of Yang et al., which demonstrated that orthotopic 9L gliosarcoma induced apoptosis of DCs delivered directly into the tumor. The investigators implicated hyaluronan on the glioma membrane via increased nitric oxide synthase (NOSi) induced by the DC-based CD44 receptor. This effect was not eliminated by stereotactic radiosurgery of the tumor, but was abrogated by pretreatment of DCs with anti-CD44 or N-mononomethyl-L-arginine (NMMA), or pre-treatment of 9L with hyaluronidase. This suggests that the efficacy of direct intratumoral injection of DCs, which has been demonstrated in other tumor models, may not translate to gliomas.

Clinical Cancer Vaccine Trials

Generation of Human DCs

Physiologically, human DCs constitute a rare but heterogeneous population that are phenotypically distinct from macrophages and represent only a small proportion of less than 1% of the circulating leukocyte pool. For therapeutic purposes large numbers of DCs are required. Three main types of DCs have been studied for use in clinical trials.

Monocyte-Derived DCs (Mo-DCs)

The best-studied human DCs are those derived from peripheral blood $CD14^+$ monocytes, which are abundantly present in peripheral blood. Monocytes can be easily obtained from peripheral blood draws or leukapheresis by several methods, including plastic adherence of Ficoll-Hypaque or Lymphoprep purified *peripheral blood mononuclear cells* (PBMCs), followed by metrizamide gradient centrifugation. Monocytes are subsequently cultured for 5 to 7 days, in the presence of GM-CSF and IL-4. Investigators have used preferentially serum-free medium or autologous plasma (1%) instead of medium supplemented with fetal calf serum, as the latter may contain trace amounts of endotoxin, TGF-β or other factors. After 1 week the yield of immature DCs generated varies from about 25–50% of the starting population. Yields of 0.5–2 × 10^6 cells per 10 ml blood are typically obtained. A representative culture will contain 95–99% $CD1a^+CD14^-CD83^{lo/-}$ cells. If cells are cultured much beyond 8 days, they will undergo spontaneous maturation with upregulation of CD83. It is not clear whether this developmental pathway of monocytes occurs frequently in vivo, or whether this represents a highly specialized stage of monocytes, expressed only under certain conditions. Development of a closed, semi-automated system for the generation of large-scale monocyte-derived DCs has been optimized by some groups.

Peripheral-Blood-Derived DCs (PBDCs)

DCs can be also generated as circulating precursors from the blood by densitybased purification techniques, after a period of in vitro culture (1-2 days) without cytokines. During this time, DC precursors undergo maturation, become larger and less dense, which allows their purification by density-gradient centrifugation. Gradient solution lacking potentially immunogenic protein such as BSA has been employed including Percoll, Nycodenz, and metrizamide. DCs isolated in this manner possess potent allostimulatory activity and the ability to prime naive $CD4^+$ T helper cells and $CD8^+$ *cytotoxic T lymphocytes* (CTLs). The use of density-based isolation is, however, limited by the low frequency of DC precursors in blood, and leukapheresis must be performed to generate sufficient numbers (on average 5×10^6 from the PBMCs of a single leukapheresis procedure) of DCs for vaccinations of humans.

$CD34^+$-Derived DCs

Human DCs can also be generated in vitro from $CD34^+$ hematopoietic progenitor cells. $CD34^+$ cells may be derived from bone marrow, cord blood, or purified directly from peripheral blood or after mobilization with cytokines such as granulocyte colony-stimulating factor (G-CSF) or GM-CSF. The generation of DCs in this way involves a positive selection using paramagnetic beads and in vitro culture with cytokines over 2 to 3-weeks. Final DC yields can be increased by expanding the progenitor pool (10–30 fold) prior to terminal DC differentiation. Some protocols include an initial expansion period [usually with Flt-3L, SCF or both, in combination with other cytokines] to boost DC progenitor cell numbers, followed by a differentiation step (which usually includes GM-CSF plus TNF-α) after culture with different combinations of cytokines, including TNF-α, Flt-3L, c-Kit, CD40 ligand (CD40L), SCF, GM-CSF or TGF-β. Both c-Kit and Flt-3L are transmembrane proteins on stromal cells that bind to tyrosine-kinase receptors and sustain DC progenitors, whereas TNF-α and CD40L block the granulocyte differentiation pathway and stimulate the final maturation of DCs. $CD34^+$-DCs appear to be more efficient in the activation of tumor-specific CTLs than those derived from $CD14^+$ progenitors. In contrast to Mo-DCs, DCs derived from $CD34^+$ cells consist of two phenotypically and functionally distinct populations. One subset is similar to the epidermal Langerhans cells, and the other termed "interstitial/dermal DCs" is similar to those derived from blood monocytes. Immune responses to these unique LC containing preparations await evaluation in humans.

In vivo Generated DCs

An alternative approach is to expand DCs in vivo. Methods of stimulating DC mobilization and trafficking in vivo, allowing the native immune environment to naturally mature DCs, may overcome the functional limitations imposed by ex vivo culture; for example, the culture conditions used to expand cells ex vivo may significantly affect their function and antigen-processing capabilities, or that DCs generated in culture may not traffic to draining lymph nodes in great numbers, thus limiting the development of systemic immunity. Treatment with the hemopoietic growth factor, Flt-3L, may potentially bypass the need for ex vivo culture and manipulation of DCs or their precursors. Results so far from the continuing human clinical studies have demonstrated that treatment with Flt-3L is well tolerated and can increase numbers of circulating DCs more than 20-fold.

Maturation of Human DCs

DCs have multiple roles and dynamically shift phenotypes relative to their environment. DC phenotype and function may be affected by the precursor cells from which the DCs are derived, as well as by the factors used to effect differentiation or maturation.

Immature DCs can be further induced to mature by co-culturing with inflammatory stimuli including TNF-α, IL-6, IL-1β, pathogen-related molecules such as LPS, bacterial DNA, T cell–derived signals and prostaglandins such as PGE2 or, alternatively, with a so-called *monocyte conditioned medium* (MCM) for an additional 3 days. The maturation process is associated with several coordinated events such as (a) expression of CD83, as well as the p55 actin-bundling protein fascin, an important controller of cytoskeleton remodeling; (b) loss of antigen-uptake capacity; (c) upregulation of T cell adhesion and costimulatory molecules (CD40, CD58, CD80, and CD86); (d) change in morphology, (e) expression of different cytokines genes; and (f) expression of chemokine receptors that guide DC migration into lymphoid organs for priming of antigen-specific T cells. Morphological changes accompanying DC maturation include a loss of adhesive structures, cytoskeleton reorganization, and acquisition of high cellular motility.

The use of DCs as adjuvants is supported by numerous animal studies with primarily mature DCs, which have shown that the injection of tumor antigen– loaded DCs reliably induces tumor-specific CTL responses, tumor resistance, and in some cases, regression of metastases. However, in the majority of pilot clinical trials reported so far for humans, immature DCs have been employed. Sporadic tumor responses are reported and the induction of tumor-specific CTLs by DC vaccination have been observed. Moreover, several reports have demonstrated that immature DCs but not mature DCs can induce tolerance to Ags used for vaccination. Therefore, mature DCs have been used in recent vaccination protocols, especially when peptides are used as a source of antigen.

In contrast to immature DCs, mature DCs are much more potent in inducing Th1 and CTL responses in vitro and are resistant to immunosuppressive effects of tumor-derived IL-10. They also become migratory and travel to the local lymph nodes, where they present antigens in association with MHC to specific T cells. Several studies have shown that DCs generated in vitro must be matured to migrate optimally and to stimulate T cells efficiently. In a small pilot trial, Jonuleit et al. vaccinated advanced, stage IV melanoma patients simultaneously with immature DCs and mature DCs loaded with different melanoma-associated peptide antigens. Both DCs populations were injected in different lymph nodes of the same patient. They demonstrated that mature DCs were capable of promoting a greater level of CTL and T helper reactivity measured in the circulating PBMCs.

Another reason some groups support adoptive transfer of mature DCs is that immature DCs may lose their efficiency for T-cell stimulation once removed from exogenously supplied cytokines. Several studies have also reported that immature Mo-DCs can reverse into a macrophage after cytokine withdrawal, whereas mature DCs cannot undergo this reversion. However, as mentioned earlier, mature DCs have a lower capacity for uptake of exogenous antigens, such as RNA, proteins, or dead tumor cells. Different maturation protocols may also produce DC populations that are functionally distinct in terms of, for example, their ability to migrate, to produce cytokines, to stimulate T cells, and to induce T-cell cytokine secretion. These differences have important implications for decisions on the most appropriate type of DCs (immature or mature) for use in clinical trials.

Antigen Loading of DCs

Several forms of DC-mediated immunotherapy are currently being investigated with great intensity in clinical trials, using a wide variety of different vaccination protocols, for numerous tumor types including melanoma, prostate cancer, AML, breast cancer, gastric cancer, lung cancer, renal cell carcinoma, gastric cancer, and others.

DCs can be pulsed with synthetic peptides or proteins derived from known *tumor-associated antigens* (TAA) such as MAGE-1 and MAGE-3, New York Esophagus (NY-ESO)-1, MUC-1, Her-2/neu, tyrosinase, *carcinoembryonic antigen* (CEA), or Melan-A/MART-1. For example, antigens of the MAGE family have been employed to induce melanoma specific immunity, first by using immature DCs and later by using terminally mature DCs. The use of defined antigens for tumor immunotherapy has the clear advantage of being able to control the amounts of antigen administered, and to monitor the emerging response. The immunogenicity of defined peptide epitopes may be substantially increased by modifying the peptide sequence at amino acid residues that are crucial for the interaction with the MHC class molecules or with the specific TCR. However, using peptides for DC loading has several intrinsic disadvantages. This approach is currently limited to that tumor type for which TAAs are identified. Moreover, the application of antigenic peptides is limited to use in patients who express a defined specific HLA haplotype. Finally, the majority of known TAA peptides are presented in association with MHC class I molecules and are recognized by tumor-specific $CD8^+$ T cells, whereas small numbers of TAA epitopes are presented in association with MHC class II molecules and are recognized by $CD4^+$ T cell.

To overcome such limitations, another approach is the use of whole proteins or multiple peptides as the source of antigen. Due to the broad spectrum of potentially recognizable peptides that can originate from each protein, this strategy allows the induction of immune responses against different epitopes that could be potentially restricted to multiple HLA alleles. Furthermore, the antigen-processing and presenting machinery could direct responses to important and immuno-dominant epitopes including both MHC class-I and class-II-restricted peptide antigens. This strategy has been followed for melanoma, using antigens against MAGE-1 and -3, tyrosinase, Melan-A and gp100 together with $CD34^+$-derived DCs.

Other approaches utilizing whole tumor cells as a source of antigen have been developed. Loading of DCs with tumor lysates or extract, obtained after repeated freezing and thawing or sonication of whole tumor cells, is one of the more established methods and has been used in a wide variety of tumor types. The studies showed induction of tumor-specific T-cell responses, including cytolytic activity and the production of immunostimulatory cytokines. DCs can also be transfected with either RNA coding for a specific tumor antigen or whole tumor RNA. The ease in generating large quantities of nucleic acids gives RNA-based vaccines an advantage over tumor lysates, especially if multiple restimulations are needed using a small tumor sample. Moreover, tumor-restricted RNA can be enriched before loading by subtractive hybridization with RNA from normal tissues. Tumor-specific immune responses are thereby augmented, and the likelihood of autoimmunity generated from self-antigens is reduced. One weakness of this strategy is the unstable, labile nature of RNA. Because DCs are very effective at presenting peptides from apoptotic cells, dying tumor cells (apoptotic bodies or necrotic cells) have also been used as sources for tumor antigens to load DCs. Another strategy designed to deliver all antigens from tumor cells directly into the cytosol of DCs is by the fusion of DCs with tumor cells. The fused DC-tumor cells obtained are thought to combine the whole antigenic spectrum of the tumor with the powerful antigen capabilities. Studies using DC-tumor cell fusions have demonstrated the generation of tumor-specific CTL in vitro and antitumor immunity in vivo. The important conceptual outcome of all these loading strategies is that tumor antigens would be processed by both the endocytic and proteosomal DC pathways and would be capable of stimulating both $CD4^+$ and $CD8^+$ T cells. Because these approaches do not require the definition of TAA or MHC haplotype of the patients they may provide for a broader clinical application.

Based on studies in a murine lymphoma model showing that vaccination with *idiotype* (Id)-pulsed DCs could generate a strong T lymphocyte anti-Id response and induce a protective antitumor immunity, several groups initiated clinical trials of Id-pulsed DC vaccination for patients with low-grade *non Hodgkin lymphoma* (NHL) and multiple myeloma. Both diseases are slowly, but inevitably, progressive malignancies, and generally express a unique immunoglobulin Id as a potential TAA. Recently, Timmerman et al. reported a long term follow-up of 35 patients with follicular NHL, treated using this approach. They described that Id-pulsed DC vaccination can induce T-cell and humoral anti-Id immune responses, as well as durable tumor regression.

The ability to manipulate DC function by gene transfer represents an attractive alternative strategy to enable some DC-based therapies, and does not require prior knowledge of the MHC type or relevant T-cell peptide epitope. The target genes transferred fall into two categories TAA and immunomodulatory proteins such as cytokines and costimulatory molecules. Available vectors include retroviruses, adenoviruses, lentiviruses, adeno-associated virus, herpes simplex virus, cationic liposomes, naked DNA and DNA-coated gold beads. The biologic effects of the transduction on DCs vary with the viral vector systems and the experimental conditions used in the studies. A comparison of various gene transfer methods in human DCs showed that adenovirus vectors was the most efficient in transducing human DCs, with transduction efficiencies exceeding 95% at higher multiplicity of infection. Potentially benefits and limitations of genetically-modified DCs for use in immunotherapy have been reviewed recently.

Evaluation of Vaccine-Induced Immune Responses

One important objective of clinical vaccine trials is to devise in vitro immunological assays that correlate with clinical outcome, for use as surrogate markers of vaccine efficacy, and to make the results from different clinical studies comparable. The most crucial end-point reflecting the efficacy of antigen-specific vaccines is the induction of responses by $CD8^+$ T cells. To date, IFN-γ ELISPOT and recombinant MHC class I multimers loaded with the respective peptide appear to be the most commonly used and sensitive detection assays to measure CTL responses following DC vaccination against a selected peptide antigen. Furthermore, tetramer staining can be used for in situ detection of peptide-specific CTL in biopsies of lesions and lymph nodes of cancer patients. An alternative approach allows the selective isolation of antigen-specific CTL by *fluorescence activated cell sorting* (FACS). However, trends towards the use of more complex immunogens, such as whole proteins, require the development of efficient and sensitive methods for monitoring more complex immunologic effects as well. In the context of a vaccination trial using full-length tyrosinase (Ty) to immunize patients with metastatic melanoma, a monitoring technique was developed in which autologous DCs infected with a recombinant adenovirus encoding the Ty protein were used to assess the Ty-specific reactivity of fresh peripheral blood lymphocytes. Quantitative real-time reverse transcription polymerase chain reaction (qRT-PCR) was used to measure the production of cytokine mRNA by T cells following a brief incubation with Ty-expressing DCs. Two out of ten patients enrolled demonstrated Ty protein-specific reactivity that increased during and after the period of vaccination. While one of these patients also reacted to an HLA-A1-compatible Ty peptide, the second did not recognize any of the known Ty epitopes, highlighting the importance of this technique for monitoring the effects of complex vaccines.

Preliminary results of clinical trials with DC immunization using ex-vivo generated DCs appear contradictory, however. Fong et al. examined in a phase I clinical trial, the ability of Flt-3L to increase the number of DCs in cancer patients as well as the ability of these expanded DCs to be harvested and used to immunize patients against CEA. They demonstrated that immunization with Flt-3L-expanded DCs loaded with an altered peptide ligand derived from CEA could lead to CEA-specific immunity and clinical responses. However, in a recent published phase II clinical trial, Rini et al. reported that Flt-3L, although capable of inducing expansion of circulating myeloid and plasmacytoid DCs in patients with metastatic renal cell carcinoma, lacked significant clinical activity at the doses and schedules examined. Further studies will be necessary to ascertain the value, if any, of Flt-3L to generate clinically effective anti-tumor immunity.

There have been few clinical trials to date of DC-based immunotherapy for malignant brain tumors involving a total of 20 patients. All have been Phase I clinical trials for the treatment of gliomas, utilizing multiple i.d. vaccinations comprised of 5-100 $\times$ 10^6 poorly characterized or immature bone-marrow derived, DCs. These DCs have been loaded with tumor antigen prepared in a variety of ways including tumor lysate, acid-eluted peptides, gamma irradiated tumor cells, and by fusion to glioma cells. Likewise, *in vitro* and *in vivo* immune monitoring was highly variable. No objective clinical responses was observed, but increased lymphocytic infiltration of tumor has been reported. Despite induction of lethal encephalitis in primates vaccinated with human glioma, treatment of humans has been well tolerated with minimal side effects, and autoimmune disease has not been reported to date. The utility of *delayed-type hypersensitivity* (DTH) and routine MRI imaging in assessing immune response and clinical efficacy has also been questioned. Preliminary reports of DC-based immunotherapy for newly diagnosed patients has been more promising, with several clinical responses observed and an extended median survival of over one year

Concluding Remark

While DCs were difficult to isolate initially, these APCs can now be generated in large numbers in vitro and manipulated in multiple ways before administered back to a patient to induce anti-tumor immunity. Studies of dendritic cell biology in the laboratory and preclinical studies in the mouse have facilitated the implantation of clinical trials using DCs in the treatment of melanoma and other cancers. Importantly, there have been no reports of serious adverse events or significant autoimmune sequelae observed with DC vaccines apart from standard Grade I toxicities. Phase I clinical trials have established the feasibility of this approach against a number of human tumors, including renal cell carcinoma, melanoma, prostate carcinoma, cervical carcinoma, breast carcinoma, ovarian carcinoma, multiple myeloma, and intracranial tumors.

Animal studies and human cancer trials have shown that specific T-cell responses against tumors as well as tumor regression can be achieved with vaccines based on DCs. One challenge to DC-based tumor vaccines remains the difficulty of measuring that a clinically relevant immune response has been induced. Thus, one would wish to detect a clinically relevant frequency of tumor-specific cytotoxic T cells and tumor-specific $CD4^+$ and $CD8^+$ T cells capable of producing inflammatory cytokines. The issues of optimal number of DCs as well as the frequency and route of administration (i.d., intranodal, s.c. or i.v.) remains uncertain, although compelling preclinical studies suggest that DCs should be administered either intradermally or intranodally, at regular intervals in the case of metastatic disease. In most published clinical trials, 4 to 70 million DCs have been administered at 2-week to 4-week intervals. DCs injected s.c. or i.d. could migrate to draining lymph nodes with varying efficiencies, although a significant number of cells remained at the injection site, whereas the i.v. route resulted in the dispersal of DCs to lung, liver, spleen, and bone marrow, but not to the peripheral lymph nodes. Unpolarized T-cell and antibody responses have been demonstrated with i.v. administration, whereas Th1 responses have been seen predominantly after i.d. and intralymphatic injections. Additional preclinical studies will be necessary to define the optimum DC population for use in clinical trials, with respect to the source and stage of maturation of DCs, and the stimuli used to generate them.

Despite unresolved issues, efforts continue to evolve DC-based antitumor vaccines. DC vaccination is currently being employed in an ever-increasing number of trials. Careful optimization of the most promising strategies, thoughtful selection of patient populations, and appropriate clinical trial design will be critical to the achievement of a reproducible determination of clinical benefit or failure of DC-based vaccines for cancer.

11

Cytokine Therapy

What is the role of the immune system in cancer? The link between the two has long been apparent, as is illustrated by the high incidence of certain cancers such as Kaposi's sarcoma or lymphoma in individuals with the *Acquired Immunodeficiency Syndrome* (AIDS). It has been hypothesized that deficits in immune surveillance must therefore permit tumor cell growth under such circumstances. This chapter discusses the role of cytokines in the immune recognition of tumor cells.

The host response to infection or malignant transformation is composed of the concerted actions of the innate and adaptive arms of the immune system. The cellular components of innate immunity are characterized by *natural killer* (NK) and phagocytic cells that rapidly and non-specifically attack foreign agents. Innate effectors subsequently provide the "*danger*" signals to activate cells of the adaptive immune system. The adaptive immune response includes B and T lymphocytes and displays antigen-specificity and immunologic memory. Central to the communication between innate and adaptive immunity are specialized "*antigen presenting*" cells (APCs) called *dendritic cells* (DCs). Immature DCs capture foreign antigens (or tumor antigens) in the periphery and migrate to lymphoid organs, where they mature and activate components of the adaptive immune system, e.g. antigen-specific $CD4^+$ helper T cells, $CD8^+$ cytotoxic T cells, and antibody-producing B cells.

The chief aim of cancer immunotherapy is to enhance the immune response against tumor targets. This can be accomplished via stimulation with tumor antigen (vaccination), provision of "*tumor-killing*" cells (adoptive cell transfer), and/or administration of growth factors called *cytokines* that regulate immune cells. Cytokine approaches for cancer therapy have three potential mechanisms of action. They can (1) directly induce cell death programs in tumor cells, (2) increase the number or activity of immune effector cells, or 3) increase the recognition of tumor cells by the immune system.

The underlying hypothesis behind cytokine therapy is that cytokines can help overcome deficiencies in the host immune response against cancer. Cancer cells escape immune surveillance through two key mechanisms. First, a state of immunodeficiency, either inherent or induced, can impair adequate anti-tumor immunity. An example of this would be a patient with AIDS and a profound T cell deficiency or a patient receiving chronic immune suppressive therapy to prevent allograft rejection by T cells. Second, the tumor or tumor micro-environment can establish a state of immune tolerance to tumor antigen and/or prevent proper tumor recognition and immune cell stimulation.

How can cytokines be utilized to correct a deficiency in tumor immunity? Systemic or local provision of specific cytokines may improve tumor antigen recognition and/or subsequent stimulation of anti-tumor immunity. For example, DCs are highly efficient APCs that can promote the antigen-specific adaptive immune response, including anti-tumor immunity. This chapter summarizes recent progress in cancer immunotherapy utilizing cytokines to enhance antigen presentation.

Antigen Presentation

A central step in the recognition of tumor cells by the adaptive immune system occurs through tumor antigen presentation. This process selectively activates tumor antigen-specific T cells or antibody-producing B cells. DCs often are called "*professional*" APCs due to their high efficiency in capturing, processing, and presenting antigens to T cells, thereby stimulating them and thus triggering the adaptive immune response. DCs first were noted by Paul Langerhans in 1868, when he identified "*Langerhans cells*" with long, thin branches in sections of human epidermis. In 1973, Ralph Steinman identified "*accessory cells*" that facilitated the induction of a specific immune response from lymphocytes in mice and named these "*dendritic*" cells for their tree-like processes. Thirty years later, investigators have further characterized DC development and the role of DCs in the immune response, with important implications for tumor immunology.

Dendritic Cells: Phenotype

DCs are derived from bone marrow progenitor cells. Fully mature DCs are highly capable of antigen presentation. Mature DCs cells have numerous membrane extensions or processes (dendrites) that facilitate physical interaction with the environment and other lymphocytes. The surface phenotype of mature DCs includes high expression of MHC Class I and II molecules, co-stimulatory molecules (CD80-B7.1, CD86-B7.2), and cell adhesion molecules (ICAM-1, LFA-3). In addition, DCs possess the intracellular machinery for processing proteins for antigen presentation, e.g. endosomes, lysosomes. DCs are negative for lineage markers CD3 (T cell), CD56 (NK cell), or CD19 (B cell).

In addition to "*danger*" signals from infectious agents, immunoregulatory cytokines can induce the expansion and maturation of DCs in mice and humans. Initial studies demonstrated that cytokines are capable of differentiating mouse and human DC populations from bone marrow or peripheral blood precursors *in vitro*. These DCs are potent stimulators of T cells *in vitro* and are capable of promoting anti-tumor immunity *in vivo*. It is now known that cytokines such as Flt-3 ligand (FL) induce the expansion and differentiation of DC precursors in the periphery. Additional cytokines such as interleukin-4 (IL-4) and *Granulocyte-Monocyte Colony Stimulating Factor* (GM-CSF) differentiate DC precursors into immature DCs that are highly capable of antigen uptake. These cytokines have some functional redundancy in the development of DCs, as evidenced by genetically targeted mice deficient for GM-CSF or GM-CSF receptor α-chain that display normal hematopoiesis. Conversely, mice lacking FL have a reduced number of DCs. Lastly, cytokines including interferons (IFN) and tumor necrosis factor-αg (TNF-α) induce maturation of DC for maximal antigen presentation in local lymphoid tissues.

Dendritic Cells: Therapy

Based on their efficient antigen presentation and ability to promote T cell activation, the potential application of DCs for cancer immunotherapy quickly was recognized. In 1996, several investigators demonstrated that DCs could be used to stimulate peptide-specific immunity *in vivo*. Bone marrow-derived DCs were loaded with ova peptide and delivered to mice that subsequently were challenged with the EL4 murine thymoma cell line expressing the ova peptide. These experiments demonstrated for the first time that peptide-loaded DC could be used to induce antigen-specific and protective immunity against tumors *in vivo*. Depletion of $CD8^+$ T cells abrogated this protective effect, while depletion of $CD4^+$ T cells had no effect, illustrating the role of DCs in tumor antigen presentation and the subsequent generation of tumor-specific $CD8^+$ cytotoxic T lymphocytes. In the same year, Paglia et al. successfully demonstrated that bone marrow-derived DCs pulsed with soluble protein (β-galactosidase) elicited protective immunity against β-gal expressing fibroblasts. Similarly, protection correlated with the expansion of $CD8^+$ T cells. This early work initiated a strong interest for developing a therapeutic strategy using *in vitro* expanded DCs that are "*pulsed*" or loaded with either tumor antigen peptides, tumor cell lysates, or transfected with tumor antigen genes. Here, we will discuss the application of cytokines to enhance antigen presentation through the *in vivo* differentiation of DCs.

Dendritic Cells: Differentiation and Maturation

While vaccines utilizing *in vitro* generated DCs have demonstrated some success, there are three key advantages to cytokine therapies that generate APCs *in vivo*. First, cytokine-based therapies are "*universal*" since they do not require the preparation of autologous cell-based therapies such as *ex vivo* generated DCs. Second, cytokine therapies do not have the time constraints and contamination risks associated with the preparation of autologous cellular therapies. Lastly, cytokine therapies may elicit a broader immune response by allowing antigen processing and peptide selection to occur *in vivo*.

The following cytokines have been shown to or have the potential to enhance antigen presentation *in vivo*.

Colony Stimulating Factors (GM-CSF, G-CSF)

GM-CSF first was identified in the late 1970s from mouse lung-conditioned medium and was capable of stimulating granulocyte, macrophage and mixed lineage colonies from bone marrow. Signaling occurs through the GM-CSF receptor α chain and common βc, shared with IL-3 and IL-5 receptors, with subsequent activation of tyrosine kinases, mainly Janus family kinases. Early work with GM-CSF revealed its ability to induce proliferation of progenitor cells from bone marrow and leukemia cell lines. In the late 1980s, several investigators demonstrated the role GM-CSF in the differentiation of human erythroid, granulocyte, and monocyte/macrophage lineages from bone marrow and peripheral blood. Witmer-Pack et al. (1987) demonstrated that GM-CSF could prolong the survival of mouse Langerhans cells *in vitro*. Migliaccio et al. (1988) used GM-CSF and G-CSF to differentiate macrophage lineages *in vitro* from human bone marrow and peripheral blood. Differentiation of macrophages is significant as these cells had the potential to become effective APCs, and further, could be differentiated into DCs. Markowicz and Engleman (1990) reported that GM-CSF could prolong the survival of peripheral blood DCs and induce differentiation of DCs from peripheral blood monocytes. In contrast, *Granulocyte Colony Stimulating Factor* (G-CSF) alone does not appear to have a significant role in the differentiation of DC precursors *in vitro*, but may have some utility when combined with GM-CSF or other cytokines *in vivo*.

Following Markowicz and Englemann's report on GM-CSF and human peripheral blood DC survival and differentiation in 1990, several other groups demonstrated that GM-CSF, alone or in combination with other cytokines, could differentiate DCs from DC precursors or progenitors *in vitro*. In 1992, Inaba et al. reported that GM-CSF could differentiate and cause proliferation of DCs from cultured mouse peripheral blood. Caux et al. induced the differentiation of DCs from human $CD34^+$ bone marrow stem cells with GM-CSF and TNF-α. Santiago-Schwarz et al. similarly induced DC differentiation from human umbilical cord blood $CD34^+$ stem cells with GM-CSF and TNF-α. In particular, the development of multiple methods for generating large numbers of DCs *in vitro* was a critical step in the study of DC biology since previous studies had been limited by the small percentage (less than 0.5%) of DCs available from peripheral blood.

GM-CSF provides protective immunity in murine models

Dranoff et al. sought to compare several cytokine gene therapies, including GM-CSF, in a mouse model of melanoma. In this model, mice were challenged with the B16 melanoma cell line and subsequently succumbed to fatal tumor burden within 15–40 days. Prior immunization with irradiated melanoma cells resulted in minimal improvement in survival and immunity. As a next step, mice were immunized with irradiated melanoma cell vaccines that had been retrovirally transduced with one of the following murine cytokine genes: IL-2, IL-4, IL-5, IL-6, GM-CSF, IFN-γ, and TNF-α. Immunization with GM-CSF-transduced tumors provided superior protection compared to all other cytokines tested. Further, the protective immunity established with GM-CSF-transduced tumor vaccination was significantly abrogated by prior depletion of either $CD4^+$ or $CD8^+$ T cells. The authors suggested that the immunostimulatory properties of GM-CSF lie in its ability to promote DC differentiation and antigen presentation, especially since the B16 tumors lacked expression of MHC Class II and thus likely were not capable of priming the CD4+ T cell response themselves. They later reported that GM-CSF-transduced tumor vaccines expanded

CD11c$^+$CD80$^+$ CD86$^+$ DCs *in vivo*, with a 40-fold increase in splenic DCs. This study was the first to make a broad comparison of cytokines as cancer vaccine adjuvants using mouse models and placed GM-CSF at the forefront of cytokine therapies for cancer. Could GM-CSF gene therapy or systemic administration of GM-CSF promote tumor immunity in patients with cancer?

Table 11.1. Cytokines and antigen presentation

Cytokine	*Effects*
GM-CSF	Proliferation and differentiation of myeloid, erythroid, granulocytic cells
	Increases antigen presentation through the expansion of DCs and DC precursors alone or in combination with other cytokines including IL-4 and TNF-α
FL	Proliferation of marrow progenitors
	Increases antigen presentation *in vivo* through the expansions of DC in mice and cancer patients
IL-4	Upregulates MHC I and MHC II in APCs
	Combination with GM-CSF promotes antigen presentation through differentiation of DCs from human peripheral blood and CD34$^+$ stem cells
IFN-α/β	Anti-viral activity
	May directly induce apoptosis in mouse and human tumors
	Activates macrophages
	Increases antigen presentation through upregulation of MHC
	Class I expression on both tumor cells and APCs
	Promotes DC maturation in combination with GM-CSF
IFN-γ	Produced by activated T cells and NK cells
	Anti-viral and anti-proliferative activity
	Major activator of macrophages
	Increases MHC Class I and II antigen processing, presentation, and expression in macrophages
TNF-α	Produced by leukocytes
	Enhances antigen presentation by monocytes
	Promotes antigen presentation through maturation of DCs in combination with GM-CSF

Clinical application of GM-CSF: gene therapy

Based on promising results from animal models using cytokine transduced cancer cells and tumor antigen-loaded DCs as vaccines, Sanda et al. (1994) sought to retrovirally transduce human GM-CSF genes into prostate cancer cells from 10 patients. They showed that these cells secreted human GM-CSF in a gene-dose dependent fashion. This early work demonstrated the feasibility of cytokine gene therapy for producing autologous cancer cell vaccines. They hypothesized that co-expression of GM-CSF with the cancer cell vaccine would induce local differentiation of DCs capable of tumor antigen presentation. Subsequently, several Phase I clinical trials initiated treatment with preparations of GM-CSF–transduced autologous metastatic renal cell carcinoma, melanoma, and prostate cancer. Each trial proved to be safe with minimal toxicity to patients with late stage or metastatic cancer. These first studies demonstrated an immunological response to the vaccines as measured by delayed-type hypersensitivity reactions and antibody titers against the autologous tumors. Local differentiation and infiltration of DCs in vaccination sites should likely have been considered as another end point of these vaccine approaches. Overall, these Phase I trials demonstrated safety and immunologic responses, suggesting approaches may be most beneficial in either in early stage cancers or in stages of minimal residual disease.

Table 11.2. GM-CSF and cancer immunotherapy

GM-CSF	*Clinical application*
Recombinant cytokine	Differentiation of DCs and DC precursors *in vitro* from peripheral blood monocytes or bone marrow/cord blood stem cells
	Alone and in combination with other cytokines (IL-4, IFN-α, TNF-α, or FL) for *in vivo* expansion of mature DCs
Gene therapy	Autologous or allogeneic-tumor cell vaccines transduced with GM-CSF to promote local differentiation of DCs and increased antigen presentation
	Poxvirus delivery of GM-CSF as an adjuvant to tumor antigen or gene

Clinical application of GM-CSF: recombinant cytokine

Systemic administration of GM-CSF is well tolerated by patients and now is indicated for neutrophil recovery following chemotherapy and mobilization of peripheral blood progenitors. Further analysis revealed that GM-CSF not only mobilizes peripheral blood progenitors, but also results in an increase in peripheral blood monocytes and DC precursors in normal healthy patients. Although recombinant GM-CSF can differentiate DCs from human bone marrow/cord blood stem cells and peripheral blood *in vitro*, GM-CSF is less effective as a DC differentiation agent when administered alone in humans. Combination treatment with GM-CSF and IL-4 efficiently expanded peripheral blood DCs (HLA-DR$^+$, CD11c$^+$, CD83$^+$) in patients with advanced cancer, while IL-4 alone does not differentiate DCs. Further, administration of GM-CSF in combination with G-CSF or FL to patients with cancer can significantly increase the number of peripheral blood DCs. Direct comparisons of GM-CSF and cytokine combinations have not yet been studied in humans. To date, GM-CSF is the most commonly used vaccine adjuvant in cancer vaccines and currently is being used in clinical trials in the form of a systemically administered recombinant cytokine or via gene therapy with GM-CSF-transfected tumor cells or subcutaneous delivery of poxviruses expressing GM-CSF.

Tumor Necrosis Factor-α (TNF-α)

TNF-α was the main component of the earliest cancer immunotherapy approach attempted in the 1890s by the surgeon William B. Coley. Coley used bacterial extracts with tumor "*necrosing*" activity in patients with advanced cancer. Today, we know that TNF-α is mainly produced by macrophages and lymphocytes in response to various infectious agents or cytokine stimuli. There are two receptors for TNF-α, TNF-R1 and TNF-R2 that are expressed ubiquitously. The main actions of TNF-α involve the direct induction of cytotoxicity and gene expression.

TNF-α and antigen presentation

In addition to the direct effects of TNF-α on tumor cells, TNF-α also regulates antigen presentation. In 1990, Zembala et al. reported that TNF-α increased the ability of human monocytes to present soluble protein antigen to autologous T cells *in vitro*. A possible mechanism for this enhanced antigen presentation was the upregulation of HLA-DR molecules after TNF-α treatment of monocytes. In 1992, two reports demonstrated that TNF-α helped to regulate the maturation of DCs from human stem cells, only in combination with GM-CSF. The combination of GM-CSF and TNF-α increased the yield of CD1a$^+$ DCs by 10 to 20-fold from CD34$^+$ hematopoietic stem cells from umbilical cord blood. Culture with TNF-α alone had no effects on the differentiation of stem cells. TNF-α now is used with GM-CSF to mature DCs derived *in vitro* from human peripheral blood or stem cells. Thus, the use of TNF-α for tumor immunotherapy could be a two-pronged attack, first by directly inducing cytotoxicity in tumors and second by potentiating antigen presentation and subsequently promoting anti-tumor immunity.

Clinical application of TNF-α

Systemic use of recombinant TNF-α for advanced cancers demonstrated little clinical benefit and caused dose-limiting toxicities that included hypotension, hepatotoxicity, malaise, fatigue, and thrombocytopenia. These toxicities are not surprising given the ubiquitous expression of TNF receptors. On a positive note, a different route of administration, "*isolated limb perfusion*," resulted in a clinical benefit with reduced toxicity for metastatic melanoma and sarcoma. Due to its toxicity, selection of TNF-α for *in vivo* cancer treatment most likely should be reserved for localized treatment and direct tumor cytotoxicity. Similarly, for cancer vaccines, TNF-α may have clinical utility if delivered locally at lower doses. One Phase I trial demonstrated that daily subcutanenous GM-CSF combined with continuous infusion of TNF-α could increase the number of Langerhans cells in the epidermis of cancer patients. However, given the higher efficacy of combined GM-CSF and IL-4 treatments to increase the number of DCs *in vivo*, recombinant TNF-α likely appears better suited for cancer vaccine strategies employing DCs generated *in vitro*, in combination with GM-CSF.

Flt3 Ligand

FL is a colony-stimulating factor that can induce proliferation, self-renewal, and differentiation of hematopoietic stem cells. FL binds its receptor, Flt3, which is a receptor tyrosine kinase belonging to the family that includes c-KIT and PDGFR. Flt3 was cloned from pro-B cell lines and also is expressed in monocytic/myeloid lineage and hematopoietic stem ($CD34^+$) cells from bone marrow or fetal liver. This pattern of expression led to the hypothesis that FL had an important role in early hematopoiesis. FL has been demonstrated to have an important regulatory role in DC biology in both mice and humans. This early work identified a rationale for the *in vivo* application of FL to promote DC expansion, antigen presentation, and subsequent adaptive (antigen-specific) immunity.

FL also plays an important role in regulating innate immunity in mice. In 1998, Shaw et al. showed that systemic administration of FL

Table 11.3. History of Flt3-ligand

Year	*Studies*
1993	Murine FL cloned
1994	Human FL homologue
1996	FL therapy expands DCs in mice
1997	FL therapy induces CD8$^+$ T cell-dependent tumor regression in mice
2000	FL therapy increased number (48 and 44-fold) of CD11c$^+$ DCs in peripheral blood of healthy human subjects
2000	FL$^{-/-}$ mice have reduced splenic DCs (3 to 12-fold)
2002	FL therapy increased number of immature DCs in patients with metastatic renal cell carcinoma, with no effect on disease
2002	FL adjuvant for HER2-neu vaccination promotes peptide-specific interferon-secreting T cells

expands the absolute number of NK cells in mice and increases their cytotoxic activity. Thereafter, in 2000, McKenna et al. reported a marked deficiency of leukocytes, including NK cells, in the FL "*knockout*" mouse. These "*knockout*" mice had reduced numbers of B lymphoid and myeloid progenitors in the bone marrow, and a marked decrease in splenic DCs (3 to 12-fold) and NK cells (5-fold).

FL expands DCs and enhances tumor immunity in vivo

In 1996, Maraskovsky et al. administered FL to wild type mice and subsequently observed a significant expansion of DCs. After only nine days of daily intraperitoneal FL, they observed expansions of CD11c$^+$ MHC Class II$^+$ DCs in the spleen (17-fold), lymph nodes (4-fold), and peripheral blood (6-fold) compared to controls. In peptide-pulsing experiments and alloantigen-stimulations, these DCs were functionally mature.

In 1997, Lynch et al. hypothesized that FL-mediated expansion of DCs *in vivo* could provide protective anti-tumor immunity. They challenged mice with murine fibrosarcomas and administered daily FL for nine days. FL-treated mice displayed marked tumor regression and retarded tumor growth. Protection provided by FL was dose-dependent and could be abrogated by *in vivo* depletion of CD8$^+$ T cells but not CD4$^+$ T cells. Further, tissues surrounding tumors in FL-treated mice displayed greater DC infiltrates than untreated mice. Immunity was transferable through adoptively transferred splenocytes from FL-treated mice that successfully had rejected tumors.

Clinical application of FL for cancer immunotherapy

Given the ability of FL to promote generation of DC precursors *in vivo*, FL was evaluated as a potential adjuvant for cancer vaccine strategies. In 2000, Maraskovsky et al. and Pulendran et al. reported the ability of FL, alone or in combination with G-CSF, to expand DCs in healthy human volunteers. Pulendran et al. reported that administration of FL alone after ten days led to a 48-fold increase in $CD11c^+$ DCs ($HLA\text{-}DR^+$ $CD86^+$) and a 13-fold increase in $CD11c^-$ DCs ($HLADR^-$ $CD86^-$) in the peripheral blood. Further, they reported that the $CD11c^+$ DCs had allostimulatory capacity when cultured with allogenenic $CD4^+$ T cells *in vitro*, while this capacity was absent in $CD11c^-$DCs. Maraskovsky's report confirmed that FL alone led to a 44-fold expansion of $CD11c^+$ DCs ($HLAD\text{-}DR^+CD86^+$), and that this population could be further differentiated *in vitro* with IL-4 and GM-CSF. $CD11c^+$ DCs expanded *in vivo* resembled immature DCs but were not as efficient at antigen uptake.

Recombinant FL was subsequently applied in patients with late stage cancer. FL was shown to be effective in mobilizing DC precursors in patients with melanoma or renal cancer. Again, FL expanded DCs (19-fold) with a partially differentiated DC phenotype, $CD11c^+$ $CD86^+$ $HLA\text{-}DR^+$, but $CD80^-$ $CD83^-$. More recently, FL has been combined with tumor antigen peptides in cancer vaccine trials. Disis et al. studied patients with HER-2/neu overexpressing malignancies and vaccinated them with HER-2/neu peptides, in combination with either recombinant FL or FL + GM-CSF. While this approach failed to promote proliferation of HER-2/neuspecific T cells, the immunization did increase the number of interferon-producing HER-2/neu-specific T cells. Infiltration and differentiation of APCs at the vaccine sites were not reported. This study demonstrated that systemic administration of FL as a vaccine adjuvant results in the mobilization of DCs capable of presenting tumor antigen and promoting T cell immunity against co-administered antigen (interferon-producing T cells).

Together, these pre-clinical and clinical data show that FL alone effectively expands DC precursors (44 to 48-fold) but that these DCs were not as effective at antigen presentation as the more mature DCs generated with GM-CSF. The most productive use of FL in cancer vaccines is in combination with other cytokines for either *in vivo* or *ex vivo* differentiation of DCs. Recombinant FL is safe, but its clinical use remains to be optimized and its production for continued clinical study in the U.S. needs to be renewed.

Interferons

Interferons (IFN) were first described in 1957 as antiviral cytokines by Issacs and Lindenmann when they demonstrated that IFN secretion could be induced by viral infection of chick embryo cells. Type I IFNs are highly heterogeneous with over 14 proteins produced in humans that include the major subtypes IFN-α, secreted by leukocytes, and IFN-β, secreted by fibroblasts. Type I IFNs signal through a Type I IFN-α or IFN-β receptor. IFN-γ is the only Type II interferon known and is secreted by activated NK cells and $CD8^+$ cytotoxic T lymphocytes. IFN-γ signals through a single IFN-γ receptor expressed on nearly all cells, including tumor cells.

The first biological activity described for IFNs was their anti-viral function in virus-infected cells. IFNs induce three pathways that regulate virus-infected cells: two pathways inhibit protein synthesis and a third inhibits viral transcription. IFNs also demonstrate anti-proliferative and cytotoxic effects on cells, which led to their early use in cancer therapy. In addition to these anti-viral and anti-tumor activities, IFNs have an important role in linking innate and adaptive immunity. Early in the immune response, innate immune effector cells (NK cells) produce abundant IFN-γ, the strongest cytokine activator of macrophages. Activated macrophages respond to IFN-γ by producing cytokines (e.g. IL-12, IL-15, TNF-α) that further induce NK cell activity. These cytokines build a positive feedback loop, wherein macrophage secreted cytokines stimulate NK cells, and NK-derived IFN-γ further activate macrophages. Cytotoxic T cells also secrete IFN-γ as an effector molecule.

Type II IFNs are also thought to have direct cytotoxic and anti-proliferative effects on tumors. Neutralization of this effector cytokine in mice limited tumor surveillance in mice chemically induced with 3-methylcholanthrene. When the IFN-γ-insensitive tumors from these mice were transferred to syngeneic mice, the tumors demonstrated lower immunogencity than IFN-γ-sensitive tumors. This process of the immune system shaping a tumor's phenotype has been termed "*cancer immunoediting*".

IFNs and antigen presentation

IFNs induce the upregulation of MHC molecules in both immune cells and tumor cells. Type I IFNs induce expression of MHC Class I molecules, while IFN-γ upregulates both MHC Class I and II molecules. In addition, IFN signaling initiates the expression of genes important for antigen processing, including genes for the proteasome enzyme complex. The proteasome is essential for the proteolytic degradation of protein products into antigenic peptides for presentation by MHC molecules. Thus, IFNs can enhance antigen processing and presentation in not only tumor cells but also host APCs, including B cells, monocytes, and DCs.

In fact, recent reports demonstrated that Type I IFNs facilitate the differentiation of DCs from either $CD34^+$ bone marrow stem cells or peripheral blood monocytes. Specifically, IFN-α can accelerate the maturation of DCs from immature DCs. Santini et al., reported that IFN-α, in combination with GM-CSF, could be used to quickly generate mature DCs from human peripheral blood monocytes *in* vitro and that these DCs were superior to those generated using IL-4 and GMCSF, with respect to stronger stimulation in mixed leukocyte reactions and greater induction of human Ig from B cells.

Clinical Application of IFNs for Cancer Immunotherapy

Type I IFNs have had extensive clinical use for infections, multiple sclerosis, and several cancers. The many effects of IFNs likely are important in the mechanism of action for each of these diseases. For example, IFN-α has been used to treat Hepatitis B or C infections, taking advantage of the anti-viral and immunological properties of IFNs. Further, Type I IFNs treatment of various tumor cell lines in vitro has shown cytotoxic and anti-proliferative effects. The effects of IFNs on antigen presentation have been studied and are most apparent in the treatment of melanoma and renal cell carcinoma. These studies, however, have focused on reactive cytotoxic and helper T lymphocytes as immunological endpoints, not activity of APCs.

One of the more successful applications of IFNs was in the early 1990s, when treatment with IFN-α was shown to induce remissions in 60–80% patients with early phase *chronic myeloid leukemia* (CML). More recently, CML-specific cytotoxic T lymphocytes and antibody producing B cells have been implicated in those patients with CML who responded to IFN-α therapy. The effects of IFN-α on antigen presentation in these patients was first suggested when Wang et al. reported that DCs derived from bone marrow of CML patients were less effective in allo-stimulation than normal bone marrow-derived DCs. Molldrem et al. identified peptides from Proteinase 3 that were highly expressed in myeloid leukemias, and recognized by cytotoxic T cells that in turn could lyse the leukemia cells. Using MHC Class I tetramers and a Proteinase 3 peptide called PR1, they demonstrated that patients responsive to IFN-α2b therapy displayed PR1-specific T cells, while non-responders lacked these T cells. Lastly, Paquette et al. reported that IFN-α and GM-CSF could differentiate DCs *in vitro* from the peripheral blood or bone marrow of CML patients, better than IL-4 and GM-CSF. Furthermore, they demonstrated that CML patients responding to IFN-α had an increase in bone marrow DCs. They hypothesized that IFN-α could facilitate antigen presentation directly from leukemic cells through upregulation of MHC molecules and other DC antigens. Additional evidence in breast and colon cancers suggests that IFN-α treatment may also directly increase expression of select antigens on tumor cells.

In contrast, cancer patients treated with Type II IFNs as single agents have had poor responses as single agents for cancer treatment. Type II IFNs have been largely studied as effector molecules of the immune response that act in a positive feedback loop to strengthen both innate and adaptive effectors. Although IFN-γ strongly increases MHC gene expression in APCs, the clinical trials completed thus far for solid and hematologic malignancies have shown little promise. Despite these results, IFN-γ has shown some efficacy for the treatment of chronic myelogenous leukemia. These studies suggest that in addition to direct cytotoxic effects on tumor cells, IFNs, especially IFN-α may mediate clinical responses through the upregulation of MHC molecules on tumor cells, increased tumor cell antigen expression, and increased differentiation and maturation of DCs.

Challenges for Cytokine Therapy

Cytokines that can increase the number of APCs and enhance tumor antigen presentation on tumor cells or on host APCs, may improve T cell recognition and responses to such antigens. While a direct role for cytokines in minimal residual disease is possible, a role in cancer vaccine strategies seems more promising. While preclinical and clinical data using GM-CSF, IL-4, FL, IFNs, and TNF-α have shown potential, however, optimal use of these cytokines may depend upon the specific cancer and tumor antigens. Successful clinical application of cytokine strategies will most likely require more preclinical and clinical studies. Mechanisms to make these cytokines available for such work should be rapidly developed by the National Cancer Institute in collaboration with industry.

12

Immune Monitoring

A fundamental aspect of developing effective cancer vaccines is the process of evaluating the immune response to such therapeutic interventions. Despite the availability of a number of immunologic assays for evaluating tumor antigen-specific immunity, no single test has emerged as an unequivocally superior metric for judging the efficacy of cancer vaccines. Nonetheless, there have been several technologic developments that will likely impact the search for the ideal biomarker for tumor-specific immunity. The available tools, major advancements, and current challenges in this quest for reliable immune monitoring techniques are the focus of this chapter.

When patients are treated for minor ailments with highly effective agents, such as the treatment of a local bacterial infection with an appropriate oral antibiotic, the initial response to treatment typically can be evaluated on clinical grounds alone. For most cancer patients with life-threatening conditions, the scenario is quite different. In many cases, the only available systemic therapies may produce a modest to poor response, and months to years may be required to confirm any survival benefit. Although clinical evaluation may include a variety of laboratory tests and imaging studies, the ability of many such tests to demonstrate a true benefit to survival is poor. Because immunotherapy remains a largely unproven therapeutic modality for the treatment of cancer, similar issues arise in the setting of cancer vaccines.

A second major obstacle in the evaluation of immune responses to vaccines is identifying the optimal patient population to be evaluated in clinical trials. Early phase studies are typically undertaken in patients with advanced disease, in part because the relative impact on patient survival and quality of life in case of an adverse event is expected to be small in a patient with a short life expectancy. If a vaccine is found to be safe, subsequent studies may also be performed in patients with minimal to no measurable disease following treatment, or in patients with earlier stage disease. Some investigators believe that tumor vaccines are not (and may never be) potent enough to eradicate extensive tumor burden, and that these patients may simply be too immunosuppressed to mount an adequate response. Patients with earlier stage disease generally have lower tumor burden and may be more immunocompetent than patients with advanced disease. They may have such long survival, however, that large numbers of patients would have to be followed over a number of years in order to prove a vaccine effective. Consequently, many investigators have focused on patients with advanced disease whose treatment has eradicated gross or "*measurable*" disease. In theory, these patients should be relatively immunocompetent despite a relatively short recurrence free and overall survival. Despite these efforts, cancer vaccines to date have exhibited at best modest clinical impact regardless of the patient population examined.

Another barrier to progress in immune monitoring is an incomplete understanding of relevant immunoregulatory mechanisms. It is likely that identification of critical signaling events necessary and sufficient for stimulating antitumor immunity will lead to recognition of reliable biomarkers for effective antitumor vaccines. Because no existing cancer vaccines induce sufficiently robust antigen-specific T cell responses, there is no standard vaccine preparation available for evaluating immune monitoring assays. Instead, investigators are left with the task of trying to optimize immunologic assays based on T cell responses that in many cases may be difficult to detect above background.

Finally, despite the publication of thousands of articles on active specific immunotherapy for the treatment of cancer, few properly controlled, prospective, randomized trials have been reported. Numerous vaccine strategies nonetheless have been abandoned as ineffective. This has made interpretation of the literature in this field difficult and has promoted skepticism about the promise of tumor vaccines. The challenge of developing and systematically testing methods of immunologic monitoring to identify promising vaccine candidates is therefore one of the most important objectives in immunotherapy at this time. This article will describe how existing strategies have been used to address this problem and will discuss technologic advancements that may facilitate the development of reliable biomarkers for clinically effective antitumor immunity.

Principles of Immunologic Monitoring

Although it is likely that many elements of humoral and cellular immunity have some influence on the ability to generate antitumor immune responses, most investigators agree that T cells play a pivotal role. Therefore, T cell biology has been a primary focus of active specific immunotherapy for a number of years and will be the focus of this chapter on immunologic monitoring. Previous chapters have described key immunologic events that appear to be critical for the induction of potent antitumor T cell responses. An open question is which of these processes most closely reflect the true clinical impact of tumor vaccines, and how such processes can be evaluated in a simple assay system.

Most assay systems designed to quantitatively measure phenotypic and/or functional properties of T cell populations contrast sharply with those used to evaluate humoral responses to prophylactic immunizations against infectious agents. In the latter case, regardless of the complex immunologic processes that ultimately lead to an antibody response, evidence has shown that a reliable biomarker for clinical efficacy of such immunizations is the titer of neutralizing antibodies present in the serum.

While it is possible that a reliable serum biomarker for antigen-specific T cell immunity exists, none has been identified thus far. Hence, most existing assays for the measurement of antitumor activity depend upon phenotypic and/or functional properties of T cells themselves. This has presented challenges along several fronts: (i) determining the most appropriate source of T cells, such as peripheral blood, the vaccination site, lymph nodes draining the vaccination site, or the tumor itself; (ii) optimizing the procurement, processing, storage and (if necessary) shipping of cells without compromising cell viability and function; (iii) identifying the phenotypic and/or functional properties of T cells that most accurately reflect antitumor immunity; (iv) establishing which subpopulations of T cells should be evaluated (e.g., $CD4^+$ [helper], $CD8^+$ [cytotoxic], $CD25^+$ [regulatory] T cells); (v) selecting the appropriate timing for immunologic monitoring following vaccination; and (vi) selecting the specific methods for evaluating tumor-specific T cell properties that most likely reflect the true antitumor response. Unfortunately, at the present time no method of immune monitoring has all these characteristics.

Table 12.1. Proposed properties of an ideal immune monitoring assay

Property
Reliable indicator of true clinical efficacy/effect on survival
Reliable indicator of true tumor-specific immunologic activity
Superior sensitivity, specificity, reproducibility
Ability to perform test on minute quantity of biological material
Adaptability to automation and high throughput analysis
Time-efficient, cost-effective

Techniques of Immune Monitoring

A variety of methods have been used to evaluate the antitumor response to immunotherapy. These may be divided into clinical and immunologic assessments, the latter being the focus of this chapter. The standard endpoint according to which all methods of assessment ultimately must be compared is overall survival. As discussed earlier, however, judging the efficacy of each individual candidate tumor vaccine on the basis of overall survival is extremely costly in terms of time and resources, and is therefore impractical. Evaluation of clinical response by measuring tumor shrinkage is common practice, and standard guidelines for this method of evaluation are available. Unfortunately, measurement of tumor shrinkage is a relatively unreliable technique for determining the response to immunotherapy, and it does not contribute to an understanding of underlying regulatory mechanisms.

The development of immunologic assays to evaluate tumor-specific T cell responses has been an area of intense investigation. Such immunologic tests comprise both in vivo and in vitro approaches. Both types of tests have been utilized extensively in the evaluation of cancer vaccines and are reviewed herein.

In Vivo Testing: Delayed Type Hypersensitivity

Delayed type hypersensitivity (DTH) testing is a classical method for measuring type IV (cellular) immune responsiveness. This technique involves administering an intradermal injection of an antigen preparation and recording the amount of erythema and induration produced after 48 to 72 hours. This response is believed to reflect antigen-specific activation of $CD4^+$ T cells to release T-helper 1 cytokines such as interferon-gamma (IFN-γ) in the region of the injection site. These cytokines recruit monocytes and other inflammatory cells to the site and cause an increase in vascular permeability and extravasation. $CD8^+$ T cells also appear to have the capacity to mediate such a response.

DTH testing requires little training, does not require sophisticated or costly equipment, and can be performed readily in the clinic or at the bedside. This technique of immune monitoring consequently has played a prominent role in the monitoring of immunotherapy trials. The procedure for applying DTH testing to immune monitoring is not standardized, however. Doses of peptide antigens, for example, may vary from the low microgram to milligram range and typically are administered in volumes of 0.1 to 1.0 ml. Preparations may contain one or more peptides, adjuvant(s), antigen-presenting cells and/or a variety of other agents designed to enhance immune reactivity. The procedure for measuring the response (erythema and induration) and the definition of a positive result also varies among studies, and there is a significant subjective component. Due to the lack of standardization of the injection procedure, measurements, and interpretation, meaningful comparison of DTH results among immunotherapy trials may can be difficult.

Another problem with DTH testing is that responses are not always antigen-specific. In one study, for example, erythema and induration were noted in response to injections with peptide-loaded *dendritic cells* (DC), but DC that were not loaded with any antigen produced a similar DTH response. In another study in which patients were injected with CEA peptide-loaded DC, some patients without apparent erythema or induration at the injection site were noted to have inflammatory infiltrates on histopathologic examination. The potential for nonspecific contributions to the DTH reaction may be particularly apparent when adjuvant agents are used. For example, GM-CSF, a cytokine included in some vaccine preparations, itself may induce a DTH response. Responses to other antigens in the vaccine preparation may also occur, as may occur when fetal bovine serum is used to cultivate cells during vaccine preparation.

Although not all studies have demonstrated DTH reactivity to be a reliable marker of antitumor immunity, some have shown concordance with other assays and/or an association with clinical response. In a study of HER2/neu peptide vaccine, a DTH induration of diameter 10 mm or greater was associated with an antigen-specific proliferative response, while lesser degrees of induration were not. Hsueh and colleagues reported that tumor-specific DTH reactivity was associated with a significantly better overall survival in stage IV melanoma patients with no measurable disease who were treated with a polyvalent allogeneic cellular melanoma vaccine.

Because DTH testing is easily incorporated into the design of immunotherapy trials and appears to have some relationship to antigen-specific immunity, it will likely remain an integral part of the immune monitoring repertoire until a superior approach is available. However, in the interim, a system of standardizing the application of this test to immune monitoring could enhance its utility.

In Vitro Methods

Sources of specimens for immune monitoring

The optimal source of specimens for use in immune monitoring assays is unknown. Most assays of antigen-specific T cell immunity are based on evaluation of T lymphocytes themselves. There are many potential sources of lymphocytes, such as the peripheral blood, tumor deposits, injection sites, or draining lymph nodes. Because the peripheral blood is the most convenient source of T cells, it has been the most widely utilized. Whether the peripheral blood T cell response to a vaccine correlates with the clinical response has been called into question, however. Lee and colleagues administered a gp100 peptide vaccine with or without IL-2 and found that the only subset of patients who showed evidence of a clinical response did *not* have detectable gp100-specific T cells in the peripheral blood. One explanation offered for this was that the tumor-specific T cells in patients with clinical responses migrated to tumor deposits or other site(s). Consistent with this hypothesis, some tumors are known to harbor tumor-specific T cells, but the presence of such *tumor-infiltrating lymphocytes* (TIL) does not necessarily correlate with clinical response.

Another potential source of T cells is the DTH (vaccine injection) site, but whether these antigen-specific T cells would have similar properties to TIL is unclear. Draining lymph nodes may also contain antigen-specific T cells, although such T cells have been found even in healthy patients without malignances. Nonetheless, this is a particularly attractive source of T cells in part because of the frequency with which regional lymph node dissections are performed for melanoma and other malignancies.

Recently, Slingluff's group reported a promising method for harvesting tumor-specific T cells from lymph nodes of melanoma patients using a procedure adapted from the sentinel lymph node biopsy technique. The lymph node directly draining the peptide vaccine site (the *sentinel immunized node*, SIN) was harvested from each of five patients. While CTL activity could be demonstrated in T cells from the SIN in 5/5 patients, similar activity was identified in only 2/5 patients with T cells from the peripheral blood. Further work will be necessary to determine whether procedures such as this will replace peripheral blood as a source of T cells for monitoring the immune response to cancer vaccines.

An alternative strategy to examining T cells themselves is to identify a surrogate biomarker for T cell activity in tissues or body fluids. Most previous studies in which serum markers were used as indicators of immune responsiveness to cancer vaccines have focused on the measurement of antibodies or immune complexes. This strategy represents an attractive option because of the difficulty of procuring, processing and storing T cells in a manner such that antigen-specific T cell activity is properly retained. One example of this approach is the analysis of serum T cell cytokine levels. While the measurement of serum cytokine levels has not yet been demonstrated to be of value in immune monitoring, this strategy could assume a more dominant role with the advent of increasingly sophisticated proteomics instrumentation and methodologies.

Regardless of the source of T cells or other specimens, the procedures for collection, processing, and in some cases storage of these samples may be critical to an accurate readout of immune assays. For example, whether and how best to cryopreserve *peripheral blood mononuclear cells* (PBMC) could have a dramatic impact of T cell activity. In part because it is generally easier to preserve molecular rather than cellular integrity and activity, a progressive shift toward molecular approaches appears likely.

Types of in vitro methods for immune monitoring

Although there is no gold standard technique for immune monitoring, a number of assays are currently in use, and there has been no shortage of novel approaches or improvements in existing ones in the published literature. Although increasingly the divisions among these categories are becoming blurred and some strategies may incorporate a combination of these features, the conceptual framework is useful.

First, these methods may be distinguished according to whether they examine *cell biological* or *molecular* properties. For example, T cell proliferation and microcytotoxicity assays reflect biological processes that may occur in response to antigen-specific T cell activation, but do not indicate the specific molecules responsible for these processes. In contrast, one can measure specific cell surface molecules or cytokines that are believed to be involved in these processes without directly examining such T cell functions. A second category applies specifically to molecular techniques and is becoming increasingly useful in light of the rapid rate of technologic advancement in this field. This regards the class of molecules that are detected by molecular techniques: *DNA*, *RNA* or *proteins*.

Finally, in vitro immune monitoring assays can be classified according to whether they evaluate *phenotypic* or *functional* properties of T cells. For example, quantitating the frequency of a T cell population based on a cell surface marker is a phenotypic assay, while cytolytic assays are functional. Although cytokine based methods in one sense could be viewed as phenotypic assays, these experiments typically involve measuring cytokines produced in vitro over a certain time period in response to antigen-specific stimulation and are generally categorized as functional assays.

A number of modifications also may be made to virtually any of these assays, but do not themselves define distinct categories. For example, in order to address the relatively poor signal-to-noise ratio of microcytotoxicity assays, one or more rounds of in vitro T cell stimulation and expansion may be carried out prior to analysis. Such manipulations may be performed prior to virtually any immunologic assay, although one could argue that this should not be necessary for the detection of truly significant antigen-specific T cell responses. Other platforms, such as multiplex and high-throughput analyses, represent additional modifications that may be applied to a variety of immune assay systems.

Assays for Immune Monitoring

Assays that measure cell biological process

Traditional immune monitoring techniques monitor cellular processes that are associated with antigen-specific T cell stimulation. Among these are T cell proliferation and microcytotoxicity assays. The use of these techniques in conjunction with *limiting dilution analysis* (LDA) enable one to obtain an estimate of T lymphocyte precursor frequency.

T cell proliferation assay

The T cell proliferation assay is generally believed to reflect the amount of $CD4^+$ T lymphocyte proliferation in response to stimulation with a specific antigen. This method involves incubation of the patient's T lymphocytes (or PBMC) and antigen with or without added antigen-presenting cells (for example, irradiated autologous or HLA-matched dendritic cells). After approximately three to five days, cells are pulsed with tritiated thymidine, and DNA synthesis is quantitated by measuring the amount of tritiated thymidine incorporated into DNA using a gamma counter. Relative proliferation may be estimated using a stimulation index, which is defined as the ratio of the [radioactivity incorporated into T cells following stimulation *with antigen*] to the [radioactivity incorporated into the control T cells in the *absence of antigen*].

The evaluation of in vitro T cell proliferation as an index of tumor antigen-specific immunity induced by vaccine therapy has been a fundamental component of the immune monitoring assessment. A major advantage of this strategy is its relative simplicity. Furthermore, it is not very labor-intensive and requires only standard reagents and equipment that are found or easily obtained at most research facilities. Its disadvantages from a technical standpoint include the lengthy incubation period of several days and its requirement for radioactivity. Of particular concern, because the proliferation assay evaluates a process (DNA synthesis) that is not associated specifically with antigen-specific activation of T cells, results may be influenced by nonspecific stimulation. Not surprisingly, proliferation assay results have not correlated strongly with clinical activity of cancer vaccines. Some of the drawbacks of the traditional proliferation assay may be circumvented with a recently described flow cytometry-based strategy for evaluating proliferation.

Microcytotoxicity

The ability of $CD8^+$ *cytotoxic T lymphocytes* (CTL) to lyse target cells may be monitored directly with microcytotoxicity assays. In this technique, effector T cells or PBMC are mixed with target tumor cells at a variety of effector:target ratios, and target cell lysis is measured after a specified time interval. The traditional approach involves using target cells loaded with a radioactive tracer such as Chromium prior to the assay and measuring the quantity of tracer released during a defined incubation period. Percent specific lysis may be calculated from the amount of tracer released using the following formula:

$$\% \text{ Specific Lysis} = \frac{\text{Total Release} - \text{Background Release}}{\text{Maximum Release} - \text{Background Release}} \times 100\%$$

where *Total Release* is the amount of radioactivity released into the medium in the presence of effector cells, *Maximum Release* is the amount released when target cells are completely lysed with detergent, and *Background Release* is the amount released in the absence of effector cells. Percent specific lysis is then plotted versus the effector:target ratio for each assay condition.

A distinct advantage of this approach is that the T lymphocyte mediated lysis of tumor cell targets in vitro is relevant to the desired effect of tumor vaccines in vivo. However, the tracers may not be taken up avidly by certain types of target cells, and the chromium-based assay requires handling of radioactive material. Although a europium-based fluorometric cytolytic assay is available, this technique has not been applied as widely as the chromium-based method, possibly due to problems with reproducibility. Due to the relatively poor signal:noise ratio of the microcytotoxicity assay, detection of tumor-specific CTL activity directly from PBMC or other sources of T cells may be difficult or impossible, and therefore one or more in vitro stimulations of T cells are often necessary prior to performing the assay. These in vitro manipulations appear to amplify, but may also distort the relative magnitude of tumor-specific CTL present in the patient. In addition, because autologous tumor cells may not be readily available for use as targets, alternative targets such as HLA-matched tumor cell lines or tumor antigen-loaded antigen-presenting cells, may be used instead. Consequently, the relevance of microcytotoxcity assays to the true tumor-specific CTL activity induced by tumor vaccines has been called into question.

Alternative methods for evaluating CTL cytotoxicity in vitro have been developed in order to circumvent some of the problems associated with the traditional chromium release assay. For example, a flow cytometry-based technique in which target cells are stained with a green fluorescent membrane dye (DiO18) and the nuclear dye propidium iodide. The percentage of target cells in each well that are lysed during an incubation period may be calculated because all cells are stained by the membrane dye, but only nonviable cells take up the propidium iodide. An alternative cytotoxicity assay is based on the flow cytometric detection of target cell Annexin I expression, which increases in response to attack by effector T cells. These alternative methods do not involve radioactive materials and are not dependent upon the ability of target cells to take up tracer material as in the release assays. Whether the results of these alternative cytotoxicity assays will predict clinical response to tumor vaccines remains to be determined.

Limiting dilution analysis

The classical approach to determining cytotoxic T lymphocyte precursor frequency is through LDA. In this technique T cells are serially diluted into a large number of wells of a microtiter plate, and cells are stimulated with an antigen of interest. A Poisson distribution analysis is used to calculate the proportion of wells with a given T cell number that contained at least one antigen-specific precursor at the beginning of the stimulation. This allows an estimate of the antigen-specific T cell precursor frequency to be calculated. LDA is labor-intensive, cumbersome, and may be difficult to reproduce. Although this method is worthy of mention as a foundation for discussion of microcytotoxicity assays, its utility in the context of cancer vaccine trials is limited.

Assays that detect molecular markers of immunity

As knowledge regarding the molecular basis of immunity and tumor immunology has grown and molecular techniques have become more powerful, there has been an increasing focus on detection of molecular biomarkers for tumor-specific immunity. Because of an incomplete understanding of these processes at the molecular level, however, it is unclear which factors would most accurately reflect the state of the immune system and would serve as the best surrogate markers of immunity. Nonetheless, several strategies already are in use, and a number of exciting modifications and entirely novel approaches have recently been described or are currently in development.

Techniques based on molecular determination of phenotype

Phenotypic and functional immunologic analyses are complementary methodologies. It appears likely that these two approaches increasingly will be used in conjunction in immune monitoring protocols and ultimately will merge seamlessly into one analysis. Purely phenotypic analyses are useful in that detailed quantitative and qualitative information can be obtained regarding a particular T cell population of interest. However, functional activity of such cell populations can only be inferred.

T cell receptor v region analysis. Antigen-specific T cells may be quantitated by examining the frequency of cells that harbor specific *T cell receptor* (TCR) V-J region sequences. The basis of this method is that a significant T cell response to a vaccine should elicit an expansion of T cells that express specific J-alpha, J-beta, V-alpha and V-beta chains that correspond to recognition of the index antigen. Flow cytometry may be used to estimate the frequency of such a T cell response with antibodies that recognize specific subfamilies of the TCR alpha or beta chains. Alternatively, polymerase chain reaction (PCR) technology may be used to derive similar information.

TCR V region analysis requires only a small amount of specimen and may be performed on T cells isolated directly from the peripheral blood without prior ex vivo expansion. Although it is somewhat cumbersome, an automated, rapid, fluorescence-based variation of the PCR technique has been developed for detecting *complementarity-determining region* 3 (CDR 3) length analysis of TCR gene families. This approach is able to distinguish among polyclonal, oligoclonal and monoclonal CDR3 distributions.

MHC-peptide tetramer analysis. An alternative approach to quantitating antigen-specific T cells is to use a flow-based technique in which fluorophor-conjugated complexes bind specifically to a TCR of interest. Tetramers consist of tetrameric complexes of a particular type of major histocompatibility complex with a defined peptide that binds to that major histocompatibility (MHC) complex. Four such complexes are bound together to a fluorophor-conjugated avidin molecule through avidin-biotin linkages, allowing for an extremely stable tetrameric unit. Such tetrameric complexes have been shown to bind stably and specifically to cognate antigen-specific T cells. An alternative reagent that may be used to detect antigen-specific T cells is a dimer of MHC-peptide complexes that is bound together through an antibody. A tetramer may be prepared for virtually any MHC class I-restricted peptide, provided the sequence of the immunogenic peptide is known and a stable tetramer can be synthesized.

MHC-peptide tetramers have proven to be a useful tool for quantitating antigen-specific T cells in the context of immunotherapy trials. One group has used tetramer staining and flow cytometry to sort antigen-specific T cells isolated from the peripheral blood or lymph nodes. They found that these T cells produced cytokines in response to antigen-specific stimulation.

Although the availability of tetramers represents a significant technologic advancement in immune monitoring, these reagents have several limitations. First, tetramers can only be developed for peptides of a defined sequence for a specific antigen, and stable tetramers may be difficult to synthesize for certain peptides. Although tetramers are available for a variety of MHC class I-restricted peptides, tetramers for class II-restricted peptides have been introduced more recently.

Therefore, far fewer tetramers are available for MHC class II-restricted peptide antigens than for class I peptides. Furthermore, tetramers are HLA class-restricted, most available tetramers being restricted to HLA-A2.01. Consequently, any particular tetramer is only useful in a minority of patients. Finally, although functional activity has been documented in antigen-specific T cells detected with tetramers, the precise composition and function of tetramer-positive cells is not completely clear at this point. One approach to circumventing this problem is the combined use of tetramer staining with other types of flow cytometry based analyses, such as cytokine flow cytometry. There also appear to be phenotypically distinct subsets, such as memory versus effector T cells, that are not evident unless appropriate markers (e.g., CD45RA/CD45RO) are examined.

Techniques based on cytokine production

Several immunological methods are available that evaluate antigen-specific T cell activation by measuring some functional property of T cells, such as the elaboration of cytokines. Although nonspecific stimulation of T cells, for example by mitogens, may induce the production of cytokines, antigen-specific cytokine production usually can be determined by cytokine-based methods if appropriate controls are incorporated. An advantage of these approaches is that the pattern of cytokines detected reflects whether the immune response has primarily a T helper 1 (Th1) or Th2 bias. In addition, cytokine-based methods can be used to quantitate T cell responses. Finally, most of these techniques are fairly sensitive and, in theory, could detect a specific antitumor T cell response at a frequency of one in 1,000 T cells or lower.

Cytokine ELISA. The *enzyme-linked immunosorbent assay* (ELISA) is a widely used immunoassay for the detection of specific proteins both in the research and clinical laboratory setting. This assay is easily standardized, is reproducible across investigators and institutions, and kits are commercially available for the detection of a variety of cytokines. In this assay, antigen-specific stimulation of T cells or PBMC is carried out in microtiter plates by the methods previously described. After a defined incubation period, usually about 24 to 48 hours, supernatants are tested for the cytokine(s) of interest using a sandwich immunoassay with a colorimetric or fluorescence based detection method. This typically involves coating nitrocellulose bottom microtiter plates with a monoclonal antibody against the cytokine of interest, adding an aliquot of each T cell supernatant, adding an enzyme conjugated form of the anti-cytokine antibody, and incubating with a substrate that is converted to a soluble colored product by the conjugated enzyme. The reaction product can be measured by colorimetric or fluorometric detection, and the relative amount of cytokine released in each well is then determined using a linear regression plot created using a cytokine standard.

In the context of cancer vaccine trials, the cytokine most frequently examined using this method is IFN-γ, which reflects a Th1 pattern of cytokine production. A number of studies have reported significant antigen-specific cytokine release by T cells from patients treated with tumor vaccines. However, experiments typically have been performed using T cells previously treated with one or more rounds of in vitro stimulation. In addition, although the quantity of cytokine released may be related to the strength of the immune response, the precise frequency of antigen-specific T cells present in a sample cannot be determined by this method. Still more concerning is the relatively poor correlation of cytokine release data with clinical response.

Elispot. The ELISpot (*enzyme-linked immunospot*) method is based on similar principles to those of the ELISA and represents a modification of the latter technique. This assay is set up in a similar fashion as the ELISA, but the T cell stimulation is performed directly in the nitrocellulose-bottom microtiter plates pre-coated with antibody against a particular cytokine. As the cytokine of interest is released during the course of the incubation period, some of it binds to the nitrocellulose in the region of the T cell of origin in a pattern reflecting its concentration gradient. This results in a "*footprint*" of bound cytokine at that site. At the end of the assay, cells are washed away with a detergent. The plate is then developed as in the ELISA, but using a substrate that produces an *insoluble* colored product, which appears as a spot on the bottom of the plate. The number of spots per well is counted and is expressed as a frequency relative to the total number of input T cells or PBMC.

Unlike the ELISA, the ELISpot allows an estimation of the antigen-specific T cell frequency. Data analysis may be more cumbersome and subjective, however, due to the large number of spots that must be counted amidst a variable amount of background staining. Special automated plate readers are available that address both of these concerns. Kits available for performing ELISA and ELISpot assays are expensive, however, and sending ELISpot plates for professional reading or purchasing an ELISpot reader represent considerable added costs. Modifications of the ELISA may circumvent some of these problems. For example, one group has developed a multiplex, fluorescence-based immunoassay that requires about 100-fold less primary antibody than the ELISA and is conducive to high-throughput analysis. The recently developed Lysispot assay represents another derivative of the ELISpot. This method enables one to quantitate cytokine-secreting T cells and cytotoxic T cells simultaneously. Interestingly, the investigators found that cytokine secretion and cytotoxicity can be independently regulated.

The ELISpot has been demonstrated to have excellent sensitivity (approximately 1 in 100,000) and specificity for antigen-specific T cell responses and to be reproducible across laboratories. A number of groups have used this technique as a method for immune monitoring in clinical trials. Consequently, the ELISpot increasingly is being touted as a standard component of the armamentarium of immune monitoring tools for cancer vaccine trials.

Flow cytometry based cytokine detection. Flow cytometry based methods also may be used to evaluate antigen-specific cytokine production by T cells following the administration of a vaccine. In *cytokine flow cytometry* (CFC), T cells or PBMC are stimulated in vitro with an antigen or cellular target of interest in the presence of stimulating anti-CD28 monoclonal antibody, which enhances co-stimulation. The secretion inhibitor brefeldin A is added so that cytokines elaborated during the assay build up within the cell of origin. At the end of the assay, the T cells are fixed, permeabilized, and stained with commercially available fluorophor-conjugated monoclonal antibodies against cell surface markers (e.g., CD8), an activation marker (i.e., CD69), and one or more intracellular cytokines (e.g., IFN-γ). Multi-parameter flow cytometry is used to analyze the frequency of T cells within the population of interest that stain positively for CD69 and the cytokine of interest. These "*double-positive*" T cells are presumed to represent functional antigen-specific T cells.

CFC has a number of advantages. It evaluates not only the relative amount of cytokine produced (i.e., relative fluorescence intensity), but also the frequency of the cytokine-producing cells. Assays are relatively easy to set up, and typical incubation periods range from four to six hours. It is also quite sensitive, allowing detection of T cells present at a frequency of one in 10,000, provided the background is adequately low. Furthermore, any T cell subpopulation of interest may be examined. In addition, with proper instrumentation, multiple cytokines may be analyzed simultaneously. The method may be even more powerful in combination with other flow-based methods, such as tetramer analysis, which enables one to precisely determine the concordance of cytokine production with the antigen-specific T cell population of interest as defined by its MHC-peptide specificity. Finally, CFC has also been adapted so that cytokine production by other immune cells of interest, such as DC, may also be examined. Therefore, the flow cytometric platform for cytokine production in principle allows for the acquisition of a large amount of quantitative and qualitative information of direct relevance to describing the T cell response to a tumor antigen of interest.

CFC unfortunately has several pitfalls. Although this technique is extremely sensitive, the background is variable and may be high enough that the limit of detection is determined more by signal:noise ratio than by the theoretical sensitivity. Like many assays of cellular immune function, it is highly dependent upon the quality of input cells and is critically dependent upon proper specimen acquisition and processing. Not only is this method dependent upon access to costly multi-parameter flow cytometry instrumentation, but the types of instruments that allow analysis of several cytokines and cell surface markers simultaneously (i.e., with more than four or five channels) are extremely expensive and are not available at most centers. Finally, cells must be fixed prior to permeabilization, and therefore live cells cannot be analyzed. This eliminates the ability to perform functional and molecular analyses on specific cytokine-producing subpopulations of cells.

Improvements in the technology for flow-based detection of cytokine-producing cells are occurring at an alarming pace and will likely increase the value of this method in immune monitoring over the next several years. For example, one modification allows the detection of cytokine-producing cells without prior fixation. This technique utilizes an anti-CD45/anti-IFN-γ bi-specific monoclonal antibody-antibody conjugate to capture elaborated IFN-γ on the surface of the T cell of origin. Application of this technology in conjunction with MHC-peptide tetramers enabled the investigators to identify live, cytokine-secreting antigen-specific T cells.

Detection of cytokine mRNA. The detection of cytokine *messenger RNA* (mRNA) is yet another approach to evaluating cytokine production by antigen-specific T cells. Quantitative reverse transcriptase-PCR (RT-PCR) represents one method of measuring the abundance of a particular transcript in a sample and has been applied to the detection of cytokine mRNA. Kammula applied this technology to the evaluation of T cell responses in a melanoma peptide vaccine trial. In this study, cytokine mRNA levels of T cells within PBMC and within fine needle aspirates of tumor tissue were examined. The authors demonstrated that this method could be used successfully to examine antigen-specific T cell immunity in response to tumor vaccines.

Proteomics in immune monitoring

Proteomics is the study of the proteome, the protein complement of the genome. The goal of proteomics is to elucidate not only protein composition, but also protein state and function and the nature of protein-protein interactions. Proteomics is increasingly being applied to challenging areas of medical research. This trend is related to technologic advancements in mass spectrometry instrumentation and software, as well as the automation and miniaturization of analytical tools for protein analysis. The application of proteomics to clinical problems already has led to the development of a promising serum test that may be useful for the early detection of ovarian cancer.

Immunoproteomics, the application of proteomics to immunologic problems, offers novel strategies for target antigen identification and for monitoring the immunologic response to therapeutic interventions. Proteomics has not yet been applied as a tool for immune monitoring in cancer vaccine trials, but offers substantial promise in this regard due to a number of theoretical advantages.

The ability to analyze serum, PBMC or other specimens that have previously been cryopreserved could increase the feasibility of multi-center trials and enhance the reproducibility of immune assays. With existing technology, multiplex immunohistochemical analysis of a wide array of cytokines and regulatory proteins simultaneously from a minute quantity of biological material is feasible. In addition, the availability of monoclonal antibodies against a variety of immune regulatory proteins phosphorylated on specific residues should enable investigators to obtain information about the regulatory mechanisms underlying tumor-specific immunity. In addition, protein profiling may allow evaluation of the immune response to a cancer vaccine from a drop of serum, and this method does not require knowledge of the identity of specific peptide species that best predict immune responsiveness. Despite the theoretical advantages of proteomics for immune monitoring, however, significant work will be necessary to establish whether this approach will have an eventual role in the context of cancer vaccine trials.

Statistical Considerations in Immune Monitoring

Without question, as the reliability and standardization of immune monitoring tests improve, the importance of proper statistical data analysis will only grow. Like the methods themselves, however, there is a lack of standardization and consensus among investigators with regard to the optimal methods for data analysis. Progress toward standardized biostatistics for immune monitoring will be expedited if several fundamental problems can be addressed. These include variability in the readout of immunologic tests, lack of consensus regarding definitions used in the interpretation of tests, and failure to apply appropriate methods of statistical analysis.

Variability in Immunologic Assays

Three sources of variability of the immunologic assay results are encountered: variability within the same specimen, variability among specimens from the same patient drawn at different times, and variability among patients. Variability in the results of a single immunologic test performed on the same specimen results largely from error that is inherent in measurements associated with each step of the assay (e.g., slightly more or less reagent is pipetted into a well). Contributions from the instrument and operator both may be minimized through proper quality control, but cannot be eliminated. Of course, it is critical to avoid systematic contributions to this variability. For example, wells on the edge of a microtiter plate may loose more volume due to evaporation over time than wells further in the center of a plate, thereby affecting the concentration of reagents and introducing a systematic error into the results obtained from those wells. Most sources of systematic error can be mitigated through standardization and automation of as many steps in immunization and immune monitoring protocols as possible.

The measure of variability of a test on individual specimens is the coefficient of variation, which is defined as [standard deviation ÷ mean] × 100%. Low coefficients of variation indicate that the reproducibility of the assay is good. The reproducibility or reliability of an assay can also be assessed by attempting to replicate the measurement on the same specimen at different times and places. In this case, variability is also introduced by differences in equipment used, differences in handling or storage of the specimen, and the analysts performing the assays. The agreement among laboratories or analysts (inter-observer), or even within the same analyst (intra-observer), can be described by the kappa statistic, which is defined as [agreement beyond chance] ÷ [amount of agreement possible beyond chance].

Characterizing the variability in the results obtained from the same patient over time is essential for interpretation of results of studies involving immunologic manipulations such as vaccines. Presently, this type of variability cannot be controlled because the immune system reacts continuously to a variety of poorly defined factors (e.g., stress or invasion by microorganisms). It is possible to vaccinate subjects with control foreign antigens, such as *kehole limpet hemocyanin* (KLH), at the same time the tumor vaccine is administered. This should allow an estimation of the temporal variability in immune responsiveness.

Finally, there is significant patient-to-patient variability. This arises, in part, from a variable degree of immune responsiveness or competence. Such differences among patients may be related to variations in tumor burden or overall medical condition. Specific characteristics of the tumors themselves also could influence responsiveness, such as the relative complement or abundance of the tumor antigens that are represented in the vaccine. In addition, some patients will have detectable base-line, pre-immunization antigen-specific T cells, while others may not. One strategy that can decrease patient-to-patient variability is the selection of similar patients for a trial, although this may not be feasible in studies restricted to uncommon malignancies or certain HLA types. Another approach to this heterogeneity among patients is to appropriately standardize immune responses during data analysis. For example, if a pre-immunization tumor antigen-specific T cell population is detectable, then one may examine the *increase* in antigen-specific T cell frequency. Standardization of responses to those against control antigens also should enable one to control for the variable overall state of immune competence among patients.

Definitions and Statistical Methods in Data Analysis

Perhaps the most important issue for the statistical analysis of results from immune assays remains the definition of what comprises a positive or negative result. Unlike many situations in medicine in which there is general agreement on how to define an entity (for example, a malignancy is defined by a number of microscopic features), there is no consensus on how to define an immune response. Because of this, there is no established gold standard against which other assays may be compared. Consequently, it has been difficult thus far to provide clear determinations of the sensitivity or specificity of a given assay.

The recent workshop by the Society for Biological Therapy intended to provide recommendations on the assays that might provide the most utility in monitoring clinical trials is an excellent first step in this regard. Nonetheless, the cut-offs chosen for positive and negative responses remain largely arbitrary. Our group has suggested that one way to empirically determine the appropriate cut-offs for positive and negative immune responses is to base them on responses to a potent immunogen, such as the *cytomegalovirus* (CMV) matrix protein, pp65. We performed ELISPOT, tetramer, and CFC assays on PBMC from CMV-seropositive and seronegative donors. This enabled us to identify a cut-off point between the two groups at which the sensitivity, specificity and accuracy were acceptable.

A final concern in the evaluation of immunologic assays is the appropriate application of valid statistical tests. This issue arises particularly often with regard to multiple comparisons. Typically, immune assays are performed at several time points during a vaccine study, and several assays may be performed at each time point. This raises the possibility that a false positive will arise by chance. Clearly, it is important to use stringent methods of adjustment to determine whether differences are truly statistically different.

Concluding Remark

A wide array of immunologic tests are available for immune monitoring in cancer vaccine trials, and the number of novel assays and technical modifications continues to burgeon. Because only a small fraction of all proposed vaccine trials tested in phase I-II trials, for practical reasons, will ultimately move forward to be tested in phase III trials, there must be a system of establishing the most promising immunization strategies. This evaluation of cancer vaccine will require standardization of the immune assays and statistical methods used in immunologic monitoring. Furthermore, the use of a systematic approach to evaluating and adopting novel technologies for immunologic assessment would likely lead to timely implementation of more reliable, practical and cost-effective methods of immune. It should be the goal and expectation that this rational approach to immune monitoring will allow the critical appraisal of the most promising vaccine candidates in the context of pivotal, multi-center trials.

13

UNDEFINED ANTIGEN VACCINE

The immune surveillance hypothesis stated that tumors arose frequently, but were recognized and then eliminated by the host immune system because they expressed *tumor-associated antigens* (TAA). This theory was questioned because immune-deficient hosts did not exhibit an increased incidence of non-virally induced tumors. However, recent experiments in genetically manipulated mice, which have been made deficient in both the innate and adaptive immune systems, revealed that the immune system does indeed alter the incidence of both carcinogen-induced and spontaneous malignancies (immunoediting). Thus, the immune surveillance hypothesis has been resuscitated and has provided renewed impetus for cancer immunotherapy.

TAA recognized by T cells consist of two distinct types: shared antigens and individual *tumor-specific antigens* (TSA). Most of the well-characterized TAA are shared tumor antigens. These include tissue differentiation antigens, such as *melanoma-associated antigens* (MAA), e.g. MART-1 and gp100; cancer-testis antigens, e.g. MAGE and NY-ESO-1; and over-expressed normal antigens, e.g. Her2/neu, telomerase and Muc-1. Shared tumor antigens are usually weak "self" antigens, which are poorly immunogenic because the high-avidity T cells that recognize strong MHC-binding epitopes derived from these shared antigens have been deleted. Very few TSA have been described thus far; and except for idiotypic determinants on malignant lymphocytes, TSA result mainly from mutations that occur in individual tumor cells within a specific patient. The lack of central tolerance to these antigens may make them more effective tumor rejection antigens. Another class of antigenic peptides comes from alternative open reading frames of mRNA that encode longer proteins, often using non-AUG as the initiation codon (e.g. CUG), or translation of introns and regions spanning the intron-exon junctions. These "*cryptic*" peptides could add a large number of TSA to the repertoire; however, it is not known whether cryptic translation also occurs in normal cells or if it is unique to transformed or virally infected cells.

A rationale for using undefined antigen vaccines to treat patients with cancer is that for the most common types of malignancy, e.g. carcinomas of epithelial origin, tumor antigens have not been well-characterized. Furthermore, in contrast to defined antigen vaccines, vaccines using intact tumor cells, or preparations derived from whole tumor cells, contain not only shared tumor antigens, but also many TSA, to which the host may not have developed tolerance.

The new immunoediting hypothesis stated that tumors arising in immune competent hosts after selection and sculpting processes would be less immunogenic than tumors that developed in immune-deficient hosts. A major challenge for the rational design of whole tumor cell vaccines will be to increase the immunogenicity of tumor cells so that the critical threshold for priming of the existing T-cell repertoire that can recognize and destroy tumor cells can be reached and to modulate host regulatory mechanisms that prevent recognition of many self antigens.

Cross-priming of T Cells

A major goal of vaccination in cancer patients is the induction of potent antitumor T-cell immune responses. Unless tumor cells metastasize to secondary lymphoid tissues, naive T cells rarely have an opportunity to interact with and be activated by solid tumor cells, even if the tumor cells express MHC/peptide complexes on their surface. The activation of tumor antigen-specific T cells relies primarily on the cross-priming pathway, which involves antigen processing and presentation of tumor cell antigens by the host professional *antigen presenting cells* (APC), particularly *dendritic cells* (DC). After they take up tumor-derived antigens DC migrate into the T-cell zones of tumor-draining lymph nodes. Although most studies indicate that the major pathways for T-cell priming by tumor cells were mediated by host APC, equally strong evidence from Zinkernagel's group indicated that localized solid tumors were largely ignored and cross-priming to antigens from solid tumors was minimal. Priming of CTL occurred only when tumor cells metastasized to or were injected directly into secondary lymphoid organs. Thus, the efficiency and physiological role of cross-priming has been challenged. The analysis of complex biological systems is greatly influenced by the model used and experimental design employed. Therefore, the generalization of any theory is difficult, and the truth probably lies between the two extremes. In fact, recent studies demonstrated that cross-priming of antigens derived from tumor cells required high levels of antigen expression, while antigens with a low level of expression were ignored by T cells. In some situations, direct and cross-priming were found to be redundant, and the absence of either pathway led to T-cell priming by the other pathway. The relative contribution of each pathway varied depending on many factors, such as level of antigen expression, and localization of tumor cells. The contribution of cross-priming to T-cell mediated immune surveillance in cancer patients may not be possible to ascertain; however, clinical trials of vaccination with whole tumor cells that are designed to increase the efficacy of cross-priming may provide clues to whether the cross-priming pathway can be co-opted to produce therapeutic activity.

This review will focus on strategies that use undefined or ill-defined antigen preparations derived from whole tumor cells as the cancer vaccines. They include the following: whole tumor cells (both autologous and allogeneic); gene-modified cells (genes encoding cytokines, chemokines, and co-stimulatory molecules); cell-derived materials (lysates, apoptotic bodies, exosomes, heat shock proteins); and tumor-APC fusion cells. The basic concepts, preclinical development, and the preliminary data from current clinical trials will be described.

Whole Cell Vaccines

Early versions of whole cell vaccines usually consisted of killed tumor cells or tumor cell lysates mixed with bacterial adjuvants such as *Bacillus Calmette Guerin* (BCG) and *Corynebacterium parvum.* Although the mechanisms of the bacterial adjuvants are still not understood very well, the innate immune responses to various bacterial components play a critical role in bridging the innate immune response and adaptive immunity to tumor antigens. In contrast to the crude bacterial adjuvants used for the generation of early cancer vaccines, more recent generations of whole cell tumor vaccines have comprised genetically modified tumor cells using defined immune-modulating genes, including cytokines, chemokines and costimulatory molecules.

Whole Cell Vaccines with Adjuvant

Bacterial adjuvants were used to boost antitumor immunity as far back as the 1890's. Studies using transplantable tumors demonstrated that the immunogenicity of whole tumor cell vaccines was enhanced by mixing tumor cells with bacterial adjuvants, such as BCG, *Corynebacterium parvum* and the streptococcal preparation OK-432. Cancer vaccines were produced from autologous or allogeneic tumor cells. For an excellent historical perspective the reader is referred to a review by Oettgen and Old. But for a few exceptions discussed below, the clinical benefits of these tumor vaccines were minimal. These studies were done before the "*modern age*" of immunology and the mechanisms for the immunopotentiation effects of bacterial adjuvants remained a mystery until the recent discovery of innate immunity receptors for bacterial-derived molecules: the *Toll-like receptor* (TLR) family of proteins. Bacterial cell wall materials (LPS, lipoproteins and peptides), unmethylated genomic DNA (CpG motif), and flagellin bind to different TLR and cause maturation of dendritic cells and facilitate antigen presentation and T-cell activation. The involvement of other innate immune cells, such as macrophages and NK cells is less defined; however, their role in antitumor immunity should not be ignored. Building a bridge between innate and adaptive immunity may well be the mechanism to improve the efficacy of whole cell vaccines, a strategy that will be tested in the near future.

A few groups have continued to study this approach to vaccination. Morton and his colleagues at the John Wayne Cancer Institute have employed a vaccine comprising three allogeneic melanoma cell lines with BCG as adjuvant and Berd et al. used autologous melanoma cells that had been chemically modified with the hapten DNP mixed with BCG. Single arm phase II studies of both vaccines indicated that vaccination improved the survival of patients with stage III disease and metastatic disease when compared to historical controls. Furthermore, clinical outcome appeared to be improved in patients who developed an immune response to the vaccine compared to patients that failed to respond. Both vaccines are being developed by private industry. Canvaxin is now being compared to BCG in a randomized study of adjuvant therapy for patients with melanoma at high risk for recurrence (state III and IV disease after complete resection). These approaches have also been tested in other diseases. For example, based on the finding that TAA can even be shared among tumors of different histology, Canvaxin was tested in patients with colon cancer. DNP-modified autologous tumor cells have been used in ovarian cancer. Two phase III adjuvant trials of an autologous tumor cell vaccine with BCG have been performed in patients with stage II and III colon cancer. One study, with 412 patients failed to detect a benefit for vaccinated patients while another study with 254 patients reported an improvement in recurrence-free survival for stage II patients, but failed to show benefit for patients with stage III colon cancer. None of the vaccines described above has resulted in an improvement in survival and therefore, they have not become part of standard therapy in the US or Europe.

Gene-Modified Tumor Vaccines Cytokines and Chemokines

Preclinical studies

The cloning of cytokine genes and development of gene transfer technology ushered in a new era of cancer vaccines. Dranoff et al. compared the efficacy of vaccination with B16 melanoma cells following gene transfer with a large array of cytokine genes using the MFG Moloney murine leukemia retrovirus as a vector. Tumor cells elicited the best protective immunity against tumor challenge if mice were vaccinated with irradiated gene-modified tumor cells that produced GM-CSF compared to cells that produced IL-1, 2, 3, 4, 5, 6, 7, 10, 12, 18, TNF-α, IFN-γ, SCF, G-CSF, M-CSF, Flt3-ligand, eotaxin, RANTES, MIP-1α, MIP-1β, or lymphotactin. The priming of antitumor CTL by GM-CSF gene-modified tumor vaccines was mediated primarily by host professional APCs. Although similar comparisons have not been performed for the ever-growing number of newly discovered chemokines, SLC appeared to exhibit potent antitumor activity when expressed by tumor cells. The immune modulating activities of cytokines and chemokines are different, and a powerful synergism of the combination has been demonstrated between lymphotactin and GM-CSF or IL-2.

Since autologous tumor cells contain both shared TAA and TSA, theoretically they would be preferable to allogeneic tumor cells, which contain only shared TAA, as vaccines. However, the wide application of autologous tumor cell vaccines has been hampered by the difficulty in obtaining adequate autologous tumor and the problems associated with the standardization of individual gene modified vaccines. Thus, allogeneic tumor cell vaccines have been pursued more actively. Although there may be a difference in efficacy between syngeneic and allogeneic whole tumor vaccines, cross protective immune responses have generally been observed. A major concern was that the development of strong allogeneic responses might override the tumor-specific responses. However, the experimental evidence strongly indicated otherwise; the allo reactions enhanced the antitumor immune responses.

Clinical trials

The results of clinical trials for tumor cell vaccines transduced with IL-2, IL-4, IL-7, IFN-γ, IL-12 and GM-CSF have been reported. Gene transfer to tumor cells has been accomplished with retroviruses, adenoviruses, lipofection or with DNA-coated gold particles. To date, melanoma has been studied most extensively, but cytokine-modified vaccines have also been used to treat patients with neuroblastoma, lung cancer, prostate cancer, ovarian cancer, kidney cancer, sarcoma, brain tumors and hematologic malignancies.

The most actively studied vaccines have been GM-CSF-transfected tumor cells. Phase I clinical trials of irradiated GM-CSF-transduced autologous tumor cells sponsored by Cell Genesys have been completed in patients with kidney cancer, prostate cancer, melanoma and non-small-cell lung cancer. To circumvent the need for transfection of autologous tumor, a GM-CSF-producing bystander K562 cell line has been developed and used in combination with autologous NSCLC cells. Allogeneic GM-CSF-transfected cell lines have been used in the adjuvant setting for patients with pancreatic cancer and to treat metastatic prostate cancer. Vaccination with GM-CSF-modified tumor cells has proven to be feasible and safe. Transduction of autologous tumors cells continues to be a challenge, but was successful in the majority of cases. The major side effect following vaccination was local tenderness at the injection site. Biopsies of vaccine sites, tumor nodules and DTH sites revealed dense dendritic cell, macrophage, granulocyte and lymphocytic infiltrates. Most patients exhibited DTH reactions to tumor cells after vaccination and individual patients developed tumor-specific CTL activity and produced high titers of antibody. None of the studies were designed to assess the clinical benefit of vaccination; however, tumor regression was observed in patients with melanoma, renal cell cancer and lung cancer. There was also a suggestion that pancreatic cancer patients treated at the highest dose of the allogeneic cell vaccine had an improvement in disease-free survival.

Costimulatory Molecules

In the two-signal hypothesis for T-cell activation, T cells are optimally activated when their T-cell receptor is engaged by a peptide/MHC complex and CD28 is engaged by a costimulatory molecule, CD80 or CD86 on the APC. In contrast to professional APCs, most cells from solid tumors do not express costimulatory molecules. Therefore, gene-modified tumor cell vaccines were produced to make tumor cells better APCs by introducing genes for costimulatory molecules. CD80 or CD86 transduction can convert tumor cells into professional APC's in vitro, although the precise role of such engineered APCs in the initiation of antitumor T-cell responses in vivo is not clear. Since naive T cells circulate primarily in lymphoid organs, and initial priming usually takes place within the secondary lymphoid tissues, direct activation of naive T cells by tumor cells could occur only when tumor cell metastasize to lymphoid tissues. Two recent studies demonstrated a redundant role for both direct-and cross-priming. Cross-priming by host APCs was more efficient than direct priming by tumor cells even when tumor cells were engineered to express costimulatory molecules. The characterizations of four additional CD28-related molecules and their ligands has not only increased the complexity of regulation of T-cell activation, but has also provided additional tools to augment antitumor immune responses. Furthermore, members of the *tumor necrosis receptor family* (TNFR) family, which not only costimulate T cells, but also exhibit additional immunomodulatory effects on innate immunity present other opportunities to evaluate costimulatory molecules in tumor immunology.

Clinical trials

CD80 gene-modified tumor cells have been used to treat patients with metastatic renal cell cancer and breast cancer. In the former study, autologous tumor cells infected with an adenoviral vector that contained the CD80 gene were used; the latter trial employed an HLA-A2-matched allogeneic breast cancer cell line lipofected with a CD80-encoding DNA plasmid. Two of the 15 patients with renal cell cancer experienced a partial remission; however, the contribution of CD80 to vaccine efficacy was impossible to discern because treatment also included low-dose interleukin-2, which has activity in this disease. Dols et al. administered their allogeneic breast cancer vaccine with BCG or GM-CSF as an adjuvant to 30 women with heavily pretreated metastatic breast cancer. At the highest tumor cell dose significant tumor-specific T-cell responses were detected, but no objective tumor regressions were observed.

Future directions

A new class of immune stimulatory receptors (NKG2D) expressed by NK cells, T cells and macrophages has the potential to modulate immune responses, including antitumor immunity. Human NKG2D binds to MHC class I-related molecules (MICA, MICB), and CMV UL16-binding proteins (ULBP1,2,3), while mouse NKG2D binds to members of the retinoic acid early inducible 1 (Rae-1) family, minor histocompatibility antigen H60 and murine ULBP-like transcript 1 (MULT1). Expression of MICA and MICB was normally restricted to gastrointestinal epithelium, but can be induced by cellular stress and is upregulated after infections, and on tumor cells of epithelial origin, such as lung, breast, kidney, prostate, and colon tumors. Members of the Rae-1 family (Rae-1α, β, γ, δ, ε) are expressed during early embryogenesis, but absent in normal adult tissues. Like MICA and MICB, expression of Rae-1 is found on several mouse tumor cell lines. MIC and Rae-1 play an important role in tumor immune surveillance. In humans, soluble MICA and MICB found in melanoma patients downregulate surface NKG2D expression on tumor-infiltrating T cells, which dampen their antitumor activity. In mice, Rae-1 expression regulates the antitumor activity of γδ T cells against cutaneous tumors.

Most importantly, mice vaccinated with tumor cells that express high levels of H60 or Rae-1 not only prevented tumor growth, but also induced CD8 T-cell dependent antitumor immunity. In another study, however, no protection was observed despite complete rejection of primary challenge with Rae-1-transfected tumor cells. While the efficacy of vaccination with B7-expressing tumor cells was dependent on inherent tumor immunogenicity, this was not the case for NKG2D costimulation. B16 melanoma cells that expressed B7 grew as rapidly as the parental line, but H60 or Rae-1 expressing B16 tumor cells were promptly rejected. Although the mechanisms by which NKG2D ligands induced antitumor CD8 T-cell responses remains to be determined, these ligands definitely add a new and potentially more powerful approach to the development of genetically modified tumor cell vaccines.

Cell-Derived Materials

Lysates

Tumor cell-derived materials, including lysates (freeze-thaw, sonication and oncolysate [lysis by lytic viruses]), shed antigens, apoptotic bodies, exosomes, and enriched or purified heat shock proteins have been pursued as alternatives to whole cell vaccines. These materials should contain most of the antigens from tumor cells; however, there have been reports that lysates were less effective than inactivated whole tumor cells at generating antitumor immune responses.

Lysates from autologous tumor cells and allogeneic cell lines, with and without adjuvant, have been tested in clinical trials. The prototype lysate vaccine that is furthest along in development is Melacine, a mixture of mechanical lysates from two allogeneic cell lines coadministered with the adjuvant DETOX. The lysate contains the following melanoma antigens: gp100, the gangliosides GD2 and GD3, MART-1, MAGE-1, -2, -3, tyrosinase, TRP-1 and HMW-MAA. The adjuvant comprises bacterial cell wall skeleton and monophosphoryl lipid A. Melacine has been under investigation since the early 1980's. It has modest antitumor activity, which may be enhanced by co-administration of interferon-alpha, in patients with metastatic melanoma. This activity in patients with stage IV disease led the Southwest Oncology Group (SWOG) to perform a phase III observation controlled trial in patients with intermediate-thickness melanoma, 1.5-4.0 mm thick or Clark's level IV. Six hundred eighty-nine patients were accrued; after a median follow-up of 5.6 years there has been no improvement in disease-free or overall survival among patients randomized to receive vaccine. However, among the 553 patients who had HLA typing performed, HLA-A2 and/or HLA-C3 positive patients who were vaccinated experienced a significant improvement in 5-year relapse-free survival (77% vs 63%, p=.004). These results suggest that HLA expression by the host may influence the efficacy of vaccine treatment. This may be due to direct effects on peptide presentation to T cells or indirectly by virtue of linkage to other polymorphic genes responsible for the actual vaccine benefit. Further evaluation of Melacine is planned in a much larger group of targeted patients who express HLA-A2 and/or HLA-C3.

Oncolysates prepared by infecting tumor cells with lytic viruses, such as Newcastle disease and vaccinia viruses, have been employed as cancer vaccines. Oncolysates may elicit inflammatory responses against viral components that could augment antitumor immunity. Phase II studies in small numbers of patients with malignant melanoma suggested an improvement in clinical outcome for patients vaccinated with oncolysates compared to historical controls. These preliminary results led to the performance of two randomized phase III clinical trials. Wallack et al. compared vaccination with a vaccinia melanoma oncolysate prepared from four allogeneic cell lines to vaccinia injection alone in 217 patients with melanoma at high risk of recurrence following surgery. Hersey et al. compared vaccination with a vaccinia oncolysate prepared from a single cell line to no immunotherapy in a similar group of 700 high-risk patients. Despite the promising results of the single arm studies, neither randomized trial demonstrated a statistically significant improvement in relapse-free or overall survival. Viral oncolysates have also been employed in the adjuvant setting for patients with completely resected colorectal cancer. Autologous colon cancer cells infected with Newcastle disease virus were used to treat 48 patients with completely resected colon cancer. The authors reported a significant improvement in 2-year survival compared to 661 historical controls. This soft clinical finding is similar to what has been observed in patients with melanoma and has not been confirmed in a controlled trial.

Another strategy employed by Bystryn and his colleagues at NYU, has been to construct a melanoma vaccine from antigens shed by tumor cells. The rationale for this approach is that a polyvalent, partially purified vaccine that contains antigens expressed on the surface of tumor cells is likely to be biologically relevant. This approach is safe and results in antibody production and CD8 T-cell responses to a variety of MAA. In single arm studies this group observed improvements in recurrence-free and overall survival of vaccine-treated stage III patients compared to historical controls. This led to a double-blind, randomized, placebo-controlled trial in which despite the small number of patients (N = 38) there was a significant improvement in median time to disease progression for patients in the vaccine arm. Confirmation of these results is needed before this treatment can be recommended in clinical practice.

Heat Shock Proteins (HSPs)

In an attempt to isolate immunogenic proteins from tumor cell homogenates (lysates) that can elicit protective antitumor immune responses, Srivastava surprisingly found that the key proteins were HSPs, ubiquitous proteins abundantly expressed in both normal and malignant cells. HSPs purified from one tumor cell line were able to elicit antitumor responses that were specific for that tumor cell line only and HSPs from normal tissues failed to induce immune responses to any tumor cells. This enigma was resolved when HSPs were shown to be molecular chaperones that bound a large collection of peptides. These peptides were proposed as the precursors to MHC-binding peptides; however, currently the definitive proof is lacking and the precise process by which these peptides are transferred to MHC molecules in vivo is still not clear. In addition, HSPs were to be able to activate host APCs via specific receptors, such CD91, LOX-1, and Toll receptors, and facilitate the cross-presentation of tumor antigens by host APCs. Thus, HSPs have the unique ability to bridge innate and adaptive immunity, and can elicit specific and potent antitumor responses in both prophylactic and therapeutic settings in multiple experimental tumor models.

Hundreds of patients with a variety of tumor types have been treated in phase I and phase II studies of autologous tumor-derived HSP-peptide complexes. The requirement for autologous tumor limits the number of patients that can be treated, but vaccine preparation at a central laboratory facilitated the participation of multiple sites. Treatment was well tolerated and two complete responses were observed among 28 patients with advanced melanoma treated with HSP gp96-peptide complexes. The same group treated 29 consecutive patients who underwent potentially curative resection of colorectal liver metastases with autologous tumor-derived HSP gp96. A significant minority of patients in both studies produced a tumor-specific T-cell response following vaccination. There was a suggestion that production of a tumor-specific T-cell response correlated with clinical response in the melanoma study and disease-free and overall survival in the patients with colorectal cancer. Tumor-derived HSP-peptide complexes are currently being tested in two phase III trials—as adjuvant therapy compared to observation following nephrectomy in high-risk patients with renal cell cancer and as initial therapy compared to standard therapy for patients with metastatic melanoma.

Exosomes

Exosomes are small membrane vesicles secreted by many different cell types as a consequence of fusion of multivesicular late endosomes/lysosomes with the plasma membrane. APCs, such as B lymphocytes and dendritic cells, secrete MHC class-I- and class-II-carrying exosomes that stimulate T-cell proliferation in vitro. Tumor-derived exosomes contain a rich source of antigens and HSP that can be transferred to DCs for cross-priming of T cells. In addition, dendritic-cell-derived exosomes, when used as a cell-free vaccine, can eradicate established murine tumors.

Dendritic Cells

Dendritic cells initiate the T-cell response to many different antigens, including tumor antigens. Because of their unique ability to activate naive T cells, DC have been evaluated by many investigators. In mice, three major subsets have been identified; $CD11b^+$ *myeloid DC*, *lymphoid-like DC* that co-express CD8, and the IFN-α-producing *plasmacytoid DC*. Similar subsets have been identified in humans. Studies of myeloid DC have been possible because large numbers of DC can be generated from GM-CSF-cultured $CD34^+$ hematopoietic progenitor cells in humans and bone marrow-derived cells in mice. Large numbers of plasmacytoid DC can also be produced from bone marrow cells following culture with Flt3 ligand. Because both myeloid and lymphoid precursors can give rise to CD8$^+$ lymphoid-like DC, CD8 expression is not a reliable marker for lymphoid DC, but serves as a maturation marker. Although mouse plasmacytoid DC can acquire CD8 expression after microbial stimulation, plasmacytoid DC are not the precursor for CD8$^+$ DC found in lymphoid tissues in mice. CD8$^+$ DC appear to be the primary APC for in vivo cross-presentation of cell-associated antigens (e.g. tumor cells, antigen-pulsed cells, cells infected with viruses and intracellular bacteria), soluble antigens, immune complexes and HSP. Cross-presentation of antigens in the context of infection results in extensive T-cell activation and expansion, while cross-presentation in a steady state, without infection, results in premature T-cell activation and deletion. Cross-presentation of antigens from growing or apoptotic tumor cells results in either tolerance, limited T-cell activation without tolerance, or priming. The vastly different outcomes might be explained by the difference in tumor immunogenicity and level of antigen expression in the tumor models used for these studies. Cross-presentation of antigens by endogenous DCs has been demonstrated to be important for optimal T-cell expansion even when mature DCs were used as the vaccine. Although the concept of cross-priming of T cells by host APC is well-accepted, its physiological significance and whether it can be manipulated for therapeutic intent in cancer immunotherapy are still hotly debated. Both GM-CSF-driven, monocyte-derived myeloid DCs and Flt3L-driven, CD34$^+$ hemopoietic progenitor cell-derived lymphoid DCs have been used for clinical trials. However, the optimal subset of DCs, and the best technique for the in vitro generation of DC to induce optimal antitumor immune responses in vivo has not been determined.

The number of clinical trials employing DCs has increased steadily in recent years. DC-based tumor vaccines have as many variations as tumor cell-based vaccines, including genetic modification of DC with cytokines, chemokines, cDNA encoding defined tumor antigens, mRNA, cRNA and genomic DNA from tumor cells, DC pulsed with recombinant tumor antigens, tumor lysates, apoptotic/necrotic cells and DC tumor fusion cells. There is also an extensive literature of peptide-pulsed DC. Only studies that employed DC in combination with undefined antigen preparations will be discussed further.

DC-Based Vaccines

Even when combined with bacterial adjuvants, direct immunization with tumor lysates was generally an inefficient method for T-cell priming. This may relate to rapid diffusion or insufficient uptake of tumor antigens by host APC. However, immunization with tumor lysate-pulsed DC greatly improved the efficacy of tumor lysates, underlining the importance of antigen presentation for efficient T-cell priming.

Presentation of exogenous proteins by APCs requires antigen acquisition, degradation, loading into MHC class I and II molecules and transport to the plasma membrane. There are at least three major routes by which DCs acquire and process exogenous antigens: receptor-mediated endocytosis, phagocytosis and macropinocytosis. Accordingly, various approaches have been used to load tumor-derived antigens, including opsonized, apoptotic or necrotic whole tumor cells, exosomes, tumor lysates or HSPs enriched from tumor lysates. Soluble antigens, such as tumor lysates, are generally acquired via macropinocytosis, however, receptor-mediated endocytosis may also be important for the acquisition of antigens included in the lysate, such as HSPs via CD91 and LOX-1, glycoproteins via C-type lectin receptors and lipoprotein via scavenger receptors.

Immature DC are more efficient than mature DC at antigen uptake; mature DC have reduced expression of antigen receptors and have down-modulated both macropinocytosis and phagocytosis. Stimulation of DC with TLR ligands leads to maturation with enhanced antigen processing and peptide-loading onto MHC molecules and transport of peptide/MHC complexes to the plasma membrane. A recent study suggests that the optimal conditions for MHC I and MHC II restricted antigen presentation are very different. Antigen-loading before DC maturation is required for optimal CD4 T-cell activation, consistent with the notion that activated DC have a decreased ability to take-up exogenous antigens. Surprisingly, cross-presentation of antigen to CD8 T cells requires DC stimulation before antigen loading. Furthermore, only a subset of TLR ligands, those associated with viral infection (TLR3 and TLR9), were able to activate the MHC I restricted cross-presentation pathway.

Clinical studies

There have been many trials of tumor lysate-pulsed DC in patients with advanced cancer. These trials include phase I studies in pediatric or adult cancer patients, and other studies that combined components of phase I and II studies by employing different doses of DCs with various schedules in patients with a single disease entity. Each study included fewer than 20 patients. Immature DCs produced by culturing peripheral blood mononuclear cells in GM-CSF and IL-4 were employed most commonly. They were cultured for 24 hours with a tumor lysate prepared by multiple freeze/thaw cycles before treatment. In other studies, TNFα or a cocktail of TNFα, IL-6 and IL-1β were used to induce DC maturation. Most investigators included KLH in the lysate, both as a reporter antigen and for its ability to provide help. Immunization was performed by a variety of routes e.g. intranodal, intradermal, subcutaneous or intravenous, and by a variety of schedules.

Some investigators employed multiple routes of administration. None of the published studies have been powered to address the issue of efficacy; however, feasibility and safety have been demonstrated. Not all patients will have adequate tumor accessible for resection, but for those that do there was a high likelihood of generating suitable tumor lysate-pulsed DC for treatment. Except for mild fever with chills and arthralgia, and local injection site reactions, treatment was well tolerated. Occasional patients produced detectable serum autoantibodies, but none have been reported to be of clinical significance. The lack of side effects indicative of autoimmune reactions after immunization with a preparation so rich in self antigens may reflect the tight regulatory controls in patients, which could in turn explain the small number of responses that have been seen in each of these trials.

A summary of the immune findings reflects the difficulty in monitoring immune responses to undefined antigens. KLH responses can be demonstrated in the majority, but not in all of the patients to whom it was administered. DTH, ELISPOT and intracellular cytokine staining were performed to determine whether patients had developed an immune response to autologous tumor antigens or peptides known to be expressed by their respective tumors. Immune responses were seen in some patients, but no correlation with clinical activity was detected. Complete responses were observed in patients with renal cell cancer, melanoma, fibrosarcoma and cutaneous T-cell lymphoma.

Gene-Modified DC Vaccines

Gene-modified DCs can be used to increase T-cell activation. The genes that have been studied include GM-CSF, CD40L and TNF, and T-cell growth factors, such as IL-7, and IL-12. Gene modification of DC with the T-cell chemotactic chemokines, SLC and lymphotactin, has also been shown to increase the efficacy of DCs pulsed with tumor-lysate or loaded with peptide. Interestingly, SLC gene-modified DCs were able to activate tumor-specific T cells without tumor involvement of draining lymph nodes, suggesting that the lymphoid neogenesis activity of SLC could induce a lymphoid-like structure in a vaccine site that enabled in situ T-cell priming.

DCs Transfected with Tumor Cell mRNA

Antigens from tumor cells can also be delivered into DC by transfection with mRNA extracted from tumor cells. One great advantage of RNA-based vaccines is that RNA can be amplified after reverse transcription, providing an essentially endless supply for vaccination. Tumor mRNA can even be prepared from single cells obtained by laser capture microdissection. Autologous DCs transfected with mRNA for specific proteins (PSA and CEA) or total mRNA from tumor cells can stimulate T-cell responses, including CTL against specific antigens or against a broad array of unidentified tumor antigens. Clinical trials using immature DCs transfected with PSA and CEA-specific mRNA have been performed, as well as a phase I study using total RNA in 15 patients with metastatic renal cell cancer. This approach, which has been employed primarily by investigators at Duke University Medical Center is feasible and well tolerated. Tumor- or antigen-specific T cells have been induced in a majority of patients but there has been little evidence of antitumor activity in patients with established tumors.

DC/Tumor Fusion Hybrid Cells

Another approach to deliver tumor-derived proteins and mRNA into DC is to fuse tumor cells and DCs in a hybrid cell. Hybrids can be created by chemical (PEG), electrofusion and biochemical (viral fusion proteins) technologies. PEG-mediated fusion is rather inefficient compared to electrofusion or *fusogenic membrane glycoprotein* (FMG) mediated fusion. Multiple vaccinations have been necessary to induce a strong antitumor immune response with fusion cells generated by PEG, whereas one immunization with hybrid cells generated by optimized electrofusion or FMG-mediated fusion was sufficient to induce a strong antitumor T-cell immune response that mediated rejection of established tumor in preclinical models. The difference in vaccine efficacy may be related to the fusion efficiency of the different methods. This underscores the importance of optimization of fusion methods. Unfortunately, like most other vaccine strategies which lack standardization, it is not possible at this time to gauge the relative superiority of the different methods. Hybrid cells have been tested in clinical trials in patients with melanoma, renal cell cancer and malignant glioma. When reported, fusion efficiency was generally

<20% using the PEG-based approach. Occasional tumor regressions were reported in patients with melanoma and glioma.

Concluding Remark

Our knowledge of the immune system and how it interacts with tumor cells continues to grow. With each advance in basic science comes a new opportunity to develop an effective treatment strategy. Many such opportunities have arisen in the past few decades and this chapter has attempted to describe how these new advances have been combined with a variety of undefined cellular antigen preparations in an attempt to develop effective cancer vaccines. None of the strategies described in this chapter have been sufficiently effective to become part of standard therapy. However, the approaches tested have generally been well-tolerated by patients with advanced cancer and the evidence of immunologic activity and examples of impressive clinical activity in a wide variety of malignancies, suggests that these strategies can be the building blocks upon which new advances are added and effective treatments developed.

14

Antibody-inducing Vaccine

Rationale for Antibody-inducing Cancer Vaccines Against Multiple Cell Surface Antigens

Antibodies Eliminate Tumor Cells In vivo

Preclinical models demonstrate that passively administered or actively induced antibodies against cancer cell surface antigens can prevent tumor recurrence in rodents. The syngeneic murine tumor models involving EL4 lymphoma are particularly informative in terms of trial design. EL4 lymphoma naturally expresses GD2 ganglioside which is recognized by monoclonal antibody (mAb) 3F8. Vaccines containing GD2 covalently conjugated to KLH and mixed with immunological adjuvant QS21 are optimal for vaccination against GD2. Relatively higher levels of mAb 3F8 administered two or four days after intravenous tumor challenge or moderate titers induced by vaccine that were present by day four after tumor challenge were able to eradicate disease in most mice. If mAb administration was deferred until day seven or ten after IV challenge, little or no benefit could be demonstrated. If the number of cells in the EL4 challenge was decreased, giving a longer window of opportunity, the vaccinations could be initiated after tumor challenge and good protection seen. These results are consistent with the need to initiate immunization with vaccines inducing antibodies in the adjuvant setting, when the targets are circulating tumor cells and micrometastases.

Comparable benefit is also seen when we use a subcutaneous foot-pad tumor challenge model which more closely mirrors the clinical setting. Vaccination or mAb administration after amputation of the foot-pad tumor results in cure of 60–80% of mice while 90–100% of control mice developed progressive disease. There are comparable syngeneic models demonstrating the anti-tumor efficacy of mAbs or vaccines against other glycolipids (GD3, GM3), mucin antigens (Tn, TF and MUC1) and a protein antigen (gp75). These experiments share one thing in common, benefit is seen primarily in minimal disease settings, comparable to the adjuvant setting in the clinic. With regard to clinical settings, naturally acquired and vaccine induced antibodies against cancer cell surface antigens have correlated with improved prognosis in several different clinical trials. Also, an increasing number of clinical trials with passively administered monoclonal antibodies (mAb) against cell surface antigens have demonstrated clinical efficacy.

Mechanisms of tumor elimination

Cancer antigens expressed at the cell surface are generally glycolipids or glycoproteins. Immunization against the carbohydrate components generally results exclusively in an antibody response, primarily an IgM antibody response. These IgM antibodies are known to induce *complement dependent cytotoxicity* (CDC), inflammation, and phagocytosis of tumor cells by the reticulo-endothelial system (opsonization). Protein antigens generally induce primarily IgG antibody responses which can also induce complement activation (with regard to IgG depending on the subclass, IgG1 and IgG3 being optimal in humans), and these same complement mediated effector mechanisms. IgG antibodies of these subclasses are also known to induce *antibody dependent cell mediated cytotoxicity* (ADCC). Antibodies are ideally suited for eradication of free tumor cells and micrometastases. This is the role of antibodies against most infectious diseases and they have accomplished this against cancer cells as described above in a variety of preclinical models. In adjuvant immunization trials, the primary targets are individual tumor cells or early micrometastases which may persist for long periods after apparent resection of all residual tumor. After surgery and completion of chemotherapy is the ideal time for immune intervention, and in particular for administration of cancer vaccines aimed at instructing the immune system to identify and kill these few remaining cancer cells. If antibodies of sufficient titer can be induced against tumor antigens to eliminate tumor cells from the blood and lymphatic systems, and to eradicate micrometastases (making establishment of new metastases no longer possible) this would dramatically change our approach to treating the cancer patient. Aggressive local therapies, including surgery, radiation therapy and intralesional treatments might result in long term control of even metastatic cancers.

Polyvalent vaccines

The basis for emphasis on polyvalent vaccines is tumor cell heterogeneity, heterogeneity of the human immune response and the correlation between overall antibody titer against tumor cells and effector mechanisms such as opsonization, CDC or ADCC. For example, using a series of 14 melanoma and sarcoma cell lines and mAbs against 3 gangliosides, we have shown that significant cell surface reactivity analyzed by flow cytometry and CDC was detected against 2–8 of the cell lines using any single mAb. This increased to all 14 of the cell lines when the 3 mAbs were pooled. The median percent CDC increased 4 fold with the pool of mAbs compared to the best single mAb. Comparable findings have been generated more recently using ten SCLC cell lines and mAbs against 4 cell surface antigens.

Selection of Cell Surface Antigens as Targets for Antibody Mediated Attack against Cancer

Cell Surface Cancer Antigens: The MSKCC Experience

We have screened a variety of malignancies and normal tissues with a series of 40 mAbs against 25 antigens which were potential target antigens for immunotherapy. Results for the twelve defined antigens expressed strongly in 50% or more of biopsy specimens of breast, ovary and prostate cancer, melanoma, sarcoma. The 10 excluded antigens (including CEA and HER2/neu) were expressed in 0–2 of the 5–10 specimens.

Our results are consistent with those from other centers with one exception, we did not find increased levels of GD2 or GD3 in small cell lung cancer (SCLC). There is a striking similarity in expression of these 15 antigens among tumors of similar embryologic background (i.e. epithelial versus neuroectodermal). Epithelial cancers (breast, ovary, prostate colon, etc) but not cancers of neuroectodermal origin (melanomas, sarcomas, neuroblastomas) expressed MUC1, Tn, sTn, TF, globo H and Le^y while only the neuroectodermal cancers expressed GD2 and GD3. SCLC shared some characteristics of each and in addition expressed fucosyl GM1 and long chains of poly-α2,8-sialic acid which were not expressed in tumors of either background.

Gangliosides GM2, GD2, GD3 and Fucosyl GM1

Gangliosides are sialic acid containing glycolipids that are expressed at the cell surface with their lipid (ceramide) moiety incorporated

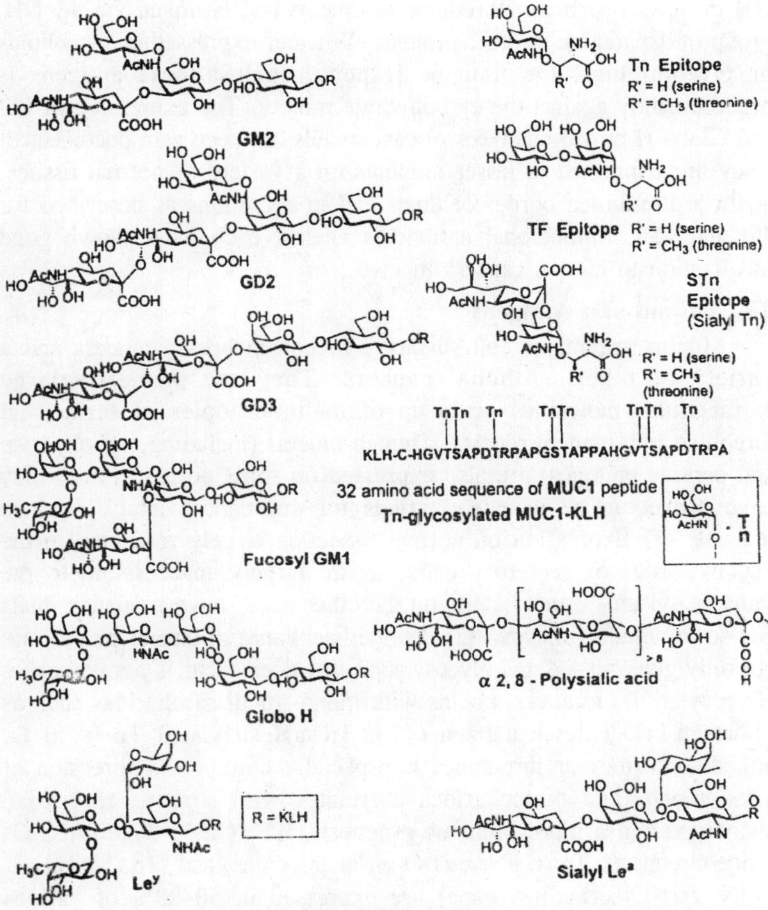

Fig. 14.1. Antigens for antibody including polyvalent cancer vaccines.

into the cell surface lipid bilayer. Most gangliosides considered as potential targets for cancer therapy are expressed primarily in tissues and tumors of neuroectodermal origin. This is true for the melanoma, sarcoma and neuroblastoma antigens GM2, GD2 and GD3, and the small cell lung cancer antigen, fucosyl GM1.Surprisingly, however, GM2 has also recently been identified in a number of epithelial cancers and at the luminal surfaces of a variety of normal epithelial tissues.

Neutral Glycolipids Lewis[y] and Globo H

Lewis[y] (Le[y]) and Globo H antigens are found at the cell surface of epithelial cancers primarily expressed as glycolipids attached to the lipid bilayer through their ceramide, but they are also O-linked via -

OH groups of serine or threonine to mucins and N-linked via the NH_2 group of asparagine in other proteins. Whether expressed as glycolipids or glycoproteins, the immune response against these antigens is predominantly against the carbohydrate moiety. The expression of Le^y and Globo H on various types of cancer cells has been well documented. They are expressed in lesser amounts on a variety of normal tissues, again at the lumen border of ducts and in secretions as described for TF and sTn. Monoclonal antibodies against each have shown good localization to human cancers in vivo.

TF, Tn and sTn Antigens

Mucins are major cell surface antigens in breast cancers and a variety of other epithelial cancers. They are primarily large extracellular molecules made up of multiple copies of serine and threonine rich tandem repeats. Though mucins (including carbohydrate and peptide epitopes) are also expressed on some normal tissues they have proved to be excellent targets for anti-cancer attack for two reasons: (1) Expression on normal tissues is largely restricted to the ductal border of secretory cells, a site largely inaccessible to the immune system. Cancer cells, on the other hand, have no patent ducts and so accumulate-mucins. (2) Peptide backbones of cancer mucins are not fully glycosylated and glycosylation that does occur is not complete. Glycosylation of cancer mucins with mono- or di-saccharides such as Thomsen-Friedenreich antigen (TF), Tn and sialylated Tn (sTn) O-linked to serines or threonines is especially common. Expression of these mono- and disaccharides correlates with a more aggressive phenotype and a more ominous prognosis. TF (Galβ1-3GalNAcα-O-serine/threonine), Tn (GalNAcα1-O-serine/threonine) and sTn (NANAα2-GalNAcα1-O-serine/threonine) are expressed in 50–80% of various epithelial cancers. STn trimer (cluster) is the epitope recognized by monoclonal antibody B72.3, and TF and sTn are closely associated with the clustered epitope recognized by monoclonal antibody CC49. Clinical trials of radiolabeled CC49 administered IP in patients with breast cancer and ovarian cancer at this center and elsewhere have shown excellent targeting. TF has also been used successfully as a target for cancer imaging. TF, Tn and sTn are expressed to a lesser extent on a variety of normal tissues, where they are expressed predominately as occasional monomers at luminal surfaces. Immunohistology performed with mAbs identifying these trimers (clusters) react strongly with a variety of epithelial cancers but only minimally, or not at all, with normal tissues, suggesting that focusing on the trimers of Tn, sTn and TF further increases the tumor specificity of the immune response. Immunization with TF and Tn has been shown to protect mice from subsequent challenge with syngeneic cancer cell lines expressing these antigens. Hence both active and passive immunotherapy trials have identified TF, Tn and sTn antigens as uniquely effective targets for cancer targeting and immunotherapy.

Polysialic Acid

The "*embryonic*" form of *neural cell adhesion molecule* (N-CAM) is expressed on the cell surface of embryonic tissues, occasional neuroendocrine cells and a variety of neuroendocrine tumors including SCLC, neuroblastomas and carcinoids. Embryonic N-CAM undergoes a series of post-translational modifications, with the acquisition of α 2,8-linked sialic acid residues as long 20–100 residue polysialic acid chains. Several monoclonal antibodies, including mAb 735 and NP-4, recognize these long polysialic acid chains and have allowed characterization of this potential antigen in both normal and malignant tissue. Zhang et al. has demonstrated that 6 of 6 SCLC tumor specimens were reactive by immunohistochemistry using mAb 735, and 5 of 6 tested SCLC tumor specimens were positive using mAb NP-4. This confirms previous results of Komminoth et al. and suggests that polysialic acid may serve as a useful target for immune attack against SCLC.

Polysialic acid is also expressed in occasional cells in the gray matter of the brain, bronchial epithelia and pneumocytes, epithelia of the colon, stomach, and pancreas, and capillary endothelial cells and ganglion neurons in the colon. The reactivity of these antibodies in epithelia is restricted to the luminal surfaces of glandular tissues, where access to the immune system is restricted. Two to five percent of normal donors have high levels of antibody against polysialic acid as a consequence of exposure to bacteria such as *Neisseria meningitidis* group B (MenB) and *Escherichia coli* K1 that also express polysialic acid. This has not been associated with any signs of autoimmunity. Consequently, vaccines against polysialic acid are being tested to combat these diseases, however polysialic acid has proved to be poorly immunogenic.

Mucin MUC1

The peptide backbones of tumor mucins may also be targets for immune attack. Mucin 1 (MUC1) is a major mucin in breast cancers and is also expressed in a variety of other epithelial cancers. It contains a large extracellular component made up of multiple copies of a 20 amino acid tandem repeat, and a cytoplasmic tail. Though mucins (including carbohydrate and peptide epitopes) are also expressed on some normal tissues they have proved to be excellent targets for anti-cancer attack for the same reasons noted for sTn, TF and Tn. Glycosylation of cancer mucins with mono- or di-saccharides such as Tn, sTn or TF O-linked to serines or threonines instead of larger, more complex carbohydrates is especially common permitting better access for antibodies to the mucin backbone. For this reason, mucin peptide specific monoclonal antibodies such as DF3 and BR2729 (against MUC1) show specificity for cancer though the amino acid sequence is apparently the same in mucins of normal cells.

Furthermore, MUC1 epitopes are known to be immunogenic in humans as a consequence of demonstrable serum antibodies in occasional patients with breast and other carcinomas. The APD-TRPA domain of the MUC1 tandem repeat is particularly immunogenic and is recognized by a variety of immune sera, monoclonal antibodies and cytotoxic T cells obtained from patients with breast or pancreatic cancer. Immunization against MUC1 has protected mice and rats from tumor challenge with syngeneic breast cancers expressing human MUC1. Other epithelial cancer mucins such as MUC2 and MUC5AC differ from MUC1 in that they do not have transmembrane domains and so are not cell surface antigens though they are secreted and form prominent components of the glycocalyx that surrounds epithelial cancer cells.

KSA

Human adenocarcinoma associated antigen (KSA), also called *epithelial glycoprotein* (EGP) and EpCAM, is a 40 kDa glycoprotein associated with the cell surface of most adenocarcinomas and with the corresponding normal tissues (once again at secretory borders). It has been recognized by a series of mAbs (17–1A, KS1/4, H99, GA733). Treatment with 17–1A has resulted in occasional clinical responses of advanced carcinomas without toxicity and when administered in the adjuvant setting to patients with Dukes C colon cancer, has prolonged disease free and overall survival compared to randomized controls. Toxicity due to antibody access to and reaction with normal tissues was not seen.

PSMA

Prostate specific membrane antigen (PSMA) is a 100 kDa integral, type II membrane protein with acidic dipeptides activity which is highly expressed in primary and metastatic prostate cancer, and to a lesser extent in normal prostate tissue. PSMA expression increases with disease progression. Recently PSMA has also been detected in tumor vascular endothelium from a variety of cancers as well as at much lower levels in some normal tissues, including duodenal mucosa and some proximal renal tubules. The relevance of PSMA as a target is emphasized by successful targeting of prostate cancer with ProstaScint, an ^{111}In-labelled anti-PSMA mAb that has been licensed by FDA for this purpose.

CA125

CA125 is amullerian duct differentiation antigen expressed in some normal secretory tissues but overexpressed in ovarian cancer and some other cancers. It has been used as a serum marker for monitoring patients with ovarian cancer since it was first identified in 1981 using a murine monoclonal antibody. It has recently been identified as a mucin (MUC16) with high seronine, threonine and proline content and many (probably >60) partially conserved tandem repeats (156aa each) at the N-terminal region. The C-terminus contains a possible trans-membrane region and a potential tyrosine phosphorylation site.

Other Potential Antigens and Vaccines Inducing T-cell Immunity

Antigens are not as abundantly expressed, nor are they expressed with the same high frequency on cancers from different patients as are the antigens described above. In addition, antigens such as the cancer-testis antigens and p53 are not cell surface antigens, which may restrict the relevant immune response to a T-cell response. This enormously complicates the analysis of immunogenicity in vaccine trials and attempts at active intervention for the following reasons:

1. Ideally, autologous cancer cells are required for testing and these are rarely available as cell lines or in frozen samples in sufficient quantities for a thorough analysis of the immune response and its specificity.
2. In vitro sensitization has in the past generally been required for demonstration of T-cell responses against tumor antigens and this adds significant risk of artifactual results and complicates the quantification of immune responses.
3. Augmentation of T-cell responses by vaccination is more difficult to induce than augmentation of B-cell responses and has yet to be clearly achieved and confirmed in a majority of vaccinated patients against any tumor antigen.
4. Vaccine design depends on the immune response desired. There are hundreds of available approaches or combinations of approaches

to inducing T-cell immunity. These include immunization with peptides or proteins with various adjuvants, dendritic cells pulsed with or transduced to express particular antigens, viruses or bacteria transduced to express antigens, and DNA or RNA vaccines. In each case these vaccines could include approaches to augmenting cytokine or second signal induction. The range of options for augmenting T-cell immunity against cancer is daunting. Unlike the picture with vaccines designed to induce an antibody response where there is one best approach (conjugate vaccines as described below), it remains unclear which is the optimal approach for induction of T-cell immunity.

5. It is unclear whether augmentation of CTLs or helper T-cells is the desired goal for vaccines inducing T-cells against cancer.
6. It is not clear which antigens should be selected as targets for T-cell attack against cancer, as no T-cell immune responses have been correlated with a more favorable prognosis as is true for antibody responses against glycolipids (GM2) and mucins (sTn).
7. Tumor cells can and frequently do fail to express relevant antigens in the context of MHC as a consequence of MHC loss or problems in antigen processing (proteosomes, TAP), or they may suppress the T-cell response or become resistant to it (by production of IL10, TGFβ, VEGF, Fas-ligand, HLA-G or Bcl-2).

Given these uncertainties, selection of a single vaccine approach for inducing optimal T-cell immunity is difficult now and will remain so for some years to come. Consequently, we have focused on antibody inducing polyvalent vaccines targeting the cell surface antigens.

Table 14.1. Cancer cell-surface targets for vaccine construction

Tumor	*Antigens*
Melanoma	GM2, GD2, GD3
Neuroblastoma	GM2, GD2, GD3, polysialic acid
Sarcoma	GM2, GD2, GD3
Small-cell lung cancer	GM2, fucosyl GM1, polysialic acid, globo H, sialyl Le^a, KSA
Breast	GM2, globo H, Le^y, TF, Tn, sTn, MUC1, KSA
Prostate	GM2, Tn, sTn, TF, Le^y, MUC1, KSA, PSMA
Ovary	GM2, globo H, sTn, TF, Le^y, MUC1, KSA, CA125 (MUC16)

Immunogenicity of these Cell Surface Antigens in Cancer Patients

Selection of KLH Conjugate Plus QS-21 Vaccines

We have explored a variety of approaches for increasing the antibody response against carbohydrate and peptide cancer antigens, including the use of different immunological adjuvants, adhering the antigens to bacteria or polystyrene beads, chemical modification of gangliosides to make them more immunogenic and conjugation to various immunogenic carrier proteins. The conclusion from these studies is that the use of a carrier protein plus an immunological adjuvant is the optimal approach. The optimal immunological adjuvant in each case was one or more purified saponin fractions (QS-21 or GPI-0100) obtained from the bark of Quillaja saponaria. The optimal carrier protein was in each case *keyhole limpet hemocyanin* (KLH). This approach (covalent attachment of the carbohydrate or peptide antigen to KLH and administration mixed with QS-21 or GPI-0100) has proved optimal for antibody induction in mice and cancer patients for most of the antigens.

Additional Variables

Two additional variables have proved critical for increasing antibody titers, the method of conjugation and the epitope ratio of antigen molecules per KLH molecule. The optimal conjugation approached has varied with the antigen. Gangliosides are best conjugated using ozone cleavage of the ceramide double bond and introducing an aldehyde group followed by coupling to aminolysyl groups of KLH by reductive amination. This approach was not as effective for conjugation of Le^y, or Globo H to KLH where an M2C2H linker arm has proved most efficient or for Tn(c), sTn(c), TF(c) or MUC1 where an MBS linker group was optimal. We have demonstrated that covalent conjugation of antigen (ganglioside GD3) to KLH is required, simply mixing the two is of little benefit. Based on our experience with GM2 and GD3 conjugate vaccines, it is our impression that within the restrictions imposed by current conjugation methods, higher epitope ratios result in higher immunogenicity. Consequently considerable effort is devoted to maximizing this ratio with each vaccine.

We have also performed a series of Phase I dosing trials to determine the impact of dose of conjugate on antibody response in vaccinated patients, and a series of experiments in the mouse to determine the impact of treatments designed to decrease suppressor cell reactivity in mice. The lowest dose of antigen in the KLH conjugates resulting in optimal antibody titers for each antigen is 10 μg for the glycolipids and polysialic acid, and 1 or 3 μg for the mucin antigens. Decreasing suppressor cell activity with low dose cyclophosphamide or anti-CTLA4 mAb had no impact on antibody titers.

Ganglioside Vaccines

We have been refining our ability to induce antibodies against GM2 in melanoma patients for fifteen years, since it was first demonstrated that patients immunized with irradiated melanoma cells occasionally produced antibodies against GM2, and that vaccines containing purified GM2 could be more immunogenic than vaccines containing tumor cells expressing GM2. Initially GM2 adherent to BCG was selected as optimal, inducing IgM antibodies in 85% of patients. Though these antibodies and monoclonal antibodies against GM2 were only able to kill 25% of melanoma cell lines by CDC, patients with natural or vaccine-induced antibodies had significantly longer disease free and overall survival. This was the basis for a randomized trial comparing immunization with BCG to immunization with GM2/BCG in 122 patients with AJCC Stage 3 melanoma. While the difference was not statistically significant, the GM2/BCG treated patients had a 12% improvement in survival and 15% improvement in disease free survival compared to the BCG patients after a minimum follow-up of 70 months. The IgM antibodies had a median titer of 1/160 and were short lived (8–12 weeks). IgG antibody induction was rare. We explored a variety of approaches to further improve this antibody response. The use of GM2 conjugated to KLH and mixed with immunological adjuvant QS-21 was consistently optimal, inducing higher titer IgM antibodies (median titer 1/640–1/1280) in all patients and IgG antibodies in most patients. Reactivity against GM2 positive melanoma cells and complement mediated lysis was seen in over 90% of patients, and the antibody duration was 3–6 months after each vaccination. Antibody titers have been maintained for over three years by administration of repeated booster immunizations at 3–4 month intervals. Antibody titers could not be further increased by pretreatment with a low dose of cyclophosphamide (300 mg/M^2) to decrease suppressor cell reactivity. As with the other carbohydrate antigen vaccines described below, no evidence of T-cell immunity detected by delayed type hypersensitivity skin test reactivity (DTH) against GM2 was found.

This GM2-KLH plus QS-21 vaccine has been tested in a Phase III randomized trial in melanoma patients in this country compared to

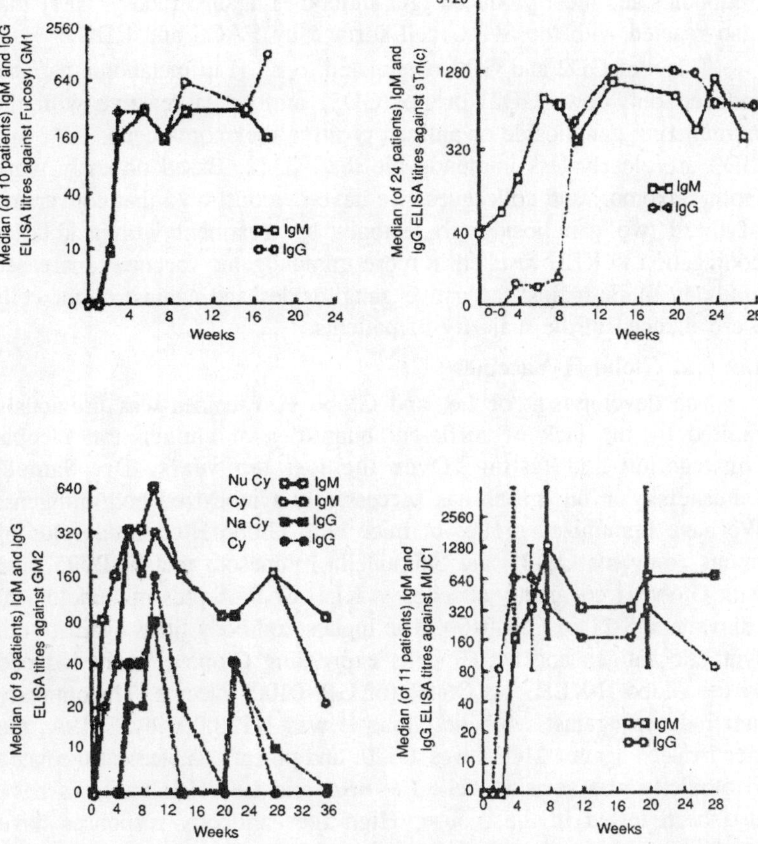

Fig. 14.2. Median sequential ELISA IgG and IgM antibody titers induced in groups of cancer patients after vaccination with KLH-antigen conjugate vaccines plus QS-21.

high dose interferon alpha. The trial was stopped because after a median follow-up of 16 months, patients receiving interferon had a significantly longer disease free and over all survival. Longer follow-up will be required to determine the long term impact, but the results to date indicate that induction of antibodies against GM2 in Stage III melanoma patients is not associated with demonstrable benefit. This may be because while essentially all melanomas express some GM2, only a minority express enough GM2 to permit cell lysis with mAbs or immune sera. This is further basis for polyvalent vaccines.

Fucosyl GM1, like GM2 is highly immunogenic. Essentially all patients vaccinated with fucosyl GM1-KLH plus QS-21 produced IgM antibodies and most produced IgG antibodies against fucosyl GM1 that also reacted with the SCLC cell surface by FACS and CDC.

Trials of GD2 and GD3 conjugated to KLH in melanoma patients induced only low (GD2) or no (GD3) antibodies reactive with the immunizing ganglioside or antigen positive melanoma cells. GD2 and GD3 are clearly less immunogenic than GM2. Based on early work from Hakomori and colleagues, we have demonstrated that conversion of these two gangliosides to lactones by treatment with acid after conjugation to KLH resulted in more immunogenic vaccines. Increased antibody titers against the native gangliosides and against tumor cells were induced in the majority of patients.

Le^y and Globo H Vaccines

The development of Le^y and Globo H vaccines was previously limited by the lack of sufficient quantities of antigen for vaccine construction and testing. Over the last ten years, Dr. Samuel Danishefsky in our group has successfully synthesized both antigens. We have immunized groups of mice with Globo H-ceramide plus or minus adjuvants QS-21 and Salmonella minnesota mutant R595, and with Globo H covalently attached to KLH or BSA plus immunological adjuvants QS-21 or GPI-0100. The highest antibody titers against both synthetic antigen and MCF7 cells expressing Globo H were induced by the Globo H-KLH plus QS-21 (or GPI-0100) vaccine. The antibody titer induced against synthetic Globo H was 1/120,000 by ELISA, the titer induced against MCF7 was 1/320, and potent complement mediated cytotoxicity was seen as well. Le^y-BSA and Le^y-KLH vaccines have also been tested in the mouse. High titer antibody responses have resulted against the synthetic epitope of Le^y and against tumor cells expressing Le^y in the majority of mice immunized. Based on these results, clinical trials with Globo H-KLH plus QS-21 and Le^y-KLH plus QS21 have been initiated in patients with breast, prostate or ovary cancer. Antibodies against the purified antigens and against tumor cells expressing these antigens were induced in most patients immunized with globo H and occasional patients immunized with Le^y.

TF, Tn and sTn Vaccines

Patients with various epithelial cancers have been immunized with unclustered TF-KLH and sTn-KLH vaccines plus various adjuvants. High titer IgM and IgG antibodies against TF and sTn antigens resulted. In our hands the majority of the reactivity was against antigenic epitopes present in the vaccine which were not present on naturally expressed mucins (porcine or ovine submaxillary mucins (PSM or OSM)) or tumor cells. Based on previous studies with Tn antigen, Kurosaka and Nakada et al. hypothesized that MLS102, a monoclonal antibody against sTn, might preferentially recognize clusters ((c)) of sTn. Studies with monoclonal antibody B72.3 and with sera raised against TF-KLH and sTn-KLH conjugate vaccines in mice and in patients resulted in the same conclusion.

The availability of synthetic TF, Tn and sTn clusters consisting of 3 epitopes covalently linked to 3 consecutive serines or threonines has permitted proof of this hypothesis. In both direct tests and inhibition assays, B72.3 recognized sTn clusters exclusively, and sera from mice immunized with sTn (c)-KLH reacted strongly with both natural mucins and tumor cells expressing sTn. Based on this background, we initiated trials with the TF(c)-KLH, Tn(c)-KLH and sTn(c)-KLH conjugate vaccines in patients with breast cancer. Antibodies of high titer and specificity, including against OSM or PSM and cancer cells expressing TF, Tn or sTn, were induced for the first time in our experience. Based on these results, we plan to include clustered Tn, sTn and TF in the polyvalent vaccines against epithelial cancers.

Several trials with TF, Tn and sTn vaccines have been reported from other centers, and a large multicenter Phase III trial with an sTn vaccine is currently in progress. Georg Springer's pioneering trials in breast cancer patients with vaccines containing TF and Tn purified from natural sources and mixed with typhoid vaccine (as adjuvant) began in the mid 1970s. DTH and IgM responses against the immunizing antigens and prolonged survival compared to historical controls were reported. MacLean immunized ten ovarian cancer patients with synthetic TF conjugated to KLH plus immunological adjuvant Detox (monophosphoryl Lipid A plus BCG cell wall skeletons) and described augmentation of IgG and IgM antibodies against synthetic TF in 9 of 10 patients. Lower levels of antibody reactivity against TF from natural sources were detected in some of these cases.

MacLean has also immunized patients with breast and other adenocarcinomas with sTn-KLH plus immunological adjuvant Detox. Induction of IgM and IgG antibodies against synthetic and natural sources of sTn was seen in essentially all patients and this response was further increased by pretreatment of patients with a low dose of cyclophosphamide. Reactivity of these sera with natural mucins and tumor cells despite the use of an unclustered sTn vaccine is probably explained by the several fold higher sTn/KLH epitope ratio achieved in the MacLean vaccine compared to our previous unclustered vaccine.

Survival appeared to be improved overall compared to historical controls and patients who responded with high antibody titers survived longer than those with lower titers. Reactivity with breast cancer cells, including complement dependent cytotoxicity, was described. This is the basis for an ongoing multicenter Phase III randomized trial of the sTn-KLH plus Detox vaccine versus no treatment in breast cancer patients with limited disease.

Polysialic Acid Vaccines

Initial attempts at preparing a vaccine against polysialic acid for use in military recruits who are at risk of group B meningococcus infection were unsuccessful. We also have completed analysis of a trial with polysialic acid conjugated to KLH plus QS-21 and found that no antibody response could be induced. Consequently, we tested a second polysialic acid vaccine that had been modified (N-propionylated) to increase its immunogenicity in collaboration with Dr. Harold Jennings who pioneered the use of N-propionylation for this purpose. This induced an antibody response against unmodified polysialic acid in five of six patients immunized. These vaccine induced antibodies also reacted with small cell lung cancer cells (and were cytotoxic for antigen positive bacteria). This N-propionylated polysialic acid vaccine is suitable for inclusion in our polyvalent vaccine against SCLC.

MUC1 Vaccines

We have immunized mice with MUC1-KLH, plus QS-21, and seen induction of consistent high titer IgM and IgG antibodies against MUC1 and human cell lines expressing MUC1, as well as protection from a syngeneic mouse breast cancer expressing human MUC1 as a consequence of gene transduction. Mice were also immunized with vaccines containing MUC1 peptides (Tn glycosylated or not) with $1^{1/2}$ or 5 tandem repeats (32 or 106 amino acids) conjugated to KLH by one of three methods or not, and mixed with QS-21 or BCG. MUC1 containing 32 amino acids, glycosylated with Tn epitopes O-linked at serines or threonines or not, conjugated to KLH and mixed with QS-21 induced the highest titer antibodies. Based on these studies in the mouse, we initiated and completed trials with these MUC1-KLH plus QS-21 vaccines in breast cancer patients who were free of detectable breast cancer after resection of all known disease. No patient had detectable MUC1 serological reactivity by ELISA or FACS prior to immunization. As was true in the mouse, the 32 amino acid MUC1 peptide conjugate, glycosylated or not, was optimal. Inhibition assays were performed to better understand this serologic response. Much of the IgM response and nearly all of the IgG response were against the immune dominant epitope, APDTRPA, preferentially with RPA at the terminal position.

Since MUC1 is a peptide, T-Lymphocyte responses against MUC1 would be expected. We have been unable to consistently demonstrate T-Lymphocyte proliferation, interferon-γ or IL4 release against MUC1 by ELISPOT or CTL assays, or positive DTH responses, after vaccination with MUC1. We have especially focused on proliferation and ELISPOT assays in the MUC1 trials. Patients were leukophoresed pre and post vaccination, providing ample lymphocytes for our studies. While occasional assays gave positive results, these were not positive on subsequent repeats or in a pattern with other assays that suggested impact of the immunizations. After 2 years of steady endeavor there has been no clear evidence of augmented T-cell reactivity against MUC1 peptides of various lengths, or in HLA A2 positive patients against heteroclytic MUC1 peptides with single amino acid changes that increased binding to HLA A2.

Several trials with MUC1 vaccines at other centers have been reported. Trials by Goydos *et al.* and Reddish *et al.* showed augmentation of CTL and/or proliferation after vaccination (with MUC1 peptides mixed with BCG or immunological adjuvant Detox) in a single blood specimen in occasional patients but assays were not repeated to confirm reproducibility. A trial was reported by Karanikas *et al.* with a MUC1-mannan fusion peptide and again occasional positive CTL or proliferation responses were seen but these were not repeated and were not both positive in the same patients. These three trials basically confirm our conclusion that vaccine induced augmentation of T-cell reactivity against MUC1 has yet to be convincingly demonstrated. The Karanikas report also described augmentation of antibody titers against the immunizing synthetic MUC1 peptide in 13 of 25 patients, but no tests against cancer cells or natural sources of MUC1 were described.

KSA Vaccines

Antibodies against KSA have been described in patients following vaccination with anti-idiotypic antibodies and some patients vaccinated with KSA of baculovirus origin. KSA is clearly potentially immunogenic in humans and these antibodies have not resulted in detectable toxicity.

PSMA Vaccines

To date, the only reports of vaccines containing PSMA involve peptides pulsed onto autologous dendritic cells. In these small studies, indications of immunogenicity were observed, and no obvious toxicity was described. Partial clinical responses were induced is some patients which were durable after one year. These trials indicate that PSMA is an appropriate choice of antigen for this patient population, even in the presence of metastatic disease. These studies are applicable only to HLA A2 positive patients and employed a technique involving *ex vivo* expansion and manipulation of dendritic cells, making them impractical for wide spread application. Antibody induction was not tested.

CA125 Vaccines

Because CA125 has only recently been sequenced, no trials with CA125 vaccines have been conducted to date. However, forty-two ovarian cancer patients have been immunized with the murine monoclonal anti-idiotype (ACA125), which imitates an epitope on CA125. While HAMA and anti-idiotype antibodies were induced in the majority of patients, reactivity of post immunization sera with tumor cells was induced in only occasional patients. There was no evidence of autoimmunity in these patients.

Glycolipids and Globular Glycoproteins are more Effective Targets for CDC than Mucins

One of several effector mechanisms thought to contribute to tumor cell death is *complement dependent cytotoxicity* (CDC). Review of the serological analysis of the series of clinical trials described above has suggested that the six vaccines containing different glycolipids induced antibodies mediating CDC whereas the four vaccines containing carbohydrate or peptide epitopes carried by mucin molecules induced antibodies that were not capable of mediating CDC. We explored whether this dichotomy was a result of properties of the induced antibodies (ie. class and effector functions), the different target cells used, or the nature of the target antigens. We compared the cell surface reactivity (assayed by FACS), complement-fixing ability (using the *immune adherence* [IA] assay) and the CDC activity of a panel of monoclonal antibodies and immune sera from these trials on the same two tumor cell lines. Antibodies against glycolipids GM2, globo H and Le^y, protein KSA and mucin antigens Tn, sTn, TF and MUC1 all reacted with these antigens expressed on tumor cells and all fixed complement. CDC, however, was mediated by mAbs or immune sera against the glycolipids and a globular protein (KSA), but not by mAbs or sera against the mucin antigens. Recently we have noted that immune

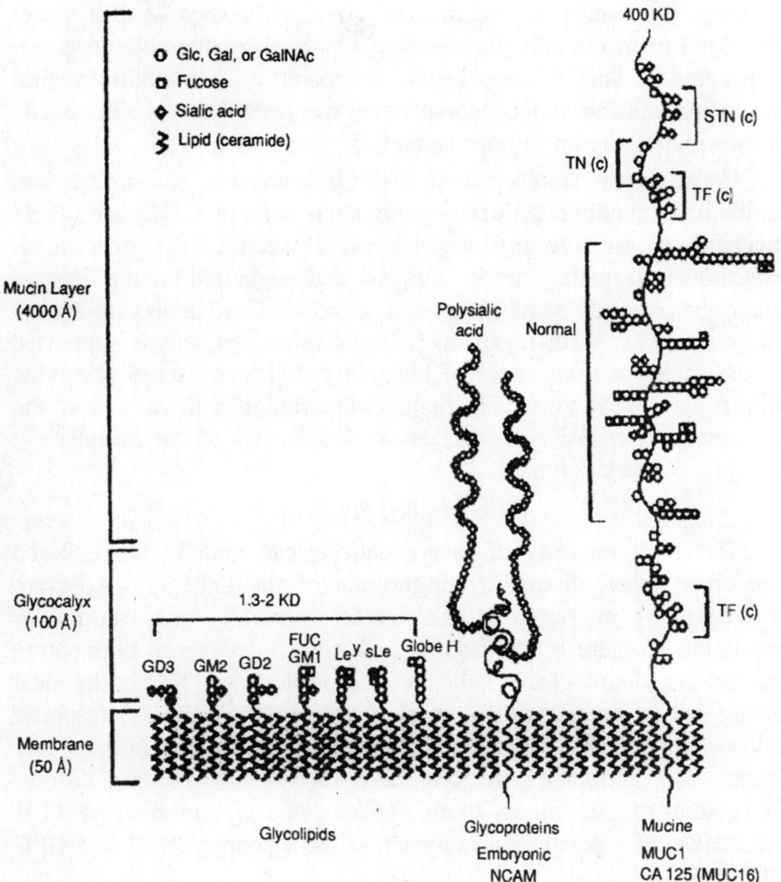

Fig. 14.3. Glycolipids and glycoproteins expressed abundantly at the cancer cell surface. Note the intimate association with the cell surface of glycolipids and the more distant association of mucins and polysialic acid.

sera and mAbs against polysialic acid are also unable to induce CDC. Like MUC1, antibodies against polysialic acid attach far from the cell surface. In the case of MUC1, this is because of the rigid carbohydrate collar that characterizes mucins. The same effect probably results as a consequence of the negative charge of both the sialic acid rich cancer cell surface and polysialic acid.

It must be emphasized that although we showed that mucins are poor targets for complement-mediated lysis of tumor cells, studies have shown that induction of antibodies against either glycolipid or mucin antigens results in protection from tumor recurrence in several different preclinical mouse models. Also, antibodies against either glycolipid or mucin epitopes correlate with a more favorable prognosis in patients. It does not appear that the inability of antibodies against mucin antigens to induce complement-mediated lysis is necessarily detrimental to the anti-tumor response.

Consequently, complement-mediated inflammation, opsonization and antibody dependent cellular cytotoxicity but not CDC are likely mechanisms for the prolonged survival seen in the preclinical experiments targeting mucin antigens and suggested in the clinical trials with passively administered and actively induced antibodies against mucin antigens. With regard to bacterial infections, this is supported by the severe consequences of hereditary deficiency states involving either the classical or alternate complement pathways and the comparatively trivial consequences to deficiencies of the complement membrane attack complex.

Concluding Remark

The great majority of cancer patients can initially be rendered free of detectable disease by surgery and/or chemotherapy. Adjuvant chemotherapy or radiation therapy are generally only minimally beneficial, so there is real need for additional methods of eliminating residual circulating cancer cells and micrometastases. This is the ideal setting for treatment with a cancer vaccine. The immune response induced is critically dependent on the antigenic epitope and vaccine design. For antibody induction there is one best vaccine design, conjugation of the antigen to an immunogenic protein such as KLH and the use of a potent adjuvant such as the saponins QS-21 and GPI-0100.

This approach alone induced strong antibody responses against the glycolipids GM2, fucosyl GM1 and globo H and the mucin backbone MUC1, and cancer cells expressing these antigens. Other antigens required additional modifications to augment relevant immunogenicity. GD2 and GD3 lactones and N-propionylated polysialic acid were significantly more effective at inducing antibodies against tumor cells than the unmodified antigens. Tn, sTn and TF trimers (clusters) were significantly more effective than the monomers at inducing antibodies reactive with the cancer cell surface. The optimal approach for Le^y, KSA, PSMA, and CA125 (MUC16) remains to be determined.

Antibodies are ideally suited for eradicating pathogens from the bloodstream and from early tissue invasion. Passively administered and vaccine induced antibodies have accomplished this, eliminating circulating tumor cells and systemic or intraperitoneal micrometastases in a variety of preclinical models, so antibody-inducing vaccines offer real promise in the adjuvant setting. Polyvalent vaccines will probably be required due to tumor cell heterogeneity, heterogeneity of the human immune response and the correlation between overall antibody titer against tumor cells and antibody effector mechanisms. Over the next several years, Phase II clinical trials designed to determine the clinical impact of polyvalent conjugate vaccines will be initiated in the adjuvant setting in patients with SCLC and several epithelial cancers.

15

THERAPEUTIC VACCINE

Many aspects of the usual paradigm for the clinical development of cytotoxic anticancer drugs are not appropriate for therapeutic cancer vaccines. In this chapter we explore some of these differences and recommend designs and strategies more suited for the development of effective therapeutic vaccines.

DOSE-ESCALATION STUDIES

Safety Studies

Phase I studies usually involve dose escalation in cohorts of three patients, starting with a very low dose, in an effort to identify a maximally tolerated dose. Phase I studies are generally conducted in patients with advanced metastatic disease who have failed all other available treatments. Tumor vaccines are often based on DNA constructs, viral vectors and cytokines that have been determined as safe in previous clinical trials. Peptide vaccines generally seem inherently safe as long as the cytokine adjuvants are used in combinations and doses previously demonstrated to be safe. Consequently, no phase I safety study should be required for most therapeutic cancer vaccines.

On the other hand, a novel virus or plasmid used as a recombinant vaccine vector for the first time should be evaluated for safety. A dose escalation design may be appropriate but patients whose immune systems have not been compromised by extensive chemotherapy are the most relevant subjects. If such vectors are proven to be nontoxic at substantial doses, then subsequent dose-escalation safety trials using the same vectors but with different recombinant inserts may not be required.

Immunogenicity Studies

Feasibility issues limit the maximum doses of certain vaccines that can be produced for administration to patients. In many cases, the dose selected will be based on pre-clinical findings or on practical considerations.

For cancer vaccines, it is not always the case that more is better. In studies of peptide vaccines based on non-mutated melanoma antigens, in vitro analysis did not reveal any correlation between peptide dose and the generation of specific T cell reactivity from the peripheral blood lymphocytes of vaccinated patients. Thus, for subsequent trials using similar peptides, an intermediate fixed dose of 1 mg was chosen for vaccination, bypassing repetitive phase I studies.

Dose ranging to find the *minimal active dose* may be feasible but the 3–6 patients per dose level used in conventional toxicity trials may not be adequate. Those small sample sizes are only sufficient to exclude high toxicity rates. Suppose that an assay is used in a binary manner to define immunogenic response. Table 15.1 shows the probability of no immunogenic responses in n patients as a function of the true immunogenic response probability. If one wants a dose at which the immunogenic response probability is at least 30% say, then if you observe no immunogenic responses in 7 patients it would be appropriate to escalate to the next dose level.

Table 15.1. Finding the minimum active dose

Probability of immunologic response	*Number of patients treated at dose*	*Probability of no immunologic responses*
0.20	11	0.09
0.25	9	0.08
0.30	7	0.08
0.40	5	0.08
0.50	4	0.06

Korn et al. defined a sequential procedure for finding a biologically active dose, although not necessarily the minimal active dose. During an initial accelerated phase one patient per dose level is treated until a biological response is seen. After the first response is seen, cohorts of 3–6 patients are treated per dose level. With 0–1 biological responses among the 3 patients at a dose level, escalate to the next level for the next cohort of patients. With 2 or 3 responses out of the 3 patients, expand the cohort to a total of 6 patients. With 5 or 6 biological responses out of the 6 patients, declare that dose level to be the biologically active level and terminate the trial. With fewer than 5 biological responses out of the 6 patients, a new cohort of 3 patients is accrued at the next higher dose level, etc. Korn et al. describe some of the statistical properties of this sequential design.

Trying to determine whether there is a dose-response relationship involves comparing immunological responses for different dose levels. Such trials, if designed properly, require larger sample sizes. Consider, for example, planning a study of two dose levels to test whether there is a relationship between dose and immunologic response. If the immunologic response probabilities at the two dose levels are 50% and 90%, then 20 patients treated at each dose level are required for a one-sided statistical significance level of 0.10 and a statistical power of 0.90. Larger sample sizes are required to detect smaller differences. Using more than two dose levels allows one to treat somewhat fewer patients at each dose level, but the total number of patients required to detect a dose-response relationship will actually be much larger than if only two dose levels are tested. This is because the two most extreme dose groups are the most informative for detecting a dose-response relationship.

Trying to characterize the shape of the dose-activity relationship or finding an optimum biologic dose is an even more ambitious objective that is rarely practical in a phase I tumor vaccine study.

Phase II Studies

The general objectives of the phase II vaccine trial are similar to those of the phase II cytotoxic trial. The primary objective is to determine whether the regimen has biologic activity that is likely to translate into patient benefit. The second objective is to optimize the regimen.

With cytotoxics, the generally accepted endpoint for phase II trials is objective tumor response; that is, tumor shrinkage by at least 50%. Tumor shrinkage is not a direct measure of patient benefit, although it sometimes is predictive of benefit. The most commonly accepted direct measures of patient benefit are survival, disease free survival and symptomatic relief. Therapeutic effect on these endpoints cannot be reliably established outside of a phase III trial with an appropriate control group not receiving the experimental therapy. Investigators sometimes like to infer that a regimen prolongs survival because the responders live longer than the non-responders, but this analysis has long been known to be invalid.

Tumor shrinkage is generally used as the endpoint for phase II trials of cytotoxics for two reasons. First, because response represents biological activity that can be attributed to the therapy (i.e. tumors rarely shrink spontaneously by 50%). Secondly, if the degree, duration and abundance of responses are sufficient, then it is plausible to hope that tumor response may translate into patient benefit. There are many cytotoxic regimens which were active in phase II trials but which subsequently had no identifiable effect on survival in phase III trials. Torri et al. performed a meta-analysis of randomized trials to quantify the relationship between improvement in response rate and improvement in survival outcome for advanced ovarian cancer studies. They found that a very substantial improvement in response rate was necessary to have any identifiable effect on survival.

For phase II tumor vaccine studies, clinical endpoints and/or immunological endpoints are commonly used. Clinical endpoints include tumor shrinkage, reduction in tumor marker levels or delay in time to tumor progression.

Single-Arm Trials Using Clinical or Immunologic Response Rate

If tumor shrinkage is the endpoint, then phase II designs used for cytotoxics can be employed. Simon's "*optimal two-stage*" designs are widely used for phase II cytotoxic trials to test whether a regimen has a response rate above a background level p_0. Frequently, $p_0 = 0.05$ is used. With clinical response, this assumes that no more than 5% of the patients will have apparent responses caused by variability in response assessment or spontaneous remissions. The 2-stage design incorporates an early termination point, which allows the investigator to discontinue patient accrual if a desired endpoint has not been achieved in the first stage of the trial.

At the conclusion of the clinical trial, the regimen will be declared active or inactive. Table 15.2 shows several designs with 10% false positive rate, 10% false negative rate and $p_0 = 0.05$. The false positive rate (α) is the probability of declaring the regimen active when the true response probability is p_0. The false negative rate (β) is the probability of declaring the regimen inactive when its true response probability is the target response rate p_1, the level of activity that we wish to be able to detect. In the first stage, N_1 evaluable patients are entered and treated. If no responses are observed, then the trial is terminated and the regimen is declared inactive. Otherwise accrual continues to a total of N evaluable patients. At that point accrual is complete. If the total number of responses is at least A, then the regimen is declared active. The last column of the table indicates the probability of early termination after the first stage when the true response probability is p_0. For example, if $p_0 = 5\%$ and the target response rate is 25%, then 9 patients are treated in the first stage of the trial. If no responses are observed, the trial is terminated. Otherwise, accrual is continued to a total of 24 patients. If at least 3 responses are seen in the 24 patients, the regimen is declared active. The probability of declaring a regimen active when it's true response rate is 5% or less is 10%. The probability of missing the activity of a regimen with a true response rate of 25% is 10%. With a regimen having a response rate of 5%, the probability of stopping after only 9 patients is 63%. This design with $p_1 = 25\%$ and $p_0 = 5\%$ seems reasonable for many initial vaccine trials using tumor regression as endpoint.

Table 15.2. Optimal two-stage designs

Target response rate (p_1)	*First stage sample size* (N_1)	*Maximum sample size* (*N*)	*Number of responses required for activity* (*A*)	*Probability of early termination*
20%	12	37	4	.54
25%	9	24	3	.63
30%	7	21	3	.70
35%	6	12	2	.74

An optimum two stage design can also be used with a binary immunologic response endpoint. In such a case, however, the values of p_0 and p_1 will generally be much higher than for a tumor regression endpoint. Optimum two-stage designs for any values of p_0, p_1, α, and β are easily generated using computer program OTSD (optimum two-stage design). The required number of patients depends strongly on the difference p_1-p_0.

A variety of alternative single-arm designs for evaluating binary endpoints have been published. For example, Garnsey-Ensign developed three stage designs, and Thall and Simon developed continuous monitoring Bayesian designs. The essential characteristics of this class of designs is that the endpoint is binary and that the objective is to evaluate the response rate of the regimen on it's own, not in comparison to the response rate for some other regimen. If the objective is comparative, then even for a single arm trial, the design and method of analysis should take into account the variability in the estimate of response rate for the external control regimen. Methods such as that of Makuch and Simon, Dixon and Simon and Thall and Simon attempt to take that variability into account.

For therapeutic vaccines, the current situation for most diseases (other than melanoma) is that few if any partial or complete tumor responses have been observed with any regimen but that varying degrees of immunogenicity have been obtained. It is usually very difficult to compare the degree of immunogenicity obtained with different regimens by different investigators because of differences in assays, variation in procedures and reagents, and differences in patient selection. It is even difficult to compare the degree of immunogenicity obtained by the same investigator in different studies with different regimens because of assay variability. There is also generally some uncertainty in what measures of immunogenicity are most appropriate. There are currently no measures that can be considered true surrogates for clinical response.

It takes fewer patients to determine whether a regimen causes any clinical responses than it does to compare it to another regimen with regard to immunologic response rate. The optimum two-stage design recommended above for evaluating clinical response rate has a first stage of only 9 patients. Consequently, a reasonable phase II development strategy is to design phase II trials using the optimal two-stage design for distinguishing a 5% clinical response rate from a 25% clinical response rate with error rates of 10%. If after accruing the 9 patients in the first stage, no clinical responses are seen, then the trial is terminated. If one or more clinical responses are seen, accrual should continue unless the level of immunologic response is so inadequate that the investigator would like to make some modifications to the regimen. In cases where accrual is terminated after 9 patients because of lack of clinical responses, the immunological activity of the regimen for the 9 patients accrued will provide information for modifications of the vaccine regimen.

Multiple Arm Screening Trials Using Immunological Response Rate

One of the complexities of therapeutic vaccine development is the many options available for attempting to enhance immunological recognition of a specified tumor antigen. In addition to the vector or mode of presentation of the antigen to the immune system, there are alternative adjuvants, preparative regimens, routes and schedules of administration. Because of the difficulty and time required for clinical trials, it is best to optimize vaccines to the extent possible using animal models. Nevertheless, there may be several vaccine candidates available for clinical trial. One approach would be to perform a two-stage 9–24 patient clinical trial on all candidate regimens, stopping at 9 patients unless partial remissions are seen. An alternative strategy is to perform a multi-arm phase II trial to optimize the regimen with regard to immunogenicity before focusing on clinical endpoints. The reason for using a multi-arm randomized phase II design is to ensure comparability of patients on the different regimens and to control for assay variability.

Factorial screening designs

Two types of randomized phase II trials are potentially relevant for optimizing a vaccine regimen. One method is the use of a phase II factorial design. Suppose that there are m binary factors that represent dimensions in which a basic vaccine may be modified. For example, one factor might be route of administration and another might be whether a specified adjuvant is administered. Since there are m binary factors, there are 2^m possible combinations of levels of the factors. For example, let the levels of each factor be denoted 0 or 1. Then with two factors the possible combinations of factors are (0,0), (0,1), (1,0), and (1,1). The study is conducted by randomizing N patients into the 2^m treatment groups. If the factors affect immunogenicity independently, then in comparing the two levels of one factor, one can ignore the other factors.

Actually, a stratified or model based analysis is more powerful than simple pooling, but the point is that the two levels of each factor are compared based on the assumption that the difference does not depend on the levels of the other factors. Consequently, comparing level 0 of a factor to level 1 of that factor involves comparing average immunogenicity for the N/2 patients with the factor at level 0 to average immunogenicity for the N/2 patients with the factor at level 1. The trial is sized, i.e. N is selected, for m independent two-arm comparisons involving N/2 patients per arm, not for one 2^m arm comparison. If there are 3 factors (m = 3), then there are $2^3 = 8$ arms to the trial. If N = 32, then 4 patients are randomly assigned to each of the arms, but the comparisons of the levels of each factor involve comparing average immunogenicity for two groups of 16 patients.

The value of N is selected based on the manner in which immunogenicity is measured (e.g. continuous scale or binary), assay and biological variability among patients, and size of difference to be detected. Suppose, for example, that immunogenicity is measured on a continuous scale, and let x denote the change in immunogenicity from base-line for a patient after treatment. Assume that x is approximately normally distributed and let σ denote the standard deviation for x for different patients receiving the same vaccine regimen. Let δ denote the size of the difference in mean value of x we wish to be able to detect in comparing vaccine groups, and let α and β denote the type 1 and type 2 error rates for the comparison. Then N/2 patients are required in each of the two groups with:

$$N = 4\left(\frac{z_{\alpha/2} + z_{\beta}}{\delta/\sigma}\right)^2 \qquad ...(1)$$

where $z_{\alpha/2}$ is the 100(α/2)'th percentile of the standard normal distribution and z_{β} is the 100β'th percentile. For 5% type 1 error and 80% power, we have $z_{\alpha/2} = 1.96$ and $z_{\beta} = 0.84$. To detect a difference in means that represents one standard deviation of inter-patient variability in immunogenicity requires N = 32 patients randomized. This gives 16 patients in each level of each binary factor. With 3 binary factors, there are 8 treatment groups. Hence randomly assigning 4 patients per treatment group will satisfy this requirement. The required sample size is very dependent on the δ/σ ratio. Reducing σ by improving the assay reproducibility will increase this ratio for a fixed δ. The quantity σ reflects both biological variability and assay variability, and so using a more homogeneous group of patients may also serve to reduce σ.

Randomized selection design

An alternative approach to optimizing a vaccine regimen is to conduct a randomized phase II trial of the variants and to select the regimen that has the best average immunogenicity in the trial. This type of approach has been described by Simon et al., Strauss and Simon and Yao et al.. The analysis does not result in any conclusions of which factors are important to immunogenicity or which regimens are significantly better than which other regimens, but merely a selection of a regimen which is most promising for further investigation. There are two approaches to establishing sample size per treatment group for such selection designs. One approach, described in Simon et al. is to require that the sample size per treatment be large enough to assure with high probability that if one treatment is superior to all other treatments by a specified amount δ, then it will have the largest sample mean and will therefore be selected. With normally distributed measures of immunogenicity, the probability of correct selection depends on the ratio of δ/σ and on the number of treatment arms. If there is one best arm and the rest are inferior by δ, then the probability of correct selection decreases as the number of arms increases. Table 15.3 shows the sample size required to have a probability of correct selection of 0.90 as a function of δ/σ and the number of treatment arms. For δ/σ values of 0.75 or greater, the design requires fewer than 15 patients per arm for up to 8 randomized arms.

Table 15.3. Number of patients per arm for randomized selection design

Number of treatment arms	*Patients per arm* $\delta/\sigma = 0.5$	$\delta/\sigma = 0.75$	$\delta/\sigma = 1.0$
2	13	6	4
3	21	9	6
4	24	11	6
5	27	13	7
6	30	14	8
7	31	14	8
8	35	15	9

Another approach to establishing sample size for randomized selection designs is based on the assumption that the true mean immunogenicity for a regimen can be regarded as a random draw from some hypothetical super-distribution of activity levels. By studying more regimens in a randomized trial, one has a greater chance of including a very active regimen. If the number of patients available for the trial is fixed, there is a trade-off between the number of arms in the trial and the number of patients per arm. If we assume that the super-distribution is normal with mean μ and standard deviation ν, then we can compute the expected mean immunogenicity level for the regimen that has the best sample mean in the randomized K arm selection trial. Table 15.4 shows the expected mean immunogenicity levels as a function of the number of randomized arms and the sample size per arm when the total number of patients is fixed at 50. Four cases are shown: 2 arms of 25 patients, 5 arms of 10 patients, 10 arms of 5 patients, and 25 arms of 2 patients. The mean μ and standard deviation ν of the super-distribution are set at 0 and 1 respectively, and the table shows results for different values of the standard deviation σ of immunogenicity measurement for patients receiving the same vaccine regimen. It can be seen from the table, that in most cases the best treatment is identified by studying 25 treatment arms, each with only 2 patients. This is not really practical and reflects the unrealistic assumption that an unlimited number of regimens are available and that the activities of these regimens are independent and can be regarded as draws from a normal distribution. Nevertheless, the model does highlight the principle that there is an opportunity cost to studying few regimens thoroughly. The approach provides some justification for screening many regimens with a smaller sample size than is used for non-selection based trials.

Table 15.4. Expected immunogenicity of selected regimen for randomized selection designs that utilize 50 patients assumes μ = 0 and ν = 1

Number of regimens	*Patients per regimen*	*Expected immunogenicity of selected regimen*		
		σ = 2	*σ = 1*	*σ = 0.75*
2	25	0.52	0.55	0.56
5	10	0.99	1.10	1.13
10	5	1.15	1.40	1.44
25	2	1.14	1.60	1.73

Controlled Phase II Trials with Time to Tumor Recurrence or Progression Endpoint

Therapeutic vaccines may be more effective in patients with lower tumor burdens, and may slow progression rather than cause regression of bulk tumor. Patients without clinical evidence of disease may have more intact immune systems and be more appropriate candidates for tumor vaccines than patients with more advanced measurable metastatic disease.

Evaluating the effect on a regimen on time to progression of sub-clinical disease is very problematic in a single arm-phase II trial. It is easy to devise a definition of disease stabilization, i.e. lack of recurrence or progression for a specified period of time, but the validity of the definition depends on the existence of data that establish that such stabilization does not occur in the absence of treatment. This is difficult to establish reliably because of the usual difficulties of identifying comparable non-randomized controls and because of special difficulties involved with measuring time to disease progression in a consistent manner for different cohorts of patients. Consequently, use of disease stabilization or time to progression as an endpoint in single arm trials should only be considered when data from a specific set of contemporaneous controls from the same institution are available. In such a case, rather than attempting to define disease stabilization as a dichotomous endpoint (e.g. present or absent based on some threshold), it is preferable to compare the time to progression for the patients in the phase II trial to the distribution of time to progression of a specific set of control patients not receiving the vaccine regimen. Dixon and Simon provide formulas for computing the number of patients required in the single arm trial.

Phase III trials are generally randomized comparisons of a new regimen compared to a standard treatment using an endpoint of established medical importance to the patient such as survival or quality of life. Phase III trials are usually planned using a 5% type one error parameter (α) because the results of phase III trials are viewed as definitive and are used as a basis for marketing approval and practice guidelines. In the development of cancer vaccines, there is a role for what might be called a "phase 2.5" trial. Such a clinical trial would also be randomized, but may use an endpoint measuring biological anti-tumor activity even though the endpoint might not be established as a valid surrogate for survival or quality of life. The phase 2.5 trial might also be based on an elevated statistical significance level since the objective of the trial would not be for marketing approval or for establishing general practice guidelines.

To detect a large effect of a treatment in delaying tumor progression in a rapidly progressive disease such as pancreatic cancer or melanoma with visceral metastases does not require many patients in a randomized trial. With exponentially distributed times to progression, a 40% reduction in the hazard of progression corresponds to a 67% increase in median time to progression. In order to have 80% power ($\beta = 0.20$) for detecting this size of effect using an $\alpha = 0.10$, only about 87 patients are required (assuming accrual rate of about 3 patients per month, median time to progression of 12 months for control group and follow-up time of 24 months after end of accrual). Hence, with 44 patients randomized to vaccine and the same number randomized to control, one can conduct a randomized "phase 2.5" trial for evaluating whether the vaccine reduces the hazard of progression by 40%. This design would be a "phase 2.5" design because of the unconventional use of a one-sided $\alpha = 0.10$ significance level and because time to progression might not be established as representing clear patient benefit. The phase 2.5 design is similar to the phase III design in the respect that it contains a control group for evaluating the experimental regimen and the intent is comparative.

Statistical power for detecting a specified reduction of the hazard of an event is determined by the number of events, not the number of patients. The number of events required to have power 1-β for detecting a treatment effect of size δ with a one-sided statistical significance level of α is approximately:

$$E = 2\left(\frac{z_{\alpha} + z_{\beta}}{\ln(\delta)}\right)^2 \qquad \text{...(2)}$$

where δ is the ratio of median time to events if the distributions are exponential. In the calculation of the previous paragraph, δ = 1.67, α = 0.10, β = 0.20 and consequently E = 35 events. The number of patients needed to obtain 35 total events depends on the accrual rate, accrual period and follow-up period. With a slowly progressive disease, it may take many patients to be entered in order to observe a specified number of events unless the follow-up time following the close of accrual is very long. If the disease is rapidly progressive and all patients are followed until progression, then only 35 patients need to be randomized to observe 35 events.

Two different vaccine regimens can be evaluated in a randomized controlled phase II trial with time to progression endpoint by utilizing a three arm design. One arm would be the control group that does not receive either vaccine. For separate evaluation of each vaccine group without adjustment of the significance level for the fact that two vaccines are being evaluated, the number of events and patients required increases by one third compared to the two-arm trial. For example, if 44 patients per arm are required for the two-arm trial above, then 44 patients per arm are required for the three arm trial.

Trials using time to progression endpoints can be terminated early if interim results are not promising. One simple strategy is to perform an interim analysis when half of the planned total number of events have been observed. Accrual can be terminated if the number of events in the treatment group is greater than the number of events in the control group at that time. This interim analysis does not effect the type 1 error rate and causes negligible loss in statistical power. More sophisticated and efficient interim analysis plans for early termination when results are not promising are also possible. For a trial with multiple vaccine arms and one control arm, the interim monitoring can be used to evaluate each vaccine arm and stop accrual to those for which results are not promising. Randomized phase 2.5 trials may be structured so that all patients first receive tumor reduction with other modalities prior to randomization.

Phase III Trails

Phase III trials are generally randomized comparisons of a new regimen compared to a standard treatment using an endpoint of established medical importance to the patient such as survival or quality of life. Phase III trials of therapeutic cancer vaccines do not differ in important respects from phase III trials of conventional treatments; a randomized trial is required in both cases with a medically relevant endpoint and an appropriate control group.

Therapeutic cancer vaccines have characteristics that require a new paradigm for phase I and phase II clinical development. Effective development plans may take advantage of some of the following observations:

1. Dose ranging safety trials are not appropriate for many cancer vaccines.
2. Dose ranging trials to establish an optimal biologic dose are often not practical. We have presented an efficient design of Korn et al. to identify an immunogenic dose.
3. Vaccine efficacy can be efficiently evaluated with tumor response as endpoint utilizing a two stage design with only 9 patients in the first stage. If no partial or complete responses are observed in the initial 9 patients, accrual to the trial is terminated.
4. Optimization of vaccine delivery by comparing results of single arm phase II studies using immunological response as endpoint is problematic because of assay variation and potential non-comparability of patients in different studies.
5. Randomized screening studies can be used to efficiently optimize vaccine immunogenicity. Efficiency in use of patients depends on having assay variation and inter-patient variability small relative to the difference in immunogenicity to be detected.
6. Phase II studies using time to progression as endpoint are most interpretable if they employ randomized designs with a no-vaccine control group. Such designs may use an inflated type 1 error rate, and need not be prohibitively large if patients with rapidly progressive disease are studied. Interim monitoring plans may effectively limit the size of the trials by terminating accrual early when results are not consistent with the targeted improvement.

Regulatory Therapeutic Vaccine

Tumor immunology began, over 100 years ago, with the observation that inflammation induced by infectious agents or their products could induce tumor regression. While numerous attempts to produce either active or passive immunity to tumors have been based on models of successful vaccines for infectious agents, graft rejection of foreign antigens, or induction of breaks in self-tolerance, the potential of the immune system to prevent and control tumor growth has yet to be fully exploited. Stimulated by the identification of human tumor rejection antigens, an emerging understanding of human immunobiology, and advances in biotechnology, the last decade has seen a marked increase in clinical trials of therapeutic cancer vaccines. Methods to identify effector T-cells and their epitopes, to augment immune responses with cytokines and costimulatory molecules, to manipulate regulatory T-cells, and to use dendritic cells to present tumor antigens, have entered the clinical arena. These advances have led to a steady increase in the number of *Investigational New Drug Applications* (INDs) filed by the *Division of Cancer Treatment and Diagnosis* (DCTD), *National Cancer Institute* (NCI), starting in 1990.

Cancer vaccines speak to the hope of biologic control of cancer with minimal toxicity. The earliest attempts to use vaccines consisted of using the patient's own killed or lysed tumor cells or tumor cell lines as a vaccine, or to create anti-sera for passive immunity. More recently, cancer vaccines often utilize well-defined, purified tumor-specific and tumor-associated antigens, in various forms including synthetic peptides and larger proteins, peptide-pulsed dendritic cells, plasmids, and virus vectors. In this chapter we provide guidance on the regulatory and clinical issues relevant to cancer vaccine trials. It should be noted that the scientific evaluation of non-cytotoxic agents is an ongoing process, with the *Food and Drug Administration* (FDA) review of investigational products evolving as clinical experience with these products is attained. Information provided in this chapter should be used as a framework or guide in considering product issues and the design of clinical trials. The FDA should always be consulted prior to the filing of an IND. One method of discussing product and clinical issues for a specific product with the FDA is the Pre-IND meeting. Reference to a FDA guidance on Pre-IND meetings is provided at the end of this chapter.

Regulatory Review Issues

In order to conduct a clinical trial with an experimental biologic agent, an IND application must be submitted to the Center for Biologics Evaluation and Research (CBER) of the FDA as well as to a local or central Institutional Review Board (IRB). Gene therapy products are also subject to further review by the National Institutes of Health (NIH).

In June 2003, CBER was reorganized and several offices were transferred to the Center for Drug Evaluation and Research (CDER). Therapeutic vaccines remain under the auspices of CBER. In particular, gene- and cell-based cancer vaccines are the regulatory responsibility of the Office of Cellular, Tissue and Gene Therapies in CBER.

Cancer vaccines range over a broad spectrum of biological products and combinations of products. These products include plasmid DNA, RNA, tumor cells, tumor cell lysates, peptides, proteins (including immunoglobulin idiotypes), recombinant viruses, peptide-pulsed dendritic cells, as well as passive immunization agents such as antibodies and adoptive cellular therapy utilizing antigen-specific T-cells. Many are combined with adjuvants such as incomplete Freund's adjuvant (water-in-oil emulsions), saponins, monophosphoryl lipid A, and aluminum salts (alum) as well as cytokines and immune stimulating agents.

Within each of the above categories many different products are being evaluated in preclinical models or are in clinical trials already. Retrovirus, vaccinia, canarypox, fowlpox, adenovirus, adeno-associated virus, herpes and lentivirus are currently being used as expression vectors to carry cytokines, costimulatory molecules, differentiation antigens and tumor-associated antigens in an attempt to generate a therapeutic immune response. For example, the DCTD, NCI has evaluated 28 different poxvirus, two adenovirus, and three plasmid vectors expressing recombinant vaccine products alone or in combination. Tumor-cell vaccines gene-modified to contain immunostimulatory molecules, dendritic cells, dendritic/tumor cell fusions, and even bacteria can be enlisted to present tumor antigens. NCI has sponsored seven INDs for whole-cell vaccines.

Peptide vaccines that represent basic tumor antigenic epitopes are well defined, relatively inexpensive, and easy to manufacture and administer. The ability to create agonist peptides by changing critical amino acids that bind to MHC or T-cell receptor molecules, adds to the potential efficacy and complexity of peptide vaccines. Passive immunization or adoptive immunotherapy clinical trials sponsored by the NCI have included the use of tumor-infiltrating lymphocytes (in some cases retrovirally-transduced with a marker gene or cytokine), autologous peripheral blood lymphocytes peptide-sensitized *ex vivo*, cloned T-cells, and expanded activated T-cells. Because cancer vaccines cover such a wide spectrum of products, they are subject to a wide variety of product-specific FDA regulatory guidelines and guidances in addition to the general FDA guidelines for all biologic products.

Often times, multiple products are used together or in sequence in order to boost an immune response. For example, a vaccinia-vectored vaccine may be used as a priming immunization, followed by boosts with a fowlpox-vectored vaccine containing a gene encoding the same antigen, given along with GM-CSF. To facilitate a multi-agent trial such as this, the original IND filing should include all of the products. A single IND might also be used to compare a number of similar candidate vaccines for the purpose of selecting the most promising one for further development.

One example would be an IND that includes multiple peptides representing CTL or $CD4^+$ epitopes of a particular differentiation antigen in the early phase of drug development (phase 1/2). By late phase 2/3, information relevant to the chosen product should be made into a new IND to support further development and eventual licensure. The DCTD's NCI's experience with the early development of vaccines and regulatory agencies is described below. Please note that the NCI's experience may not be universally applicable as each vaccine brings unique issues that should be considered on a product specific basis.

Gene-based Vaccine Products

Cancer vaccines that contain *recombinant DNA* (rDNA) such as DNA plasmids and viral-vectored vaccines are a special case, which may be subject to NIH review. Cancer vaccines are included in this category for review by the Office of Biotechnology Activities (OBA) in the NIH Guidelines for Research Involving rDNA Molecules. A footnote states that, "Human studies in which induction or enhancement of an immune response to a vector encoded microbial immunogen is the major goal, such an immune response has been demonstrated in model systems, and the persistence of the vector-encoded immunogen is not expected to persist are exempt". Since this footnote identifies agents that are not subject to OBA submission, this is meant to imply that cancer vaccines containing *human* genes are subject to the NIH Guidelines and therefore require submission to OBA for review.

This applies to studies that utilize any federal funding for recombinant DNA research and those for which the sponsor or institution conducting the study receives such funding. Protocols plus supporting documentation must be submitted to the Office of Biotechnology Activities (OBA), NIH per the NIH Guidelines for Research Involving Recombinant DNA Molecules. These protocols must also be submitted to the Institutional Biosafety Committee (IBC), as well as to the Institutional Review Board (IRB). IRB, IBC and FDA review and approval are not required prior to OBA submission, but are necessary prior to the start of the clinical trial.

Product Issues

FDA guidance on the manufacture of biological products is based on ensuring the identity, potency, purity, stability, bioavailability and safety of the product prior to human use. In general, there should be an adherence to the current Good Manufacturing Practices (cGMP), with full cGMP adherence by the time clinical studies reach phase 3. These general principles apply to all cancer vaccines. Below, we will discuss select issues most relevant to cancer vaccine development.

An important product issue that is frequently overlooked in early trials is the development of a potency assay. This assay should be an *in vivo* or *in vitro* measure of the biological function of the product. While such a potency assay is not mandatory for early clinical development, in our experience, an assay measuring the intended biologic activity is essential for interpreting clinical results, especially those based on individualized products such as cellular vaccines. Prior to phase 3 clinical trials or, for that matter, any clinical trial that is intended to support product registration, a validated potency assay based on biological function must be utilized. The assay must be robust, sensitive, specific, quantitative, and reproducible.

As biological agents, many cancer vaccines are manufactured using animal-derived reagents including fermentation broth, serum, amino acids, transferrin, albumin, enzymes, and lipids. Since 1991, the FDA has issued several guidances and Letters to Manufacturers, regarding the use of ruminant-derived reagents and the FDA's concern about potential transmission of classic and variant Creutzfeldt-Jakob disease. There is evidence that variant Creutzfeldt-Jakob disease may be associated with the causative agent of *bovine spongiform encephalopathy* (BSE). Therefore, the FDA has requested that, materials derived from ruminants that have resided in countries where BSE has been diagnosed, or where they are unable to assure that BSE does not exist, not be used in product manufacture.

The United States Department of Agriculture (USDA) maintains a list of countries at risk for BSE. Because this list continues to grow as more and more ruminants infected with BSE are identified, it may be preferable if no ruminant-derived (or even animal-derived) products are used in the manufacture of cancer vaccines, regardless of their country of origin. Regarding products manufactured prior to the issuance of FDA guidance on BSE, FDA advisory committees acknowledged that risks posed by the use of bovine materials are theoretical and negligible, but they also advocated that there should be public disclosure regarding these risks and that materials from countries on the FDA BSE list be replaced as soon as possible. In general, if any animal-derived reagents of unknown origin were used during product manufacture, the Informed Consent should contain this information as well, noting the unlikely but possible risk of BSE transmission.

Gene-based Vaccine Products

Individual categories of cancer vaccine agents have particular product issues worth specific mention. Gene-based vaccines less than 40 kilobase pairs in length must be entirely sequenced prior to phase 1 clinical trials. For vectors 40 kilobase pairs or greater in length, the insert plus flanking regions (e.g., 500–1000 base pairs upstream and downstream), as well as transcriptional control regions for the inserted transgene, any other portion of the vector genome manipulated during derivation of the vector, or any regions with known toxic effects should be sequenced prior to phase 1 clinical trials. A comparison of the sequence with existing human sequences using the Basic Local Alignment Search Tool (BLAST) is also recommended in order to detect any potentially harmful sequences and homology with human proteins.

Whole Cell and Tumor Lysate Products

Whole cell and tumor lysate vaccines are complex mixtures and as such present challenges with respect to lot-to-lot consistency. Lot-to-lot reproducibility must be demonstrated with respect to identity, purity, and potency. To achieve consistency, one must have a defined isolation, culture and expansion procedure that yields a well-defined cellular product. Products must be characterized with respect to morphology, immuno-phenotype, and function.

It is desirable to identify several immunologically relevant antigens on the tumor cells and demonstrate their consistency from lot-to-lot. The proportion of irrelevant contaminating cells may need to be quantified in order to assess purity. Where appropriate, contamination with live tumor cells must be quantified. If cells or lysate are cryopreserved, validated assay methods should be used to demonstrate that there has been no change in viability, phenotype, and function upon thawing. Criteria for standardization are still in development for most products.

Other Issues for Gene- and Cell-based Products

In March 2000, the Office of Therapeutics, CBER sent out letters to sponsors of all gene-based INDs and Master Files requesting specific manufacturing information in an attempt to determine if current standards for the manufacture and testing of products were being followed. In particular, they requested manufacturing data, a summary of quality control/quality assurance (QC/QA) procedures, and a description of the clinical oversight and monitoring programs. Requested manufacturing data included product characterization and testing (methods, specifications, results), disqualification of lots, stability program, and a listing of all products made in the facility. These issues should be addressed in any gene transfer or cellular therapy IND and updated in subsequent Annual Reports. More recently, similar types of letters have been sent to sponsors of cell therapy INDs. Amongst other items the FDA requested a description of the QC/QA programs for cellular therapy products that included the qualification program for cells, critical reagents, and equipment; and product tracking/labeling, as well as personnel qualifications and procedures for auditing contractors.

Long-term follow-up of patients is required for all gene-based products. The FDA's Biological Response Modifiers Advisory Committee has recommended that long-term follow-up extend over 15 years and should focus on the collection of clinical information pertaining to *de novo* cancer, neurologic, autoimmune, and hematologic disorders. Unexpected medical problems including information on hospitalizations and medications should be collected. For retrovirus-based products in particular, testing for replication-competent retrovirus should be conducted on patient samples. In some cases, the clonality of vector integration sites should also be assessed using patient samples.

Preclinical Safety/Efficacy Issues

Preclinical studies must support the safety and rationale for the proposed clinical dose and schedule. Studies should be conducted in the most relevant species and model available utilizing a dosing schedule close to or identical to the proposed clinical use. There are many biologic products that are species-specific and, therefore, may be best tested in a pharmacologically relevant species, not necessarily a traditional toxicology species. For some agents, such as human cytotoxic T-lymphocytes, there may be no relevant animal model. In such cases, extremely cautious phase I safety testing may be most appropriate. Pharmacokinetic studies should also be conducted where appropriate.

Preclinical toxicology studies should be designed to determine a dose range and potential dose-related toxicities in order to monitor safety in human trials. Animal models of disease can be utilized to address efficacy and, at the same time, some safety issues. For cancer vaccines, immunological activity should be studied, either *in vitro* or *in vivo*, depending on feasibility. Murine models expressing human transgenes for MHC molecules or tumor antigens are available to examine MHC restriction and tolerance. Cancer vaccines are intended to stimulate the immune system so one must separate intended effects from aberrant, toxic effects (immunotoxicity).

If there is prior human experience that demonstrates the safety of a class of agents, then this may be sufficient to support entry of a new member of this class into clinical trials. For example, extensive clinical data demonstrating the safe use of a tumor antigen plus extensive experience with vaccinia and avipox vaccines may allow a new poxvirus vaccine product containing the gene for the same tumor antigen, to enter into phase 1 clinical trials without further *in vivo* toxicity testing. However, additional non-clinical safety studies in relevant animal models may be needed prior to large-scale clinical trials in, for example, less critically ill or a more heterogeneous patient population. The FDA should be consulted regarding this option. Toxicology studies are required for first generation vectors, those with new molecular entities and for agents when adverse events have been observed with a similar vector or transgene construct. Compliance with Good Laboratory Practice (GLP) regulations is generally expected for all non-clinical studies supporting safety.

The FDA will be reviewing the pharmacology/toxicology studies to assess the risk versus benefit of the product. The patient population, the severity of the disease, as well as the availability of alternative therapies will be considered during this process. Particular categories of cancer vaccines will have particular pharmacology/toxicology issues and these are discussed below.

Gene-based Products

Bio-distribution studies to evaluate the tissue distribution, persistence, and integration potential of a vector must be conducted with gene transfer agents. Such non-clinical safety studies can identify potential target organs for toxicity (distribution of vector to non-target sites) in addition to determining the potential for germline transmission. Information regarding the level and duration of gene expression *in vivo* should also be obtained whenever possible.

A biodistribution study would be expected pre-phase 1 for a first generation vector or a new molecular entity, a change in formulation, a change to systemic route of administration, or if the transgene has the potential to induce toxicity if expressed in non-target tissue. A biodistribution study does not necessarily need to be performed prior to phase 1 studies if there is already extensive human experience with that class of vectors and the inserted product or expression cassette is not expected to influence the toxicity or the biodistribution of the product. A bridging study comparing the pharmacological activity and transfection efficiency of two related vector preparations, may supplant the need for toxicology testing as well.

Peptide Vaccine Products

Peptide vaccine products are often considered to be of low risk. Since peptides themselves do not usually have any biological activity except for their intended immunogenicity, there is often more concern about the toxicity of the adjuvant rather than the peptide. For novel adjuvants, preclinical studies should be conducted with the adjuvant, using single and repeat dosage with the route used in clinical studies, and usually in more than one species. If toxicology studies exist and there is previous human experience with a particular adjuvant alone and in combination with other antigens, then a complete toxicology study may not be needed, if the antigen-adjuvant combination does not pose a special risk.

Introduction to Clinical Trials

As we begin the 21st century, there are still no therapeutic cancer vaccines licensed for use in the United States. This reflects the fact that no phase 3 clinical cancer vaccine trials have been consistently successful in demonstrating a clinical benefit. There are currently 15 or more phase 3 clinical trials in progress in a variety of cancer types and which utilize different therapeutic approaches. The wide variety of vaccine products and approaches also reflects the fact that there is no consensus regarding the best way to produce an effective anti-tumor response and no clear understanding of how best to develop cancer vaccines that are very likely to be effective.

The development of an effective therapeutic cancer vaccine presents a difficult problem. Due to the number of combinations of potential tumor-specific and tumor-associated antigens, adjuvants, and varieties of strategies for immunization that could be used for a therapeutic cancer vaccine, it is impossible to test them in a systematic manner using clinical end points while immunologic endpoints still require validation. In addition, current stratagems for designing and producing vaccines are often based as much on intellectual property owned by individual companies or investigators as on experimental data. In our experience, independent clinical investigators have initiated most therapeutic cancer vaccine development.

Sponsoring companies, the majority of which are biotechnology companies, usually have a limited number of products in development and are relatively new to therapeutic vaccine development. With a few exceptions, the pharmaceutical industry has limited experience in the development of therapeutic cancer vaccines. The few companies that specialize in vaccines develop prophylactic vaccines intended to protect against infection. Effective methods for choosing potential candidates based on pre-clinical data and for conducting phase 1 and phase 2 trials in an efficient manner are progressing along with our ability to manipulate the human immune system. Toward this end some standardization of study methods and immunologic evaluation is essential in order to compare and contrast results from different studies.

In one respect there is a currently approved vaccine for cancer. A vaccine already exists that prevents cancer by preventing infection by the cancer-causing virus, Hepatitis B (hepatoma). In addition, a vaccine for the human papilloma virus (cervical cancer) has had clinical success. Also, there is interest in a vaccine for the bacteria, *H. pylori* for the prevention of ulcers, which would also have the benefit of preventing gastric cancer. Licensing guidelines for a papilloma virus vaccine discussed at a November 2001 meeting of the Vaccine and Related Products Advisory Committee follow more generally the path of traditional vaccines with the most significant discussion centered on the use of virologic measures as surrogate end points for tumor prevention rather than reduction of the incidence of dysplasia as a clinical end point.

There is much less experience to guide the development of therapeutic vaccines. At least one vaccine, Melacine for prevention of recurrence of resected stage II melanoma, was approved for use in Canada but not approved by the U.S. FDA as clinical trials failed to meet primary end points. Further interest in the Melacine vaccine was stimulated by a retrospective subset analysis showing a 30% survival advantage for patients who are HLA A1 and/or C3 positive. Further clinical studies will need to be conducted to determine efficacy in this patient subset. The complex biologic, clinical, and regulatory questions raised by the development of this whole cell lysate vaccine were extensively discussed at an ODAC meeting. One comment deserves close attention by anyone engaged in therapeutic cancer vaccine development.

Ultimately, it is prudent to get FDA input before putting in 7 to 10 years, tens of millions of dollars, and hundreds of patients in clinical trials to make sure it will satisfy not only the Agency but also what expert advisors feel is appropriate. Prior to study implementation, the FDA will provide a special protocol assessment upon request. This is a procedure whereby the FDA will review a proposed phase 3 study whose data will form the primary basis for an efficacy claim. They will assess whether it is adequate to meet the scientific and regulatory requirements identified by the sponsor.

Regulatory guidelines perhaps have most impact at two stages of clinical trials. The first is during the pre-clinical development and the safety evaluation of the product in order to meet the requirements for filing an IND and conducting a phase 1 trial. The second is for the design and interpretation of phase 3 trials to meet the statutory requirements for demonstration of safety and efficacy and providing labeling information required to license and define the use of the drug.

Phase 1 Clinical Trials

Phase 1 trials are typically designed to test the safety of an agent and to determine a recommended phase 2 dose to evaluate efficacy. The typical dose escalation trial of cytotoxic drugs is premised on determining the maximum dose of any agent or combination that can be given. Phase 1 clinical trials with cancer vaccines on the other hand are designed to determine not only the safety of the vaccine but the optimal dose for eliciting the measured immune response which may involve a threshold as well as an upper limit.

Since immunologic responses are generally not dose-dependent beyond a threshold response, demonstration of an immunologic response in a significant proportion of patients might be a reasonable end point for phase 1 trials. There are two significant ways that, in our experience, vaccine trials differ from more traditional trials of phase 1 cytotoxic drugs. First, the direct toxicity of vaccines and adjuvants is often minimal; the most frequent toxicities include local reaction, adenopathy, and constitutional symptoms such as fever, headache, and fatigue. Systemic toxicity when observed is most often associated with cytokines such as GM-CSF or IL-2, which are often given to enhance immunologic responses. Second, autoimmunity is a consideration for any vaccine that enhances immunologic responses. For example, IL-2 is frequently associated with autoimmune hypothyroid disease. Recently an agent thought to enhance immunologic responses, anti-CTLA-4 antibody, has been administered in conjunction with cancer vaccines, and has been reported to be associated with autoimmune reactions, sometimes severe.

The patient population selected for phase 1 trials has typically been patients with incurable or otherwise untreatable metastatic malignancy and this tradition has been maintained for vaccine trials. Since immune responses may be impaired in patients with advanced disease, it is possible that safety and efficacy questions may require studying patients with less advanced disease. The ability to administer high doses of vaccines and the understanding that the largest dose may not be the optimal dose requires an evaluation of the targeted immunologic response to determine a biologically active dose. Beyond safety, phase 1 (or early phase 2 trials) may be very useful to identify appropriate phase 2 end points, obtain and validate immunologic studies or surrogate end points, and evaluate factors in patient selection (including the presence of the target, the ability of the patient to mount an immune response, and the immunologic susceptibility of tumor). The average phase 1 trial may take between 6 to 24 months to complete depending on size, accrual, immunization schedules, and the time required between patient cohorts to allow dose escalation.

In our studies, phase 1 trials have ranged from very simple dose escalation designs requiring no more than 12–18 patients to more elaborate phase 1/2 designs that gather significant information on immunologic efficacy and clinical activity of both single and combination agents. Clinical studies should have a study design, end points, defined patient population, and correlative studies that can be related to clearly identified objectives. The more information that is obtained regarding the biology and potential anti-tumor mechanisms in early trials, the more likely meaningful information would be obtained to support later trials. The number of currently active phase 1 trials of therapeutic cancer vaccines is difficult to estimate but probably represents the introduction of 50–100 new products over the past two years.

Phase 2 Clinical Trails

Phase 2 clinical trials are usually disease and stage specific since it is assumed that this would identify a reasonably uniform population and provide consistent results in larger trials. Since most phase 2 trials are not randomized, the selection of patients may be the critical factor in trying to establish efficacy based upon historic comparison and in the failure to replicate apparently successful trials in larger settings. The primary objective of phase 2 trials defines the range of responses at an optimal dose and schedule from phase 1 trials. For conventional cytotoxic drugs this is most conveniently accomplished using measurements of decreases in tumor size to define an objective response as a decrease in overall tumor burden. The *Response Evaluation Criteria in Solid Tumors* (RECIST) defines an objective response as a 30% or greater decrease in the sum of long diameters of measurable tumor. Other disease specific criteria are available for lymphoma, myeloma, and PSA responses in prostate cancer. Whether or not these objective criteria represent the most appropriate way to evaluate the clinical benefit of vaccines is a matter for continued analysis.

The presence of partial responses may demonstrate activity but often not clinical benefit, while mixed responses, with some lesions resolving while others progress, perhaps reflects local determinants of the ongoing battle between tumor and T-cell. Occasionally pathologic complete response can be determined when biopsy shows absence of viable tumor but lesions are still measurable. While vaccines for infectious diseases are evaluated after a single course there is reason to think that therapeutic vaccines would require continued boosting or even retargeting of antigens as part of maintenance regimens for patients with responses or stable disease. Such long term protracted approaches remain to be evaluated. And, while complete responses are most frequently associated with the potential for long-term survival for an individual patient, the lack of objective responses may not capture ongoing anti-tumor activity that could be reflected by increases in time to progression and overall survival.

Since tumors may initially progress while patients are being vaccinated, trials should attempt to allow sufficient time for the patient to develop an immunologic response before concluding a vaccine is not effective. In addition, there are clear examples reported in which a tumor may respond after initial progression if enough time is permitted to complete a vaccine regimen and observe a response. An effective vaccination is most likely to be completed in the adjuvant setting. In patients with advanced disease, progression may limit the therapy. Modifications to allow continued treatment after limited progression need to be evaluated.

Designs for cancer vaccine trials that could be used for efficient evaluation of candidate vaccines have been reviewed. Randomized phase 2 designs have been suggested that could serve to identify promising agents and regimens, utilizing clinical progression endpoints or surrogate markers. The appropriate sizing of phase 2 trials may vary from small trials that demonstrate large treatment effects to larger trials intended to show smaller differences. Asking phase 3 efficacy questions that require randomization, survival endpoints, and appropriate controls of smaller phase 2 designed trials may be highly misleading.

For example, a randomized design in patients with renal cell cancer using monoclonal anti-VEGF antibody, bevacizumab, while demonstrating only a 10% objective response rate succeeded in demonstrating a significant increase in time to progression in patients receiving the antibody. The critical factor that made this study successful was a carefully constructed, conducted, credible study design, but all depended on the strong effect of the agent, representing a hazard ratio of 2.5 compared to placebo. However, it is clear from this illustration that a less active agent would not have been likely to have a significant result.

Phase 3 Clinical Trails

Phase 3 trials intended to support regulatory marketing approval require, substantial evidence of efficacy from adequate and well-controlled investigations. Studies must allow a valid comparison to a control group and adequate quantitative assessment of the drug's benefit, which is interpreted as prolongation of life, a better quality of life or an established surrogate. An application must also provide sufficient information to allow the product label to describe the effective and safe use of the agent in a defined population. The Federal Food Drug and Cosmetic Act requires that drugs be safe for intended use and an amendment in 1962 to that Act codifies the efficacy requirements.

In 1992 an addition, Subpart H (Accelerated Approval of New Drugs for Serious or Life Threatening Illnesses), to the new drug application regulations allowed accelerated approval on the basis of a surrogate end point such as response rate or time to progression, if it appears to provide benefit. The accelerated approval requires post-marketing studies to demonstrate the treatment is beneficial. Of 57 drugs approved between 1990 to 2002, about one third were approved based on survival and almost one half were approved based on response rate.

Concluding Remark

What is the appropriate end point for a therapeutic vaccine? Although we have begun to see objective tumor responses in some patients, response rates of 10 to 20% are not generally adequate to use as end points in phase 2 trials. In order to see reliable differences in survival in a phase 2 trial, a very striking treatment effect in a well-controlled setting is probably required. As a practical matter, to show benefit, most phase 3 studies of therapeutic vaccines have used overall survival in advanced disease or time to recurrence either in the adjuvant setting or following complete resection with a high risk of recurrence. It is important to understand some of the reasons phase 3 vaccine trials have consistently failed to meet expectations following promising phase 2 trials. Phase 2 trial results may be strongly influenced by patient selection and retrospective analysis of subgroups, which may contribute to inadequate phase 3 trials even when based on positive phase 2 data. However, even with well designed trials, rational vaccine development beyond the empiric evaluation of individual products will require a deeper understanding of human tumor immunobiology.

INDEX

H

I

J

K

L

M

S

T

U

V

W

X